A Featured-Based Syntax of Functional Categories

Studies in Generative Grammar 79

Editors

Mouton de Gruyter
Berlin · New York

A Featured-Based Syntax of Functional Categories

The Structure, Acquisition and Specific Impairment of Functional Systems

by

Michael Hegarty

Mouton de Gruyter
Berlin · New York

Mouton de Gruyter (formerly Mouton, The Hague)
is a Division of Walter de Gruyter GmbH & Co. KG, Berlin.

The series Studies in Generative Grammar was formerly published by Foris Publications Holland.

∞ Printed on acid-free paper which falls within the guidelines of the ANSI to ensure permanence and durability.

Library of Congress Cataloging-in-Publication Data

Hegarty, Michael, 1959–
A feature-based syntax of functional categories : the structure, acquisition and specific impairment of functional systems / by Michael Hegarty.
p. cm. – (Studies in generative grammar ; 79)
Includes bibliographical references and index.
ISBN 3-11-018413-3 (cloth : alk. paper)
1. Grammar, Comparative and general – Grammatical categories.
2. Functionalism (Linguistics) 3. Grammar, Comparative and general – Syntax. 4. English language – Grammar, Historical. 5. Language acquisition. 6. Language disorders. I. Title. II. Series.
P240.5.H44 2005
410'.1'8–dc22
2005011296

Bibliographic information published by Die Deutsche Bibliothek

Die Deutsche Bibliothek lists this publication in the Deutsche Nationalbibliografie; detailed bibliographic data is available in the Internet at <http://dnb.ddb.de>.

ISBN 3-11-018413-3

Cover design: Christopher Schneider, Berlin.
Printed in Germany.

Preface

Alongside lexical content items such as nouns and verbs, natural languages feature functional elements such as tense, negation, agreement elements, and complementizers. But standard treatments of functional elements, assigning them to functional categories posited as primitive items of phrase structure, have some basic conceptual problems associated with them. The present work develops ideas of Minimalist syntax to derive functional categories from the morphological and semantic features expressed by functional elements, thereby dispensing with functional categories as primitives of the theory. It generalizes some attempts to do this in the literature, while introducing constraints to ensure that workable systems of functional categories emerge naturally from the derivation, rather than through stipulation. The resulting theory of the construction of functional categories is then applied to the analysis of some disparate syntactic phenomena, including patterns of verb-second in Germanic languages, variation in the form of existential constructions across Germanic languages, the placement of weak (clitic) pronouns in some Romance languages, and some previously unexamined coordinate structures in colloquial English.

The feature-based derivation of functional categories directly accounts for the forms of expression of functional elements in early child language as resulting from the projection into phrase structure of feature matrices composed of individual features and non-adult combinations of features. Furthermore, the theory developed here provides a basis for developmental stages in child language acquisition characterized, at each stage, by the number of adult functional categories which can be represented together within a clause, depending on the representational resources of the child's grammar at that stage. This leads to empirical predictions which are close to those of a theory proposed in the literature ("bottom-up structure building"), on which functional categories emerge one after another in a fixed sequence, but crucially different in that the present theory limits only the number, not the actual inventory, of the functional categories exhibited at each stage. The predictions of this and various prominent theories of the acquisition of functional categories in the literature are spelled out in the text, and compared with the results of a quantitative study I undertook using data available on the CHILDES website. The results of this study support the feature-based construction of functional categories, and indicate that the development of the functional category system is characterized not by the emergence or maturation of specific grammatical formatives, but by the growth of more basic representational resources of the child's grammar.

Finally, the theory makes explicable the results of another quantitative study I conducted, concerning the lag in the production of multiple functional elements within the clausal system exhibited by children with Specific Language Impairment (SLI). My study shows that children with SLI lag not only behind their language-matched normally developing peers (as previously discovered in the literature), but they lag behind what they should be capable of producing given the individual functional elements which they have acquired, and the phrase structure complexity they have attained. Using phrase structure complexity as a control on limitations of working memory and processing capacity, it is argued that this lag cannot be attributed to these other factors. The results are interpreted to show that children with SLI are not just slower to acquire classes of functional elements, or particular functional categories, but that they have a deficit in the representational resources required to project multiple functional categories within a single clause.

Baton Rouge, April 2005 Michael Hegarty

Acknowledgements

The ideas in this book have developed through three stages. The earliest stage was an attempt to provide an account of clitic placement in Romance languages as a product of verb and clitic movement to functional heads, along the lines explored by Richard Kayne and others, with the aim of deriving the intricacies of the data entirely from independently motivated principles for the projection of functional categories. For opportunities to present those ideas, and for feedback which was encouraging but suitably critical, I would like to acknowledge audiences at the University of Pennsylvania, the CUNY Graduate School, the 1994 Minimalism Workshop at the University of Maryland, the University of North Carolina at Chapel Hill, the University of Connecticut, the 1994 Workshop on Greek Syntax at the Humboldt University in Berlin, and the University of Minnesota. The middle stage of this work pursued the same goal in light of the reduction of functional categories to matrices of functional features. This opened up connections to work other people had done on the comparative analysis of Germanic verb-second, and it opened up a new avenue of investigation of child language acquisition of functional categories, greatly widening the scope of the project. For opportunities to present this stage of the work, and for helpful comments and suggestions, I am grateful to audiences at the University of Arizona, Louisiana State University, and at the 2002 joint meeting of the International Association for the Study of Child Language and the Symposium on Research in Child Language Disorders in Madison, Wisconsin. The third stage of this project involved quantitative work on child language acquisition and Specific Language Impairment, using data posted on the CHILDES website, and solidification and extension of the theoretical concepts. For support of this stage of the work, I am particularly grateful to Louisiana State University for a Council on Research summer grant, a Manship Summer Fellowship awarded by the College of Arts and Sciences, and a research leave for the fall semester of 2003. A special thanks to the English Department at LSU, for welcoming a generative linguist into their midst, and to the Interdepartmental Linguistics Program, for keeping linguistics going at LSU.

I am extremely grateful to people who have taken time to discuss the ideas in this book (or their precursors) with me, especially (in rough chronological order) Sabine Iatridou, Alexis Demitriadis, Tony Kroch,

Richard Kayne, Howard Lasnik, Janna Oetting, and Matthew Rispoli. They wouldn't necessarily agree with what I have done here, but their questions and comments have spurred development of the ideas in this book and improved the presentation and argumentation.

In many instances, my initial foray into a topic area of this book was in teaching a graduate seminar. I am most grateful to students and visitors in these seminars who tolerated my lack of expertise and enthusiastically joined with me in exploration. Students in my seminar in syntactic theory at the University of Pennsylvania in 1993 joined me in comparing Minimalism, and the ideas I had at the time about the projection of functional categories, with Tree Adjoining Grammar. A special thanks to Owen Rambow for discussing his own version of feature-based syntax with us, and to Tony Kroch for enlightening contributions. Students in my seminar in comparative syntax at the University of Connecticut in 1994 joined me with great patience in exhaustively playing out my early ideas on verb and clitic movement; special thanks to Željko Bošković, Roger Martin, Kazumi Matsuoka, and Masao Ochi for the time they spent with us. Students in my seminar on the acquisition of syntax at the University of Minnesota in 1997 joined me in a survey of the literature on the acquisition of functional categories, recasting the results in light of a feature-based syntax of functional categories. By the time of my syntax seminar at the University of Minnesota in 1998, the feature-based account of clitic placement was more developed, and I was lucky to have students specializing in Romance syntax and pronominal clitics in the class; special thanks to Laura Colantoni, Tonya Custis, and John Halligan. Finally, students in my seminar on the syntax of Old and Middle English at Louisiana State University in 2004 enthusiastically joined me in drawing full-blown feature-based phrase structure trees of Old English sentences, and in devising alternate derivations of Old English word order from variant base orders; special thanks to Danielle Alfandre and Sarah Ross.

Finally, I would like to thank Ann Mulkern for the index, and much more importantly, for sharing everything with me, including her perspectives on linguistics, politics, art, music, and life, for the better part of the past decade.

Contents

Chapter 1
Introduction

1. Aims and approach

Different approaches to a generative syntactic theory pursue different goals. All approaches share the goal of constructing a grammar for each natural language L which generates the grammatical sentences of L and distinguishes them in some way from linguistic forms which are not grammatical sentences of L. (Realistically, L is a register of a dialect, typically conceived under some degree of idealization.) In some theories of grammar, this distinction is made directly by generating all and only the grammatical sentences of L. Other theories of grammar make the distinction more indirectly by seeking to specify a generative system which assigns different statuses to different classes of linguistic forms in such a way as to capture salient properties of these forms, whether or not they are grammatical. Other goals which approaches to syntactic theory might pursue include the following: attaining formal simplicity and elegance, mathematical explicitness, or computational tractability; providing a vehicle for explicating syntactic variation and change; accommodating accounts of language acquisition, and accounts of syntactic deficits and language impairment; and formulating a theory with a plausible neurological instantiation.

An aim for maximum coverage of data at the expense of regard for the form of the theory presents a danger of achieving little more than facile description, without attaining any deeper understanding of the phenomena. It's a fact about syntactic theory (as opposed to syntactic description) that tighter formalisms which can account for a range of facts using limited theoretical resources make possible epistemological scenarios in which one domain of data can be predicted or derived from the formulation of theory based on examination of another domain of data. The logical relationships involved in these epistemological scenarios, together with the high ratio of fact covered to theory expended, are the basis for the judgment that some degree of understanding has been achieved, over and above description. This is not likely to happen if coverage of data is the only desideratum of a syntactic theory.

In contrast, syntax from the perspective of Platonic linguistics embraces a concern not just for data coverage, but also concern for the mathematical form of the theory, possibly united with concerns for accommodating accounts of syntactic variation and change. But Platonic syntax typically disregards concerns for learnability, neurological instantiation, and the goal of understanding syntactic deficits or impairment.

Finally, syntax from a biological or cognitive science perspective strives for maximum coverage of the data in the best and most convenient formalism, while striving to accommodate accounts of language variation and change, and at the same time to provide for insightful accounts of learnability, deficits and impairment, and the possibility of neurological instantiation. From this perspective, the basic goals of syntactic theory are essentially reconfigured. The goal is not simply to construct a single grammar of a language L which meets some set of desiderata. Rather, the goal is to construct a syntactic theory which equally well provides grammars of all sociolinguistic and historical varieties of a language, coherently relating them to one another in terms of principles of language variation and change; and which provides grammars of various stages of child language and coherently relates them to one another and to the adult target in terms of principles of language development; and which provides grammars of a language under various types of deficits, coherently relating them to normal grammars and normally developing grammars in terms of what is understood about language impairment; and to do all this, as much as possible, across all the languages of the world, since language, on this perspective, is a biological property of the species.

It was mentioned above that when coverage of data takes total precedence over other concerns, the theory tends toward facile description. But exclusive concern for the form of the theory at the expense of data coverage poses a contrary danger of a priori theorizing. And concern for facts of acquisition and syntactic deficits without sufficient attention to how these facts relate to the form of the theory of syntactic structure poses a danger of achieving a description of acquisition and impairment facts uninformed by the nature of the syntactic system which is being acquired or which suffers the impairment. For these reasons, different frameworks of syntactic theory (even ones pursuing the same set of goals) make different moves, and accept different trade-offs or compromises, in maneuvering to achieve a theory of grammar which will embody the right degree of generative power and finesse to generate grammatical forms of the language and make relevant distinctions among different classes of forms, grammatical or ungrammatical, while satisfying whatever desiderata for formal properties, psycholinguistic utility, or utility in accounting for syntactic variation and change which they might have.

Progress in syntactic theory often comes through exploitation of the tension between these various concerns, by taking a theory which is well developed up to a point, taking recalcitrant phenomena seriously, and seeking to accommodate them by enlarging our understanding of the domain at hand. Work influenced by this tension tends to be animated by a sense of a deeper underlying system to be discovered. Syntax, on this view, is not simply a matter of tweaking a formalism until data fall into line (although that can sometimes be an advance), nor simply a matter of constructing the most conceptually satisfying theory. The expectation is rather that one understands some portion of the reality of syntactic structure, but by no means the whole of it, and that in struggling with recalcitrant data, one is attempting to expand or rectify one's understanding.

The point of mentioning these basic issues is to counter the notion that ongoing work in syntax must be concerned primarily with enlarging the body of known data on a topic, or concerned primarily with a particular framework of syntactic theory and the development of its full theoretical apparatus. It is possible for a new work to primarily concern itself with the relationship between known data and a given theoretical framework, taken as fixed at least in outline form, or theoretical frameworks of a given type. The goal might be to improve this relationship by making elements of the theory more conceptually basic and sound, and explanations of the data more efficient through the elimination of special circumstances of application. Such is the case with the work presented here.

The present work is a study of the nature of functional categories in a feature-based formulation of syntactic theory such as Minimalist syntax (but equally applicable to any Principles and Parameters syntax, and with suitable reformulation, to other frameworks). It is concerned with the way in which functional projections are defined or constructed in terms of morpho-syntactic and semantic features, and in particular, with the formulation of constraints on these construction operations to ensure that the structures created in particular contexts are few, or unique. The construction of functional categories at issue, and the proposed constraints on this construction, have application to some quite varied problems of syntactic analysis of adult language data. Furthermore, they are applied to achieve a better understanding of child language acquisition of functional categories, and a better understanding of the role of knowledge of the functional category system in at least some cases of Specific Language Impairment.

The choice of topics and the range of theory addressed here are chosen to maintain a particular degree of tension between the tendencies described above. In particular, although the present work seeks to refine and improve the formulation of the syntax of functional categories in a feature-based syntax such as Minimalism, it is not a devoted development of Minimalist syntax in its own right. The basic constraints on the projection of functional categories which will be developed here are ones which should be embodied in any feature-based framework of syntactic theory, including Head-Driven Phrase Structure Grammar (HPSG) and Tree Adjoining Grammar. For this reason, the present work will take pains over the exposition of a handful of critical ideas of Minimalist syntax, but will not strive for a comprehensive investigation of the full range of properties of that framework. But likewise, on most points addressed, it will not constitute a comprehensive study of the relevant empirical domain. For many of the topics discussed here, the aim will be to show that a limited body of well known data can be accounted for much more straightforwardly within a feature-based syntax than on other known or proposed accounts. For others, the empirical boundaries of the topic will be expanded through the presentation and discussion of new items of data.

2. Elements of Minimalist syntax

There are several different ways to use morpho-syntactic and semantic features to condition syntactic representations and/or derivations. Feature conflicts can be generated on an elementary tree, to be resolved through the insertion of an auxiliary tree, blowing the structure up from the inside-out, as in Tree Adjoining Grammar. Features on lexical items can be checked off against matching features entered onto functional categories in highly local configurations obtained through syntactic movement, as in Minimalism. Feature matching can be achieved through unification employed as a static well-formedness condition on syntactic representations without any overt derivation of phrase structure, as in HPSG. The fact that all of these frameworks rely on operations on morpho-syntactic and semantic features to generate or verify phrase structure does not mean that they are all equivalent in empirical coverage, generative power mathematically defined, or general theoretical import. But it represents a striking convergence in the belief that these features have a role to play in determining syntactic phrase structure.

The present work will investigate a syntactic theory in which aspects of syntactic structure follow from feature-matching under syntactic movement, focusing on the ways in which matching features are deployed.

Following, in broad outline, Chomsky (1993, 1995a), and, in most essentials, Chomsky (1995b, 2000, 2001), the syntactic structure of a sentence will be constructed by selecting the lexical items w_i ($i = 1, 2, \ldots, n$) which enter into the sentence, where each w_i is accompanied by a feature matrix, $[F_i^1, \ldots, F_i^{k_i}]$. A partial linear ordering is defined on the features, such that $F_j^s < F_i^r$ holds just in case the checking of F_i^r must precede the checking of F_j^s (for $i, j \in \{1, 2, \ldots, n\}$; $r \in \{1, 2, \ldots, k_i\}$, $s \in \{1, 2, \ldots, k_j\}$). These features include the so-called φ-features of person, number, and gender agreement (whichever are marked in the language at hand). They also include case features on nominals, which on this formulation of the grammar must originate on a sub-phrasal head, which might be taken to be K(ase), in a KP-DP-NP structure for nominals, otherwise on D^o. The features include inflectional features on verbs and adjectives. Using terminology from Chomsky (1995a, 1995b), we will call this set of lexical items with associated feature matrices the lexical array; adding features to check the features on lexical items, the numeration of a sentence is derived, from which the phrase structure of the sentence will be constructed. To handle distinct tokens of a single type, each w_i $[F_i^1, \ldots, F_i^{k_i}]$ will be accompanied by an index for the number of times which that lexical item is to be used. Although multiple use of an item type is not particularly common, it is not exceptionally rare, and accounts for the term 'numeration' to characterize the materials out of which the syntactic structure of a clause is built.

Matching features are projected onto a suite of functional categories. The inventory of functional categories, and the degree and nature of functional category variation across languages, is a substantive matter of current research; see Cinque (1999, 2002) and Rizzi (2004) for recent proposals. Most work assumes that a fixed inventory of functional heads, such as C, Agr_S, T, Agr_O, Asp(ect), and possibly others, is in effect within a given language. Assuming this inventory, for purposes of exposition, agreement φ-features matching the φ-features on nominals are projected onto Agr_S and Agr_O. Tense features are projected onto T, as is a nominative case feature, given the association between nominative case and finite tense. Following Chomsky and Lasnik (1995) and Martin (1996, 2001), a null case feature for PRO is projected on the T node of a control infinitive. The EPP feature, effecting the Extended Projection Principle, which requires a clause to have a subject, will be projected onto Agr_S as well. It will be assumed here that the EPP feature can be checked by any suitable XP constituent (depending on what constituents the language permits as subject of the predicate involved), and that it is not projected to match an EPP feature in the lexical array. This reflects the fact that the EPP is a property of the clause, not of a lexical item occurring within the clause.

The [WH] feature of an interrogative nominal (NP or DP) is matched by a [WH] feature projected onto an interrogative C node. This drives the movement of the lexical [WH] feature, which (depending on the language) may or may not pied-pipe the phonological content of the *wh*-phrase, resulting in the effects of overt or covert *wh*-movement, respectively. In addition, it will be assumed that an interrogative feature [Q] is projected in C^o of an interrogative clause, typing the clause as interrogative. The feature [Q] can be specified as morphologically dependent, requiring checking, in which case it can be checked by the nearest verb under head-to-head movement. But as an interpretable feature, it doesn't delete under checking. As with the EPP feature, it will be assumed that [Q] is not a match to a lexical feature since being interrogative is a property of the clause, not of the highest verb, which checks the feature.

Lexical phrase structure is built by merging lexical items one-by-one with the previously constructed phrase marker, as determined by selectional properties of the items. Phrase structure will be built using the Minimalist merge operation, in which a phrase marker K with label α is merged with a phrase marker K′ with label β, to form a phrase marker K*, with label β. The object constructed through this merge operation will be construed here simply as a binary branching category which, using the labels, can be represented as in (1) below.

(1)

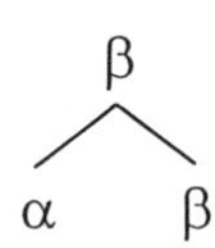

The bar-level of the resulting category in (1) is determined by the status (XP or X^o) of the merged element α, which, in turn, depends on whether or not α is syntactically derived, and if so, how it is derived. In typical formulations of Minimalist syntax, functional categories are merged into phrase structure in the same way, with the label α chosen from the standard, fixed stock of functional categories, C, Agr_S, T, Agr_O, and perhaps Asp. The present work will modify the formulation of functional categories in a syntactic framework of the sort sketched here.

The only levels of representation admitted by Minimalist syntax are PF, the interface with articulatory-perceptual systems, and LF, the interface with the interpretive systems (which Chomsky calls intentional-conceptual systems). The derivation of phrase structure from a numeration through merge operations obviates the need for a "base structure", or level of D-structure, as in other (earlier) varieties of Principles and Parameters syntax. The point, Spell-Out, at which one copy of the derived structure is sent to PF, and a separate and, on most accounts, independent copy is sent to LF, is not a level of representation, but merely a point at which the copy sent to PF becomes (largely or wholly) inaccessible to further merge operations (except perhaps cliticization), and the copy sent to LF becomes (largely or wholly) inaccessible to merge operations which use items from the numeration. (See Bošković 2000 for proposals which, if correct, necessitate the "largely" qualification on the lack of lexical insertion in the derivation to LF after Spell-Out.) The machinery of Minimalist syntax regulating the differences between movement and feature checking in the overt syntax, before Spell-Out, and movement and feature checking covertly, on the way to LF after Spell-Out, includes distinctions in feature strength, along with constraints (Greed, or Enlightened Self Interest) which assure that some instances of feature checking occur in the overt syntax, and other constraints (Procrastinate) which assure that others occur in the covert syntax. Phenomena discussed in the present work rely on merge operations (including movement) in the overt syntax, and not so much on distinctions between overt and covert movement. Furthermore, a number of phenomena which were previously analyzed in terms of covert movement have more recently been cast partly or entirely in terms of overt movement, including *wh*-movement in *wh*-in-situ languages (Watanabe 1992), checking of case and φ-features on an object in English (Koizumi 1993, 1995), and quantifier scope phenomena (Hornstein 1995, 1999; Kitahara 1996). For these reasons, the Minimalist machinery involved in distinguishing overt from covert movement will not be given much consideration here.

The grammar is further constrained by economy conditions, the most basic of which will be adopted here. Assuming that feature movement (and any associated pied-piping of lexical items) is driven by attraction by a matching feature (Attract-F), the "shallowness" condition on attraction will be assumed: that a feature attracts the nearest matching feature which could check it. This effects an economy condition on derivations. Economy conditions on representations include the Full Interpretation condition, which requires that undeleted features present at LF be semantically interpretable. Some new economy conditions will be introduced in the course of the present work.

3. Feature-based projection of functional categories

The merge order of functional categories cannot be determined by semantic selectional relationships (s-selection) in the way that the merging of lexical items can. Furthermore, the stock of functional categories seems to vary, depending on the morpho-syntactic and semantic features expressed by a language, and, on some accounts, seems to vary somewhat across constructions within a single language. These considerations motivate the derivation of the functional categories within a clause to meet the feature-matching needs of lexical items in the numeration, a view developed by Chomsky (1995a) and Giorgi and Pianesi (1996, 1997). Functional categories on this view, rather than being primitive formatives of the syntax, would be merely vessels for, or bundles of, morpho-syntactic (and semantic) features. Features can be bundled together onto functional categories in different ways in different languages, and, in some cases, in different clause types within the same language. The bundles must, however, respect the partial linear checking order defined on the features: a feature which must be checked earlier than another cannot be bundled onto a functional category which is merged later (higher) in the phrase structure of the clause than the category on which the other feature is bundled.

The derivation of functional categories in this way stands in need of some constraints. In certain cases, it is clear that a feature F on a lexical item will check multiple copies of matching features on functional categories; a subject which agrees both with a subject-attribute adjective and with a copular verb in Spanish is a case in point. If features on lexical items were matched one-to-one with matching features projected onto functional categories, then the projection of matching features would be limited to the introduction of one matching feature per lexical feature. But the possibility of multiple checking by such a feature introduces the possibility of introducing matching features without bound, and thus of generating structure which is excessive and redundant without bound, in a way which is fully contrary to any plausible conception of Economy of Representation. The projection of matching features should therefore be subject to an economy constraint requiring that the matching features be minimal in a suitably specified sense. A constraint along these lines, given below, is motivated in Chapter 2 and applied to the analysis of particular linguistic phenomena in subsequent chapters.

(2) *Economy of Feature Projection*
Given the lexical categories in a numeration, a minimal suite of matching features is entered into the numeration to be projected onto functional categories.

In the simplest case, a minimal suite will contain a single matching feature for each feature in the lexical array. In cases in which a single lexical feature is used to mediate more than one instance of NP-head agreement, the matching features will be required to be no more than required to perform this task.

More technical considerations serve to motivate a further constraint on the features projected onto functional heads (whether they are projected to match features on lexical items or are clause-defining features associated with the EPP, negation, or mood), one which concerns not the number of matching features which are projected, but the combinations in which they are projected. In grouping matching features into bundles (more technically, feature matrices) to project as functional categories in the clausal system, there is reason to require that each projected feature matrix serve as a landing site of head movement, thus preventing the projection of a clausal functional head devoted entirely to N-features. The initial formulation of such a constraint, developed in Chapter 2 and applied and refined thereafter, is the following.

(3) *Economy of Projection of Infl-Categories*
If features F_1, F_2, ..., F_n are projected together onto a functional head X within the Infl-system of a clause, then at least one of F_1, F_2, ..., F_n must be a clausal feature.

Clausal features include the EPP feature, a feature such as [Q] which types a clause according to its mood, or a feature matching the lexical feature on a verb or adjective (or other predicative head) within the clause.

Since the analyses developed in this work depend so much on the partial linear checking order of features projected onto functional heads, it turns out that empirical advantage can be gained through an economy constraint on the specification of this ordering relation. The most general formulation of such a constraint is the Minimal Feature Ordering principle below. Two corollaries of this constraint, given in preliminary formulations in (5)–(6) below, limit the ordering of N-features in a numeration and limit the specification of the checking order to features within a clause or at a clausal boundary. (A phase is a derivational episode effecting the derivation of a clause or complex nominal; see Chomsky 2000, 2001. Projection of F_i and F_j across a phase boundary means there are phases α and β such that β immediately follows α, and one of F_i and F_j is the last feature matrix projected in α, and the other is the first feature matrix projected in β.)

(4) *Minimal Feature Ordering*
The partial linear order defining the checking order of features in a numeration is minimal to determine a convergent derivation of a syntactic structure from the numeration.

(5) *Minimal Feature Ordering: Corollary 1*
The partial linear order defining the checking order of features in a numeration does not specify the checking order of N-features with respect to one another, but only with respect to V-features.

(6) *Minimal Feature Ordering: Corollary 2*
Feature matrices F_i and F_j within a numeration are ordered with respect to one another only if they are projected together within a phase, or if they are projected, one immediately after the other, across a phase boundary.

The principles in (2)–(4), and the two corollaries of (4) given in (5)–(6), are not merely plausible instantiations of the Economy of Representation and the Economy of Derivation; they earn their keep by making certain numerations from a given lexical array possible, and by ruling out others, and by making certain derivations of a sentence from a given numeration possible, and ruling out others. In doing so, they play a major role in providing a theoretical distinction between grammatical and ungrammatical forms, permitting the derivation of grammatical forms, and preventing the derivation of (otherwise very similar) forms which are ungrammatical.

The derivation of functional categories as hierarchically structured matrices of grammatical features lends some new perspectives to the study of child language acquisition of functional categories. Previously, the concern was whether a particular functional category (say T) is present, and whether it is innate or has been acquired, to support a paradigm of associated functional elements (morphemes or words) once they have been acquired. Under the derivation of functional categories as matrices of features, this concern is replaced with a concern for the acquisition of the distribution of features into feature matrices to be projected as functional heads. The focus on whether functional categories within a fixed stock (C, Agr_S, T, etc.) have been acquired, or are innate, is replaced by new concerns, including (1.) the inventory of functional features available to the child at a given point in child language development; (2.) the feature matrices which can be constructed out of these features and projected as functional heads; and, (3.) the development of the adult functional category system in which multiple feature matrices are projected together within a clause. From this perspective, the forms of expression of functional elements in early child language can be seen to result from the projection of individual features, or of non-adult combinations of features, as functional categories which don't occur in the adult system. Turning to constraints on the projection of adult functional categories, it is easy to demonstrate that, quite early in the age range investigated here, children can represent phrase structure complexity (measured in terms of the number of heads involved in selectional chains within a sentence) sufficient to represent a full set of functional categories. Thus, it is possible to eliminate concern with the capacity to represent phrase structure in general, and to focus specifically on the capacity to represent matrices of functional features, projected as functional categories. This leads to an investigation of child language acquisition of functional categories which measures something different from what is measured in existing studies. Specifically, it leads to a study which counts the functional categories which can be represented within the clausal system at a given time, and tracks the maximum of this count over time, looking for an increase in the capacity to represent multiple functional categories within a single clause, without any particular regard for the identities of those categories.

Likewise, the derivation of functional categories as matrices of features lends a new perspective to the study of the role of functional categories in language impairment. One question to be asked in these studies, on both the old perspective and the new, is whether a particular type of language impairment involves a failure to acquire or use particular classes of functional elements (such as complementizers, or auxiliary verbs), or whether it involves a limitation in general phrase structure complexity. But on top of those concerns, the new perspective leads to a concern with the number of matrices of matching features which can be projected together within a clause. In the present work, this question is pursued for the cases classified as Specific Language Impairment (SLI), where there are language deficits despite normal intelligence and the absence of any articulatory or hearing difficulties, or any identifiable neurological trauma.

Chapter 2 reviews the role of functional categories in generative syntax, focusing on movement-based frameworks in the Principles and Parameters tradition. A derivation of functional categories as matrices of morpho-syntactic and semantic features is then presented, elaborating on proposals made by Giorgi and Pianesi (1996, 1997) and, in a rather different formalism, by Rambow (1994) and Rambow and Santorini (1995). The Economy of Feature Projection and the Economy of Projection of Infl-Categories, given in (2) and (3) above, are motivated and formulated here.

Chapters 3–8 present substantive new applications of this theory to problems in syntactic analysis, child language acquisition, and the study of Specific Language Impairment.

Chapter 3, on Germanic verb-second, accounts for patterns of verb-second in Germanic languages in a way that is quite parallel to the account in Rambow and Santorini (1995), but implemented within the notation developed here. This account is then extended to cross-linguistic variation in the distribution of expletive subjects in these languages, and to some intricacies of verb-second in Old and Middle English.

Chapter 4, on the placement of pronominal clitics, accounts for relative orders of verb and clitic, and the possibility of clitic climbing in restructuring contexts, providing a novel execution of patterns of verb and clitic movement to obtain the relevant facts, one which is argued to be better grounded than those proposed by other researchers. Within this domain, the present account does not expand coverage of data, but achieves the effects of existing accounts of clitic placement by orchestrating verb and clitic movement through feature-matching associations driving such movements, and by appealing to constraints on these associations which are less ad hoc than were previously available, as a foundation for the account.

Chapter 5, on tenseless clauses and coordination, investigates a form of coordination in colloquial English which has received little (or no) attention in the literature, and shows that it can be explained using the representation of functional categories, along with the constraints on these representations, developed in Chapter 2. It is then shown that this approach to the new data can be directly adapted to account for the structure of small clause complements of perception verbs.

Chapter 6, the first chapter on child language acquisition, investigates forms of clause structure distinctive to early child English and shows that they follow from the projection of functional features, individually or in non-adult combinations. On this account, the functional category system of early child language is produced by the same operations of functional category construction which are employed in the adult grammar, but operating on more limited inventories of functional features, in the context of a more limited capacity to project multiple functional categories within a clause, producing functional category systems in early child language which are different from the adult system.

Chapter 7, on child acquisition of adult functional categories, shows that the facts concerning the development of the system of adult functional categories do not match the predictions of most of the standard theories of this process, but reflect instead the growth or development of more basic representational resources of the child's grammar. In particular, it is shown that the use of clausal functional categories lags behind the development of the phrase structure complexity required to represent multiple functional categories per clause. The results obtained in this chapter to some extent match the effects found by Guilfoyle and Noonan (1992) and Vainikka (1993/94), which they interpreted in terms of a sequential acquisition of the fixed stock of standard functional categories, I and C. But the present account reduces these effects to more basic developments in the growth of the child's grammar.

Chapter 8, on Specific Language Impairment (SLI), shows that children with SLI lag in their production of multiple functional elements within the clausal system, and specifically, that they lag not only behind their language-matched normally developing peers, but they lag behind what should be possible given the individual functional categories which they seem to have acquired and the phrase structure complexity they have attained. The results are interpreted to show that children with SLI are not just slower to acquire classes of functional elements, but that they have a deficit in the representational resources required to project multiple functional categories within a single clause.

Chapter 2
A feature-based derivation of functional heads

1. The syntactic utility of functional heads

Functional elements include markers of tense and modality, clausal subordination and mood, subject-verb agreement, negation, and aspect, each of which can be expressed in the morphology or in the syntax. But the syntactic significance of the functional systems, which consist of the syntactic structures associated with functional elements, goes beyond what is directly expressed in the syntax. The functional systems are implicated by syntactic theory in a variety of syntactic processes and relations, including the assignment or realization of structural grammatical case, the derivation of word order differences between interrogatives and declaratives, and between finite and infinitival clauses, the derivation of verb-second effects in most Germanic languages and of clitic-second effects in many modern and historical languages, and in the placement of pronominal clitics in Romance languages and languages of the Balkan peninsula.

A simple system of functional categories reserves a head Infl (or I) for tense features and/or morphemes, for subject-verb agreement features and/or morphemes, and charges it with the case assigned to the subject (since this usually depends on whether the tense is finite or non-finite). When a subject is placed within its specifier, this category projects to a maximal projection IP. The periphery of a clause is marked by complementizer elements marking mood or clausal subordination; a functional C(omplementizer) position is reserved for such elements. Adding elements for the expression of sentence negation, projected between I and VP, a simple representation of functional categories for a left-headed language such as English is given by the tree structure in (1a), equivalent to the labeled bracketing in (1b). The functional systems are frequently (or on some formulations of syntactic theory, primarily) landing sites for head movement and XP-movement. Some examples will be reviewed here in order to illustrate the use of functional categories, and to introduce basic data in areas which will be examined more closely later. To take the most standard example, the association of C with mood implicates C in the analysis of

Aux-fronting and *wh*-fronting in root interrogative forms in languages with overt *wh*-movement.

(1) a.

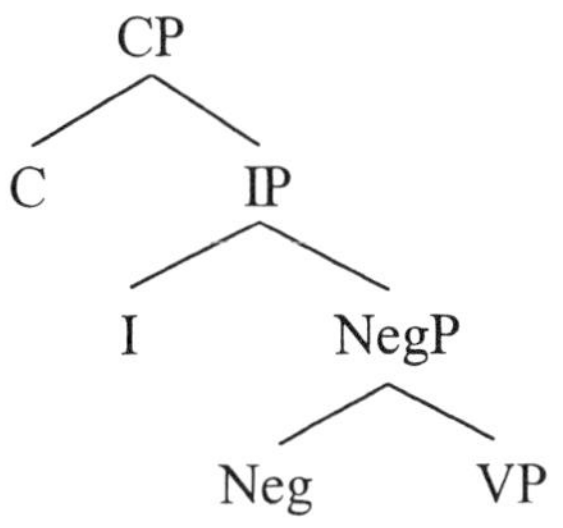

b. $[_{CP}$ C $[_{IP}$ I $[_{NegP}$ Neg $[_{VP}$ . . .]]]]

The word order in the *yes/no*-question in (2) below can be related to the normal declarative order through a syntactic derivation involving head movement of I to C, provided the interrogative feature [Q] in (3) attracts Aux in I, with the result shown in (4).

(2) *Have you fed the dog?*

(3) $[_{CP}$ $[_{C[Q]}$] $[_{IP}$ *you* $[_{I}$ *have*] $[_{VP}$ *fed the dog*]]]

(4) $[_{CP}$ $[_{C[Q]}$ $[_{I}$ *have*]] $[_{IP}$ *you* $[_{I}$ t_I] $[_{VP}$ *fed the dog*]]]

Likewise, the word order of (5) is related to that in the declarative by Aux movement coupled with *wh*-movement, as shown in (6), where the feature [WH] attracts the *wh*-expression to the specifier of CP.

(5) *Which dog have you fed?*

(6) $[_{CP}$ $[_{DP[WH]}$ *which dog*] $[_{C[Q, WH]}$ $[_{I}$ *have*]] $[_{IP}$ *you* $[_{I}$ t_I]
$[_{VP}$ *fed* t_{DP}]]]

The verb-second (V2) phenomenon can be explicated using the same theoretical resources. As shown in the German data in (7)–(8) below, the finite verb – an auxiliary in (7) and a main verb in (8) – is in second position, preceded by an element which is displaced from the neutral SOV order displayed in non-verb-second contexts.[1]

(7)

a.	*Karl*	*hat*		*das*	*Buch*	*gelesen.*
b.	*Das Buch*	*hat*	*Karl*			*gelesen.*
c.	*Gestern*	*hat*	*Karl*	*das*	*Buch*	*gelesen.*
	Top	has	Karl	the	book	read

(8)

a.	*Karl*	*liest*		*das Buch.*
b.	*Das Buch*	*liest*	*Karl.*	
c.	*Heute*	*liest*	*Karl*	*das Buch.*
	Top	read	Karl	the book

The role of the functional category C is indicated by the pattern that obtains in embedded clauses, where V2 is in complementary distribution with an overt complementizer.

(9)

a. *Sie sagt, daß Karl dieses Buch gelesen hat.*
   She says that Karl this book read has

b. *Sie sagt Karl hat dieses Buch gelesen.*

c. *Sie sagt dieses Buch hat Karl gelesen.*

d. *Sie sagt gestern hat Karl dieses Buch gelesen.*
   She says yesterday has Karl this book read

The alternation in (9) between V2 and the complementizer *daß* follows directly, along with the basic V2 pattern in (7)–(8), provided that the finite verb is attracted to C just in case C is empty, in which case the topic element is attracted to spec-CP, as shown in (10).[2]

(10)

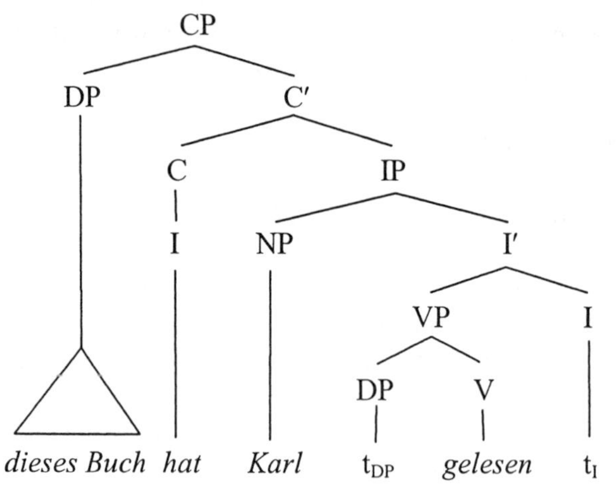

The reliance on the C-system by both V2 and question formation yields a straightforward explanation of the rather intricate interactions between V2 and question formation shown in (11) below (from Vikner 1995: 114–115).

(11) *Welchen Film hat sie gesagt ...*
which film has she said

a. ... t_{wh}' *daß die Kinder* t_{wh} *gesehen haben?*
that the children seen have

b. * ... *in der Schule haben die Kinder* t_{top} t_{wh} *gesehen?*
in the school have the children seen

c. * ... *die Kinder haben* t_{top} t_{wh} *gesehen?*
the children have seen

d. ... t_{wh}' *haben die Kinder* t_{wh} *gesehen?*
have the children seen

In (11a), with an overt complementizer introducing a non-V2 complement clause, the direct object *welchen film* extracts from the direct object position before the verb, through spec-CP of the complement clause, to spec-CP of the main clause, a prototypical example of successive cyclic movement; the subordinate clause with traces of movement is represented in (12).

(12)

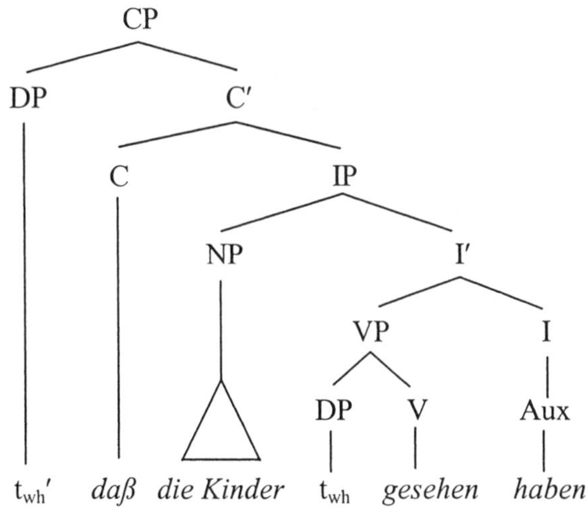

In (11b), where the complement clause is V2, the adverbial PP *in der Schule* has moved to spec-CP as the topic element, thus blocking extraction of *welchen film*; see (13).

(13)

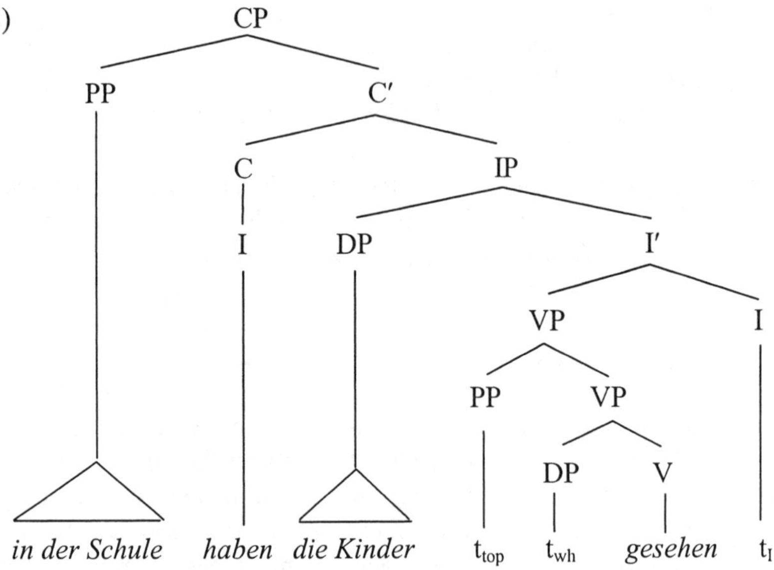

In (11c), the lower subject *die Kinder* has become the topic element in the V2 structure, blocking extraction of the direct object, just as in (11b). Finally, in (11d), the direct object *welchen film* has itself moved to spec-CP as the topic element of the V2 structure; as a result, it is in position to be attracted to the main clause spec-CP, completing a *wh*-question over the direct object in the lower clause, which is represented in (14). The tight interaction between the derivations of V2 and question formation in this account of the data in (11) gives the account a degree of explanatory power.

(14)

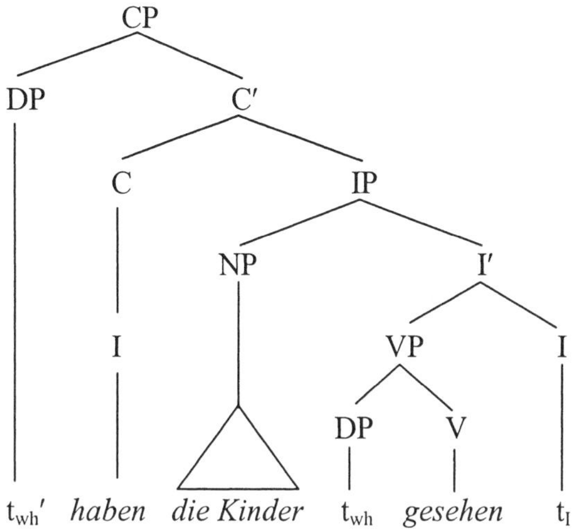

Similar processes can be observed to operate in Tohono O'odham, an Uto-Aztecan language of Southern Arizona and Northern Mexico. To begin with, in declarative root clauses, the O'odham "auxiliary" element (as it is called in the literature), which is inflected for person and number agreement with the subject and for perfective or imperfective aspect, appears almost invariably in second position, with a wide variety of elements as options for first position, including arguments of the verb, the verb itself, and the negation marker. (See Zepeda 1983.) This is illustrated in (15)–(20) below, with imperfective auxiliaries in (15)–(19), and perfective auxiliaries in (20)–(22).[3] (Examples (15)–(18) are from Zepeda 1983: 20, 31–33; (19)–(22) are from Langacker 1972: 150–151. 'SPRON' = subject pronoun; 'PERF' = perfective; 'IMPF' = imperfective; 'SG' and 'PL' on subject pronouns and the auxiliary mark singular and plural number of the subject, respectively; 'OPL' marks plural number of the object; and numbers indicate the first, second, or third person.)

(15) a. *'a:ñi* *'añ* *s-hottam* *cipkan.*
SPRON.1.SG IMPF.1.SG quickly work
'I am/was working quickly.'
b. *S-hottam 'añ cipkan 'a:ñi.*
c. *Cipkan 'añ 'a:ñi s-hottam.*

(16) a. *'a:pi 'ap s-ba:bigi him.*
SPRON.2.SG IMPF.2.SG slowly walk
'You are/were walking slowly.'
b. *S-ba:bigi 'ap him 'a:pi.*
c. *Him 'ap s-ba:bigi 'a:pi.*

(17) *Ban 'o g totobi ha-huhu'id.*
coyote IMPF.3.SG the rabbits OPL-chase
'The coyote is/was chasing the rabbits.'

(18) *'a:cim 'ac g ki: kegcid.*
SPRON.1.PL IMPF.1.PL the house clean
'We are/were cleaning the house.'

(19) *Hegai ceoj 'o ge'ej.*
that man IMPF.3.SG big
'That man is/was big.'

(20) *'a:ñi 'ant wu: g wisilo.*
SPRON.1.SG PERF.1.SG rope.PERF the calf
'I roped the calf.'

(21) *Ceoj 'at ha-cecpos g wipsilo.*
man PERF.3.SG OPL-brand.PERF.OPL the calves
'The man branded the calves.'

(22) *'a:cim 'att cepos g wisilo.*
SPRON.1.PL PERF.1.PL brand.PERF the calf
'We branded the calf.'

The second-position property of the auxiliary bears some resemblance to Germanic verb-second, but there are some significant differences, and the "Aux-second" property of O'odham will simply be taken for granted for the moment. What is striking about O'odham in terms of what we have seen above is the behavior of the auxiliary element in subordinate clauses and *yes/no*-questions, shown in (23)–(28), with *yes/no*-questions in (23), a complement clause in (24), and relative clauses in (25)–(28). (Example (23) is from Zepeda 1983: 14, 21; (24) is from Zepeda, 108, and (25)–(28)

are from Langacker 1972: 151. 'INT' marks interrogative mood, and 'COMP' is a complementizer, introducing subordinate clauses.)

(23) a. *No g mi:stol ko:s?*
INT-IMPF.3.SG the cat sleep
'Is the cat sleeping?'
b. *Nap 'a:pi cipkan?*
INT-IMPF.2.SG SPRON.2.SG work
'Are you working?'

(24) *Hegai ceoj 'o kaij mo cipkan*
that boy IMPF.3.SG say COMP.IMPF.3.SG work
g huan.
the Huan
'That boy says that Juan is working'

(25) *Hegai ceoj mo g husi ñi:d*
that man COMP.IMPF.3.SG the Husi sees
'o ge'ej.
IMPF.3.SG big
'The man José sees is big.'

(26) *Hegai wisilo mant 'a:ñi wu:*
that calf COMP.PERF.1.SG SPRON.1.SG roped.PERF
'o ge'ej.
IMPF.3.SG big
'That calf that I roped is/was big.'

(27) *Hegai ceoj mat ha-cecpos g*
that man COMP.PERF.3.SG OPL-brand.PERF.OPL the
wipsilo 'o ge'ej.
calves IMPF.3.SG big
'That man that branded the calves is/was big.'

(28) *Gogs 'o huhu'id hegai wisilo matt*
dog IMPF.3.SG chase that calf COMP.PERF.1.PL
'a:cim cipos.
SPRON.1.PL brand.PERF
'The dog is/was chasing the calf that we branded.'

In these, the auxiliary element is displaced out of the clause and morphologically joins with a bound morpheme at the clause periphery, the *yes/no*-question particle *n-*, or the subordinate clause marker, *m-*; the initial glottal stop [ʔ] of the auxiliary phonologically deletes upon affixation of *m-* or *n-*.

(29) *n-* + *'o* → *no*
n- + *'ap* → *nap*
m- + *'o* → *mo*
m- + *'ant* → *mant*
m- + *'at* → *mat*
m- + *'att* → *matt*

Since the clause-introducing particles mark mood and/or subordination, and occur clause-peripherally, they should be generated in a clause-initial C^o. The facts cited above then follow if the auxiliary (*'o*, *'ap*, *'ant*, etc.) occupies the highest clausal head prior to movement to C, and is attracted to C^o by the bound complementizer morpheme, with the order of the complementizer element with respect to Aux determined by the affixal properties of the complementizer.

The pattern in *yes/no*-questions and subordinate clauses is not Aux-second since, although the auxiliary element does appear in second-position, the element in first position is fixed, and is, moreover, morphologically united with the auxiliary, rather than concatenated syntactically. In *yes/no*-questions and subordinate clauses, the auxiliary might be moving out of an Aux-second structure, and thereby obscuring it, or there may be no Aux-second structure in these examples. We leave it open here whether the auxiliary normally appears in the highest inflectional head, or in a supra-Infl head Z^o required to produce the Aux-second order in examples such as (15)–(22). Similarly, it is left open whether the movement in the *yes/no*-questions and subordinate clauses in (23)–(28) are straightforward cases of I-to-C movement, or whether the auxiliary moves out of an additional head Z^o, as an instance of Z-to-C movement in these examples.[4]

With these considerations in mind, the structure of the subordinate clause CP in (24) can be represented as shown in (30) below, and the relativized subject DP in (26) can be diagrammed as in (31).

(30)

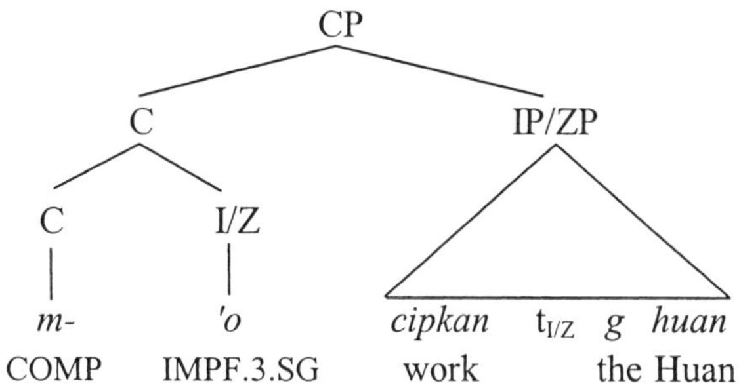

(31)

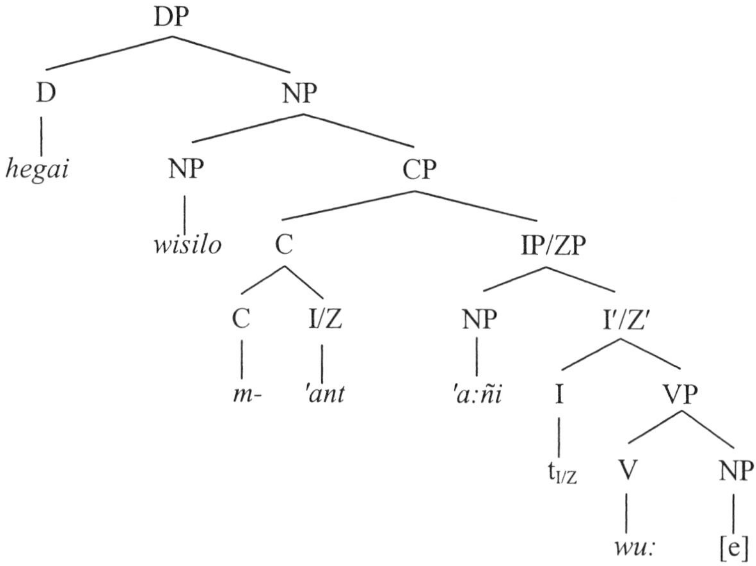

V-to-C movement involves the periphery of the clause and either alternation with clausal subordinators (as in German embedded V2) or morphological union with them (as in O'odham). Verb movement within a clause (such as V-to-I movement) is evidenced by alternations in verb position with respect to negation and clause-medial adverbials. A prototypical case is French V-to-I movement in finite clauses, discussed by Emonds (1978) and Pollock (1989), and shown in (32). (Data in (32)–(35) from Pollock 1989.)

(32) a. *Marie embrasse souvent Jean.*
Marie kisses often Jean.

b. *Pierre parle à peine l'italien.*
Pierre speaks hardly Italian
c. *Jean (n') aime pas Marie.*
Jean (NEG) likes not Marie

Alternation is observed between the position of the main verb in (32) with its position in infinitives, where an auxiliary may move to I, as in (33b), or not, as in (33a), but the main verb cannot move to I, as shown in (34).

(33) a. *Ne pas être heureux est une condition pour écrire des romans.*
NEG not be happy is a prerequisite for writing novels
b. *N'être pas heureux est …*
NEG-be not happy is

(34) a. *Ne pas posséder de voiture en banlieue rend la vie difficile.*
NEG not own of-a car in suburbs makes the life difficult
b. * *Ne posséder pas de voiture en banlieue …*
NEG own not of-a car in suburbs

French infinitives exhibit the possibility of an optional short movement of the main verb to a position below negation, as in (35b), implicating a functional category below the landing site of verb movement in finite clauses.

(35) a. *À peine parler l'italien rend la vie difficile.*
hardly to-speak Italian makes the life difficult
b. *Parler à peine l'italien rend …*
to-speak hardly Italian makes

Pollock (1989) advances this as evidence that Infl is split, constituted of a component T with tense, above negation, and another component below negation. Pollock identifies the lower component as Agr, the projection site of subject agreement features and/or morphemes, but the subject agreement projection (Agr_S) is more commonly located above TP since subject agreement morphemes are external to tense morphemes in morphological ordering of affixation to the root. The lower inflectional head, below T, might therefore be identified as an object agreement head, Agr_O.

Baker (1991), Williams (1994), and others, have proposed alternative analyses of the French verb, adverb, and negation ordering facts in (32)–(35), accounting for them with language-specific phrase structure expansion rules. This packs cross-linguistic diversity into the phrase structure rules instead of into the triggering conditions for verb movement. But this isn't an even trade-off in complexity since the V-movement account appeals to basic and quite regular principles of clause construction (such as adverbs of specific types having particular loci of attachment within the clause for reasons depending, in part, on their interpretations), plus a basic general-purpose syntactic operation (head movement), whereas the language-specific phrase structure expansion rules in the alternative account do not put theoretically constrained bounds on the resulting cross-linguistic variation in clause structure. See Iatridou (1990) and Pollock (1997) for further discussion of Pollock's (1989) arguments for verb movement.

Allowing for the positioning of a subject agreement head above a head for tense, as argued by Belletti (1990), and allowing for a head to perform a symmetric function for the object(s), the particular form of split Infl shown in (36), proposed by Chomsky (1991), is obtained.

(36)

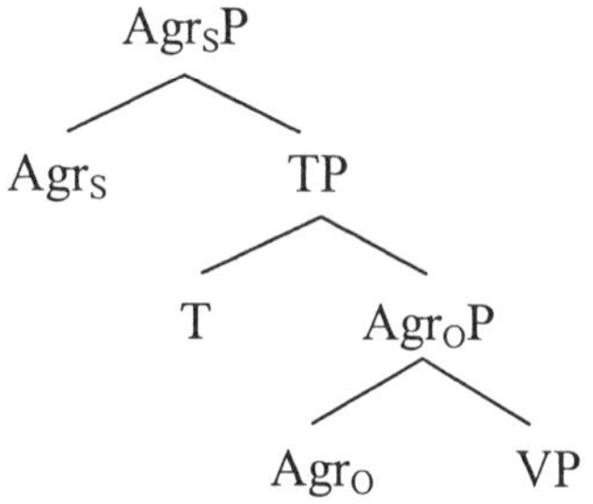

2. Derived functional heads

2.1. Derived functional heads in the literature

As illustrated above, the systems of functional categories play a critical role in explanatory accounts of a variety of phenomena across languages, explanatory in that the facts are derived from the interaction between general syntactic movement operations in the context of general functional category systems, rather than from language-specific and construction-specific conditions. But there are conceptual problems in taking functional categories to be primitive. Most pressing are questions about where functional categories come from, and what determines their order with respect to one another.

Grimshaw (1991) proposed an answer to these questions in terms of semantic function and a partial reduction of functional category placement to semantic selection. Assuming that a VP denotes an action, Grimshaw proposed that I, in taking VP as its complement, maps an action to a corresponding event or situation, and that C, in taking IP as its complement, maps the event or situation to the proposition that this event or situation is realized at a time, or within a time interval, specified by the tense and aspect of the clause. One limitation of this proposal is that it doesn't address the order of Agr with respect to other categories, since Agr nodes don't enter into the sort of semantic composition invoked by Grimshaw. Furthermore, it has a drawback in that infinitival clauses without a *for* complementizer, occurring in complement position to verbs such as *expect*, have referents which can more readily be construed as propositional than as events or situations; yet, as Bošković (1995, 1996, 1997) argues, infinitivals without an overt complementizer seem to be of category IP, not CP.

In another attempt to address these questions, Hegarty (1993) proposed that functional heads are interpolated as needed to match features on lexical items, following the construction of a skeletal phrase structure with projections of lexical categories. On this approach, the functional heads needed were determined by feature-matching needs on lexical items (following Chomsky 1991, 1993 on this point, though not on other points related to the account), and the positions of functional categories were determined by economy constraints on the movements required to meet the needs of lexical items, computed across alternative positions assigned to the relevant functional heads. This led to difficulties with functional elements such as overt complementizers, which, by virtue of their lexical material, should be generated as part of the lexical structure of the sentence, rather than interpolated later; furthermore, it invoked a quite unconstrained set of alternative derivations, posing issues for the complexity of computation of the most economical derivation.

In the meantime, the idea of having a fixed stock of pre-identified functional categories, such as those in (36) or any elaborations thereof, was being challenged in localized ways by a variety of researchers, and in a wholesale fashion by Chomsky's (1995a, distributed 1993) framework of bare phrase structure; out of these developments, there arose an entirely different way of posing the questions at hand. To review these briefly, van Gelderen (1993) and Giorgi and Pianesi (1996, 1997) argue for certain instances of non-standard bundling of features, where a tense or agreement feature normally projected on an inflectional head is exceptionally projected on C instead, to handle particular syntactic data. Heycock and Kroch (1993) propose that in certain cases, specifically in German subject-initial verb-second clauses, the functional heads C and I should be fused into a single head C/I performing the functions of both C and I. Rambow (1994) and Rambow and Santorini (1995) provide a construction of functional heads out of verb, inflectional, mood, and complementizer features, {+V, +I, +M, +C}, in which distinct (though possibly overlapping) sets of such features define distinct functional heads. Specifically, feature values drawn from this set are specified on verbs and complementizers among the lexical items, and a set of features on a verb results in projection of a functional category with that feature set as a landing site for the verb upon verb movement; and a set of features on a complementizer projects a functional category with that feature set when the complementizer is inserted.[5] Van Gelderen (1996) proposes that functional structure be derived from feature structure, and not stipulated as given, but resorts to an extreme form of feature scattering – one feature per head.

Giorgi and Pianesi (1996, 1997) provide an illustration of the utility of alternate feature bundlings provided by a feature-based construction of functional heads. They address complementizer deletion and interrogative data in Modern Italian, including the problem of accounting for the distribution of subjects in subjunctive complement clauses which are not introduced by a complementizer, as in (37) below (from Giorgi and Pianesi 1996: 138, 144).[6]

(37) a. *Tutti credevano fosse arrivato Gianni.*
they-all believed had(SUBJ) arrived Gianni
'Everyone believed that Gianni had arrived.'
b. * *Tutti credevano fosse Gianni arrivato.*
c. % *Tutti credevano Gianni fosse arrivato.*

As shown in (37), the complementizerless subjunctive complement cannot take a full nominal (NP or DP) subject between the raised auxiliary and the participle; it can only take a nominal subject postverbally, or, for some speakers, before the auxiliary. In Rizzi (1996), building on proposals for

French by Rizzi and Roberts ([1989] 1996), these are analyzed as involving Aux movement to Agr, in the C – Agr – T phrase structure of Belletti (1990), followed by [Aux-Agr] movement to C, with the configuration resulting from Agr-to-C circumventing assignment of nominative case to a subject in spec-AgrP. But, Giorgi and Pianesi point out, this would lead us to expect that there should be a similar failure of nominative case assignment in Aux-to-Comp structures such as that in (38) below (Giorgi and Pianesi 1996: 138).

(38) *Avendo Gianni perso il treno, arrivammo in ritardo.*
having Gianni missed the train, arrived-we late
'Gianni having missed the train, we arrived late.'

In order to solve this problem, Giorgi and Pianesi appeal to general processes for bundling features on elements (lexical or functional) in syntax. They observe that features cluster in language-particular ways on lexical categories. In the extreme cases of highly agglutinative and highly analytic languages, the mapping from morphemes to inflectional features might be one-to-one. But in a language like Italian, a single morpheme might be syncretic, carrying values for multiple features. The inflection *-a* of an adjective like *bella* 'beautiful', for example, expresses features for gender and number, feminine singular. Against the backdrop of these considerations, Giorgi and Pianesi frame the issue of how features come to be associated with items in a numeration (a set of elements out of which to build a sentence) based on an array of lexical choices, in the framework of Chomsky (1995a). For lexical categories, there is not much for the syntax to say in this regard. The lexical categories present in a numeration N are selected by the speaker or writer based on what they intend to say, and the distribution of features on lexical categories is determined by lexical properties of the language. Thus, the extent to which these categories are syncretic is determined by lexical/grammatical properties of the language. In the specification of the feature content of functional categories, Giorgi and Pianesi argue that there is some limited room for the language to maneuver, in order to provide multiple options. Specifically, instead of assuming that there is an invariant (language particular) distribution of features on functional categories in a numeration, Giorgi and Pianesi propose that features are given as ordered in a numeration, and that they are gathered into distinct bundles (not violating this ordering) and the bundles are projected onto functional categories in the numeration, subject to general constraints.

(Rizzi 1996 made a proposal in the same spirit in order to account for differences between embedded and root interrogatives in Italian; Giorgi and Pianesi develop and systematize the idea within the Minimalist framework.) To illustrate with examples pertinent to this and subsequent chapters, tense and nominative case features are typically bundled together and projected onto T^o, with the tense feature checked upon verb movement to T, and the nominative case feature checked upon movement of T to $Agr_{(S)}$ and the subject nominal to spec-$Agr_{(S)}$P. Similarly, given the presence of a nominal element among the lexical categories in a numeration, to be projected as an object of a verb, a set of N-features matching those on the nominal will appear as a feature matrix, $F_{N\text{-}o}$, which will typically be combined with a feature matrix, $F_{V\text{-}o}$, of V-features matching those on the verb, to form a larger matrix, $[F_{V\text{-}o}, F_{N\text{-}o}]$ to be projected onto an Agr_O node.

Giorgi and Pianesi propose the following principles to constrain the projection of features onto functional categories:

(39) *Universal Ordering Constraint*
The features are ordered [in a numeration] so that $F_2 < F_1$ iff the checking of F_1 precedes the checking of F_2.

(40) *Feature Scattering Principle*
Each feature can head a projection.

The scattering of features expressed in (40) is an extreme case; the intent is to allow all clusters of features on a single head consistent with the universal ordering constraint, up to the extreme case of one feature per head. This allows for syncretic categories in which a single head carries more than one feature.

A further constraint on the projection of features onto functional categories is expressed by Giorgi and Pianesi in the following passage (1996: 142):

(41) Finally, the actual number of projections is defined according to economy considerations, that is, the shortest derivation compatible with the initial array is selected (cf. Chomsky [1995a], section 3).[7]

This conception of Minimalist syntax will be considered further below. Turning back to the empirical problem posed by subjunctive complements in Italian, Giorgi and Pianesi propose that features within the subjunctive complement clause can be projected onto functional categories in the numeration in the relatively scattered form given in (42a) below, yielding ordinary C – Agr – T structures with an overt complementizer, or in the more highly syncretic form given in (42b), which leads to a syncretic "amalgamated" category C/Agr (which Giorgi and Pianesi call 'Mood/Agr').[8]

(42) a. ⟨+Mood⟩, ⟨+φ, +Nom⟩, ⟨+V, –N, +φ, +Nom, +Mood⟩
b. ⟨+Mood, +φ, +Nom⟩, ⟨+V, –N, +φ, +Nom, +Mood⟩

In the phrase structure tree resulting from (42a), an overt complementizer is projected in C, and the auxiliary does not move to C; the subject appears preverbally in spec-AgrP. The form in (37a) is derived from the alternate bundling of features given in (42b). In the derivation of (37a), ⟨+Mood, +φ, +Nom⟩ are projected onto C/Agr, taking VP as its complement, and Aux moves to C/Agr, leaving no possible source for the structure in (37b) with *Gianni* between the auxiliary and the participle.

(43) $[_{\mathrm{C/AgrP}}$ C/Agr $[_{\mathrm{VP}}$ Aux $[[_{\mathrm{VP}}$ V] $\mathrm{NP}_{\mathrm{subj}}$]]]

The postverbal subject is not affected by the choice of (42a,b) and is available in either case.[9] Ordinary Aux-to-Comp in (38) results from movement of [Aux-Agr] to an ordinary C^{o}.

The syncretic categories of Giorgi and Pianesi permit a more fine-grained separation of features than could be expressed with category labels drawn from any common system of functional heads. These more fine-grained capabilities will be required for some of the applications in subsequent chapters of the present work. Hence, although the notation for features and feature bundles adopted below is substantially different from that of Giorgi and Pianesi, the essence of their idea will be pursued.

2.2. Feature matrices and constraints

A derivation of functional categories along the lines proposed by Giorgi and Pianesi will be developed here, with particular attention to constraints on the bundling of features and the projection of functional heads derived from feature bundles.

A sentence will be derived from an array of lexical items, shown in (44), in which each lexical item w_i is accompanied by a feature matrix, $[F_i^1, \ldots, F_i^{k_i}]$.

(44) $A = \{\ w_1[F_1^1, \ldots, F_1^{k_1}], w_2[F_2^1, \ldots, F_2^{k_2}], \ldots, w_n[F_n^1, \ldots, F_n^{k_n}]\ \}$

The checking order is a partial linear order defined on the set of features in (44), as in (45).[10]

(45) $F_j^s < F_i^r$ iff the checking of F_i^r must precede the checking of F_j^s.

The feature matrices associated with each word in (44) are not necessarily sequences of individual features; each of the F_i^r ($i = 1, \ldots, n$; $r = 1, \ldots, k_i$) may itself be a hierarchically structured matrix of features. The constraints on these feature matrices are that for each w_i ($i = 1, \ldots, n$), $[F_i^1, \ldots, F_i^{k_i}]$ should contain all the individual features associated with w_i, and should be structured so that each sub-matrix, F_i^r, is either an individual feature or is a morphologically coherent matrix of features which all have the same checking order. For example, the features marked on a subject pronoun in English will typically consist of a hierarchically structured matrix of person and number agreement features, together with a separate nominative case feature, as in (46) below.

(46) *we*

[NOM] ,	[1PER] [PL]

For convenience, the feature matrix in (46) will normally be written out as in (47).

(47) *we* [[NOM], [[1PER], [PL]]]

The notation embodies the constraint that, while [[1PER], [PL]] and [NOM] may be checked at different points in the derivation, [1PER] and [PL] must be checked together.

Matching features to those on each lexical item in (44) are added with the same linear order defined on them as that defined on the originals. This forms a complete numeration, which provides the starting point for a derivation, and for all derivations in its comparison class under the Economy of Derivation. Since all the features within an immediate sub-matrix, F_i^r, in (44) must be checked together, it follows that the matching features to those in F_i^r should be structured into an identical matrix to F_i^r, so that they will be checked together against their counterparts within F_i^r.

Negation and complementizers are functional elements which occur in the lexical array. They instantiate their own features, rather than projecting features which match features on other lexical items. Features instantiated by functional elements, together with those added to the numeration to check features on lexical items, will be called functional features. Features instantiated by negation or complementizer elements participate in the partial linear order defined on features in the numeration. These elements can be assumed to check the features they instantiate, in which case the ordering on these features is a checking order, as it is with features projected to match features on lexical items. Alternatively, the ordering on features instantiated by negation and complementizers can be considered to be the merge order of these elements in the construction of the functional category system.

It will be assumed that phrase structure is composed by the merge operation of Minimalist syntax; see Chomsky (1993, 1995a, 1995b, 2000, 2001). When a head X is merged with a non-head target K, the result [X K] is X′, a projection of X, with K its complement. When a non-head constituent Z is merged with X′, the result [Z X′] is a higher projection of X, designated XP; the constituent Z is then the specifier of X, spec-XP. It will be assumed as well that a non-head Z can be merged with XP to form a higher segment of XP, thus producing multiple specifiers. Features are checked under two configurations: (1.) head-head, when a newly merged head Y attracts a lower head X, which moves and merges with it to form $[_Y$ X Y], whereupon features in the feature matrix associated with Y can be checked against their counterparts in the feature matrix associated with X; and, (2.) spec-head, when the most recently merged head Y attracts a non-head constituent Z to form a specifier of Y, whereupon features in the feature matrix of Y can check against their counterparts in the feature matrix associated with Z. Typically, a lexical VP or AP predicate is constructed as the lexical core of a clause, and the functional structure is constructed on top of the lexical core through successive merger of functional heads. In cases of clausal complementation (as well as with complex NP or DP complementation), the complement is constructed first, with its functional and lexical projections, and the higher head (typically, verb or adjective), of which it is the complement, is subsequently merged with it.

The functional architecture of a sentence is determined by the matrix structure and partial linear ordering of the functional features. The features matching features on lexical items in the lexical array for a clause, or instantiated by functional elements (such as negation or a complementizer) in the lexical array, are used to construct the functional structure of that clause. (Exceptions to this are quite special in character, and will be a particular focus of later chapters.) For each clause, in the normal case, the functional features are distributed into separate feature matrices, respecting the sub-matrices F_i^r in (44), and in general respecting the linear order defined on all the features within the matrices in (44). (Further constraints on this distribution will be presented later in this chapter.) Returning for illustration to the example of the subject pronoun in (46)–(47), the matching features to [1PER] and [PL] will occur together within a sub-matrix and will be projected and checked together, but the matching feature for [NOM] will not necessarily be included in a feature matrix with [1PER] and [PL], and will therefore not necessarily be projected onto the same functional head as [[1PER], [PL]]. In addition to these nominal features (N-features) there are associated verbal features (V-features) on the finite verb, which express verb inflection; a matching suite of V-features will be projected onto functional categories and will drive verb movement, whether overt or covert.

A theoretical goal for many of the researchers mentioned in section 2.1 above, and for the present work, is to identify functional categories as much as possible with the matrices formed of the functional features. That is, the minimal answer to the question, "What is a functional category?" would be that it is merely a matrix of features, added to the numeration to match features on lexical items, or (in the case of negation and complementizers) instantiated by a functional element in the lexical array. To a large extent, this identification can be made, but there is a residue of difference. However much we might be able to simply identify a functional category with a particular matrix of features, we must still distinguish the matrix of features as such, sitting by itself in the numeration, from the same matrix of features functioning as a functional head, capable of being merged into the syntactic phrase structure. To this end, if $[F_1, \ldots, F_n]$ is a matrix of functional features, where each F_i may itself be a sub-matrix of features, let ^$[F_1, \ldots, F_n]$ be the functional category projecting $[F_1, \ldots, F_n]$; let ^$([F_1, \ldots, F_n])'$ be the result of merging ^$[F_1, \ldots, F_n]$ with a target phrase structure K; and let (^$[F_1, \ldots, F_n]$)P be the result of merging a constituent with ^$([F_1, \ldots, F_n])'$ or with (^$[F_1, \ldots, F_n]$)P. If no specifier element is merged with ^$([F_1, \ldots, F_n])'$, then ^$([F_1, \ldots, F_n])'$ can be identified as ^$([F_1, \ldots, F_n])$P, the maximal projection of ^$[F_1, \ldots, F_n]$. Clearly, functional heads must be merged into phrase structure in an order respecting the checking order of their component features: if $F_j^s < F_i^r$, then F_i^r must not be projected onto a higher functional head than F_j^s. For convenience, it is useful to simplify notation by letting M = $[F_1, \ldots, F_n]$, from which the head ^M is defined, with projections (^M)′ and (^M)P, but in doing so, we should keep clear that 'M' designates a feature matrix, and is not a standard functional category label.

Given a matrix M of functional features, if M contains all and only the features represented on one of the standard functional categories, such as C, Agr_S, T, Agr_O, Asp, or the like, then we can identify ^M as the feature-based construction of that functional category. In this case, ^M will indeed correspond to the standard functional head, but a very different conception of functional categories still underlies its derivation, and as we will see through the course of this work, this has consequences for many instances of syntactic analysis, and for accounts of how functional category structure is acquired and how this acquisition can be impaired.[11]

It is explicitly proposed above that the matrices of functional features are added to the numeration, and that this is conceptually distinct from the projection of a feature matrix M as a functional head ^M. It should be noted that the same points hold for lexical categories. A word, represented in (44) as an item w_i $[F_i^1, \ldots, F_i^{k_i}]$ of the lexical array, is not itself a syntactic head, but is projected into the syntax as a syntactic head, which we might designate as ^w_i $[F_i^1, \ldots, F_i^{k_i}]$. Note that the word consists of more than its morpho-syntactic feature matrix, $[F_i^1, \ldots, F_i^{k_i}]$; it also consists of its pronunciation (in the form of an extensive autosegmental representation), its syntactic category label, its subcategorization frame and selectional properties, among other things. So a word cannot be reduced to the feature matrices given in (44). But the point is that the numeration consists of words and matrices of matching (or instantiated) features, and that each of these must be projected onto a syntactic head in its turn before it can be merged into the syntactic structure.

An illustration is provided by the Spanish sentence in (48), for which the lexical array is represented in (49).

(48) *María está alt-a.*
Maria be.PRES.3.SG tall-FEM.SG

(49) { *está* [$F_{V\text{-}T}$, $F_{V\text{-}s}$], *María* [$F_{N\text{-}s}$, NOM], *alta* [F_A] }

When matrices of matching features are constructed, the complete numeration in (50) is obtained. The brackets and the traditional functional category labels, Agr_A, Agr_S, and T, in the first line of (50) are not part of the numeration, and the lexical category labels are actually features in the representation of the lexical item; the first line of (50) is included entirely for expository convenience, and is therefore enclosed in double quotes. The numeration is not ordered, but the elements of the numeration are presented here in merge order (going right-to-left) for convenience; the merge order is actually determined by selectional properties of lexical items and the checking order of features.

(50)

"Agr_S	T	V	[Agr_A	[NP	A]]"
		está		*María*	*alta*
$F_{V\text{-}s}$	$F_{V\text{-}T}$	$F_{V\text{-}T}$	F_A	$F_{N\text{-}s}$	F_A
$F_{N\text{-}s}$	[NOM]	$F_{V\text{-}s}$	$F_{N\text{-}s}$	[NOM]	

The features in (50) reflect adjective agreement with the subject, the verification of verb tense, subject-verb agreement, and the verification of nominative case on the subject. The derivation begins by merging the subject *María* to the adjective *alta* to form the small clause *María alta*, given in (51). Complete syntactic representations of the lexical categories in (50) and (51) would be extensive feature matrices representing all relevant syntactic information, including the syntactic category label represented as a feature, as well as the morpho-syntactic features given here. In (51) and subsequent tree diagrams in this discussion, lexical categories are indicated for convenience using traditional lexical category labels rather than complete representations.

(51)

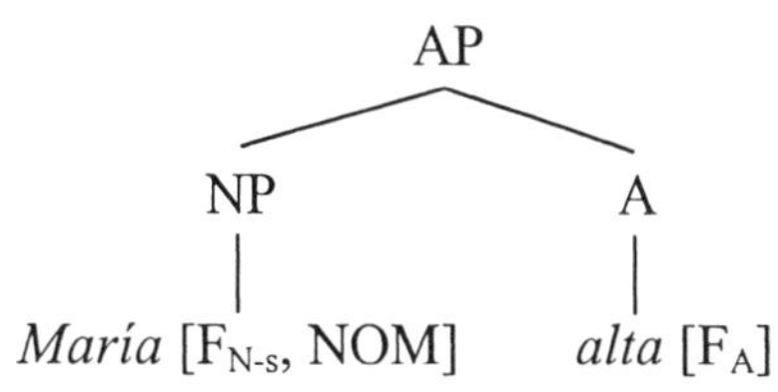

Adjective agreement with the subject is mediated by ^[F_A, $F_{N\text{-}s}$], which is merged into a position taking the small clause AP as its complement. The feature matrix F_A attracts the adjective, which moves and merges with ^[F_A, $F_{N\text{-}s}$], checking the F_A features in the head-head relation. The result is shown in (52), where checked features are indicated by strikethrough.

(52)

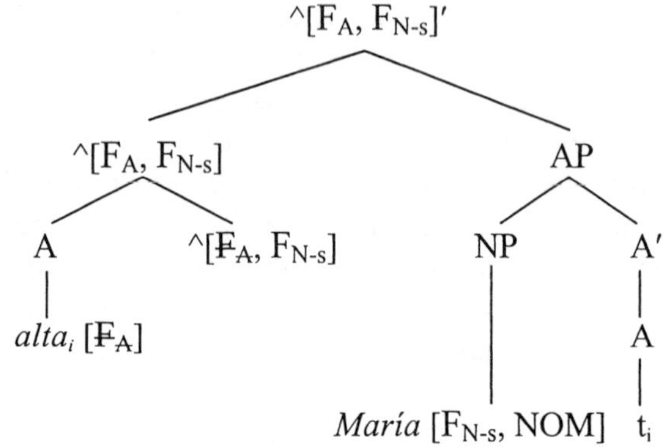

Then $F_{N\text{-}s}$ matrix attracts the subject which moves and merges with ^[F_A, $F_{N\text{-}s}$]′, effecting construction of spec-^[F_A, $F_{N\text{-}s}$]P; the features $F_{N\text{-}s}$ are then checked against the functional head, with the results shown in (53). (The checked features on lexical items maintain the capacity to check additional copies on higher functional categories which attract them.) Thus, adjective agreement with the subject is effected through a combination of feature checking in the head-head and spec-head configurations.

(53)

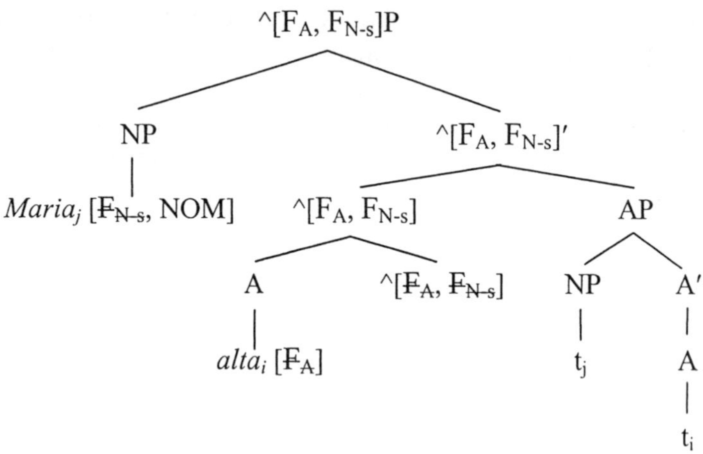

After the verb *está* is merged into the phrase structure to form a projection of V, the functional head ^[$F_{V\text{-}T}$, [NOM]] is merged with VP, and the verb tense is checked by merging the verb *está* with ^[$F_{V\text{-}T}$, [NOM]], with the result shown in (54).

(54)

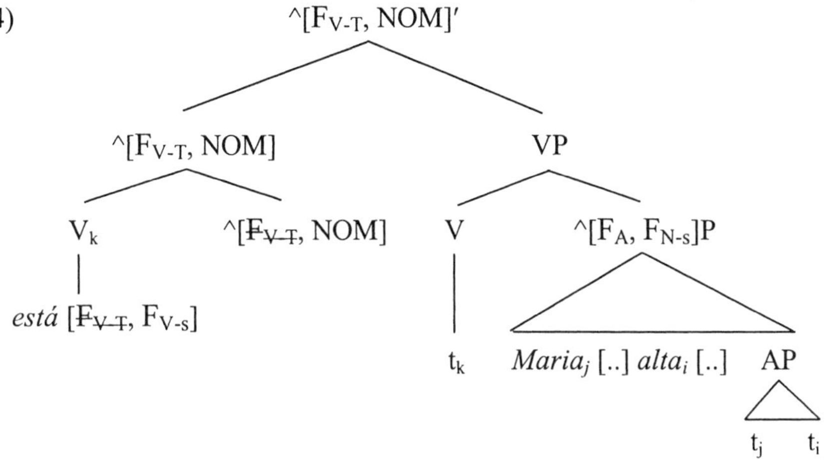

Finally, the functional head ^[$F_{V\text{-}s}$, $F_{N\text{-}s}$] is merged with "TP", that is, with ^[$F_{V\text{-}T}$, [NOM]]P whereupon $F_{V\text{-}s}$ attracts the head [V-^[$F_{V\text{-}T}$, [NOM]]], which moves and merges with ^[$F_{V\text{-}s}$, $F_{N\text{-}s}$], and $F_{N\text{-}s}$ attracts the subject NP to move and merge with ^[$F_{V\text{-}s}$, $F_{N\text{-}s}$]′, to form the specifier of ^[$F_{V\text{-}s}$, $F_{N\text{-}s}$]P, allowing $F_{V\text{-}s}$ to be checked under head-head agreement, and $F_{N\text{-}s}$ and [NOM] to be checked under spec-head agreement.[12] The results of these final stages of the derivation are shown in (55). This example illustrates more than the mechanics of the projection of feature matrices as functional heads and of feature checking under movement. It shows that a typical instance of NP-head agreement is mediated by a matrix of matching features which contains a V-feature or A-feature attracting the head, as well as a N-feature attracting the NP. For example, the penultimate step in the derivation of (52) above merges ^[F_A, $F_{N\text{-}s}$] with the AP to set up movements which permit checking of the features in the matrix F_A, and the derivational step which sets up the final round of feature checking in (55) merges ^[$F_{V\text{-}s}$, $F_{N\text{-}s}$] with TP to set up checking of $F_{V\text{-}s}$, $F_{N\text{-}s}$ (as well as [NOM] on T). This seems to be the "normal case"; the question is whether there exist cases that do not conform to this pattern.

(55)

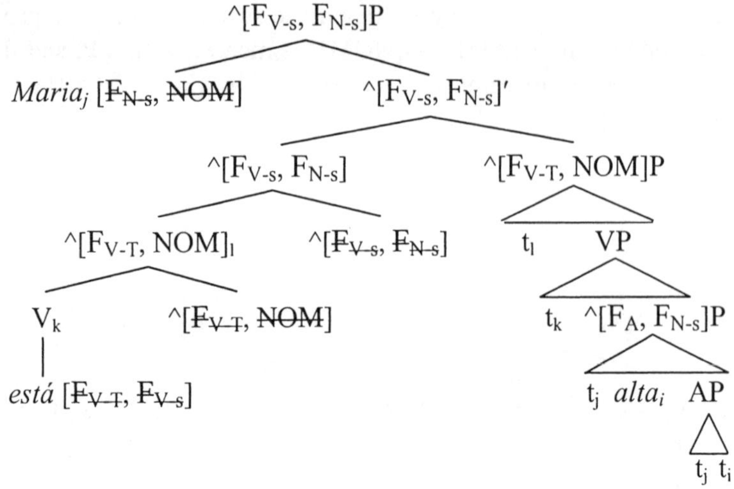

The supposition that there are not – that matrices of matching features are constrained to conform to the pattern illustrated above – is worth entertaining as a general principle of the grammar. The pattern exhibited is that agreement between a NP and a lexical head is accomplished through checking N-features of the NP and features of the lexical head against matching features projected together on a functional head, ^M. This prevents N-features from being projected in separate feature matrices, on their own, which means that the projection of a functional head ^M within the Infl-system should be blocked in principle when the feature matrix M carries no verbal features (V-features or A-features). The requirement that functional heads within the Infl-system should carry verbal features blocks the projection of extraneous functional categories within the Infl-system to check N-features on their own, as a plausible implication of the Economy of Representation. We provisionally adopt it as such, in (56) below.

(56) *Economy of Projection of Infl-Categories*
If features F_1, F_2, ..., F_n are elements of a feature matrix M projected as a functional head ^M within the Infl-system of a clause, then one of F_1, F_2, ..., F_n must be a V/A-feature matching some $F_{V/A}$ on a verb/adjective within that clause.[13]

The more compact projection of N-features with clausal (verbal or adjectival) head features should be preferred by the principle that Giorgi and Pianesi state in the passage quoted in (41) above, on which "the actual number of projections is defined according to economy considerations, that is, the shortest derivation compatible with the initial array is selected."

The real import of the Economy of Projection of Infl-Categories is that a functional head within the clausal system should contain at least one clausal (verbal or adjectival) feature, and should not consist solely of nominal features. By symmetry, a functional head within the nominal system, should contain at least one nominal feature to be checked by a D or N head within the nominal. In some applications of this principle in later chapters, it will be necessary to distinguish N-features not just from V-features and A-features, but from any features which are projected onto functional heads in order to drive the construction of the clause, rather than to satisfy the checking requirement of features on nominals. In particular, the EPP feature, which is an intrinsic property of a clause (whether a full clause or a small clause), and not an intrinsic property of any NP or DP, is projected onto a functional head in order to drive clause construction, not to check a morpho-syntactic property of a nominal. A slightly revised reformulation of (56) embodying this distinction is formulated in (57).

(57) *Economy of Projection of Infl-Categories*
If features F_1, F_2, ..., F_n are elements of a feature matrix M projected as a functional head ^M within the Infl-system of a clause, then at least one of F_1, F_2, ..., F_n must be a clausal feature (matching some $F_{V/A}$ on a predicative head, or an EPP feature); that is, not all of F_1, F_2, ..., F_n can be N-features matching some F_N within the numeration.

These considerations raise anew the question of where features on items in a numeration come from. Following Chomsky (1995b), the set of lexical items from which a sentence is constructed determines a numeration containing these lexical items together with matching features chosen to check features on the lexical items. (To this, we have added features instantiated by functional elements in the lexical array, such as negation and complementizers.) Formal features are entered on lexical categories at the point at which they are selected for a numeration.[14] For example, the choice of a third-person feminine singular subject in (48) lies beyond the computational system. For the purposes of the computational system, therefore, the lexical categories that appear in the numeration, and the formal features on them, are given. If we adhere to this strictly, then subject-verb agreement and subject-adjective agreement in (48) are not guaranteed within the numeration; they are ratified by feature checking within the syntactic tree in the course of the derivation. What about the functional categories? In the course of a syntactic derivation producing a sequence of syntactic objects (σ_1, σ_2, ..., σ_n), merge operates by projecting an element of the numeration and merging it with σ_i to produce σ_{i+1}.[15]

But given that features on lexical items can successively check multiple copies of matching features, if feature projection were not constrained in some further way, it would permit the construction of elaborately excessive numerations for a given sentence. For example, for the sentence *Sam read the book*, it would permit construction of a numeration in which an indefinitely large number of copies of $F_{V\text{-}o}$ matching the object V-features on the verb are sorted into separate feature matrices and projected onto an equal number of functional heads, perhaps accompanied by an equal number of copies of $F_{N\text{-}o}$ matching the N-features of the object NP, as in the numeration fragment given in (58) below; the multiple copies of the feature matrix [$F_{V\text{-}o}$, $F_{N\text{-}o}$] in this structure project to multiple copies of a feature-based counterpart of an Agr_O node.[16]

(58)

			Sam	*[the book]*	*read*
$F_{V\text{-}o}$	$F_{V\text{-}o}$	$F_{V\text{-}o}$	$F_{N\text{-}s}$	$F_{N\text{-}o}$	$F_{V\text{-}o}$
$F_{N\text{-}o}$	$F_{N\text{-}o}$	$F_{N\text{-}o}$			

In the derivation from (58), as the verb raised through the ^[$F_{V\text{-}o}$, $F_{N\text{-}o}$] functional heads, the feature $F_{V\text{-}o}$ on the verb would check off the copies of $F_{V\text{-}o}$ on the functional heads. Likewise for the copies of $F_{N\text{-}o}$, as the object raised. In this way, a wild profusion of entirely useless copies of object V-features and N-features could be entered into the numeration, giving rise to a profusion of equally useless derivations. Since there is no bound on the number of [$F_{V\text{-}o}$, $F_{N\text{-}o}$] matrices which could be entered into the numeration as in (58), the class of numerations produced in this way is unbounded. Pursuing all possible derivations from these numerations, the grammar is committed to evaluation of an infinite class of derivations for the sentence *Sam read the book*. The derivation of this simple sentence is thus rendered intractable by the generation of numerations such as that in (58). This contrasts with the parallel but finite computation involved in the derivational ratification of feature values described in footnote 15.

Contrast this with the Spanish example (48), with adjectival and copular agreement with the subject, and consider again the numeration for (48) given in (50) (repeated below).

(48) *María está alt-a.*
Maria be.PRES.3.SG tall-FEM.SG

(50)

		está		*María*	*alta*
$F_{V\text{-s}}$	$F_{V\text{-T}}$	$F_{V\text{-T}}$	F_A	$F_{N\text{-s}}$	F_A
$F_{N\text{-s}}$	[NOM]	$F_{V\text{-s}}$	$F_{N\text{-s}}$	[NOM]	

In (49), $F_{N\text{-s}}$ is projected in conjunction with F_A, as the functional head ^[$F_{N\text{-s}}$, F_A] in order to establish NP-adjective agreement. A duplicate copy of $F_{N\text{-s}}$ is projected in conjunction with a copy of the $F_{V\text{-s}}$ of the copular verb as [$F_{V\text{-s}}$, $F_{N\text{-s}}$], in order to establish subject-verb agreement. Turning to the undesirable numeration, in (58), the copies of $F_{V\text{-o}}$ and $F_{N\text{-o}}$ on the lowest matrix [$F_{V\text{-o}}$, $F_{N\text{-o}}$] are needed to check features on the verb and direct object, but the copies included in the two higher [$F_{V\text{-o}}$, $F_{N\text{-o}}$] matrices are not needed by any lexical item. The additional ^[$F_{V\text{-o}}$, $F_{N\text{-o}}$] functional heads which would be projected from (58) are thus not needed. These examples motivate an economy constraint which, given features on a lexical item, constrains the projection of matching copies of features onto functional heads. Specifically, they suggest that one matching copy of features can be allowed to check the features of the lexical item, and additional copies may be projected only in conjunction with V-features (or A-features) as needed to establish instances of NP-head agreement. The most general form of such a constraint is formulated in (59) below.[17]

(59) *Economy of Feature Projection*
Given the lexical categories in a numeration, a minimal suite of matching features is entered into the numeration to be projected onto functional categories.

The requirement that the matching features be a minimal suite in (59) is intended to assure that one copy of $F_{V/A}$ is projected to match an instance of $F_{V/A}$ on a lexical item and that one copy of F_N is projected to mediate each instance of NP-head agreement. In a minimal suite of matching features, given a feature (or feature matrix) F on a lexical item α in the numeration, a matching F can be projected onto a functional category without constraint if there is no higher ranked F already in the numeration; if one or more higher ranked copies of F exist on functional categories in the numeration, then an additional copy of F can be projected only in conjunction with features F_L matching F_L on another lexical head L, in order to establish agreement between α and L.

In the examples at hand, given agreement φ-features F_N on a nominal element α, matching F_N can be projected once without constraint, in order to check the F_N on α, but additional set(s) of matching F_N can only be projected in conjunction with other features F_L, such as F_V or F_A, in order to establish agreement between α and L. Furthermore, since the Economy of Feature Projection prevents the unnecessary duplication of the F_V features in (58), the Economy of Projection of Infl-Categories will block the projection of the superfluous copies of the feature matrix [$F_{V\text{-}o}$, $F_{N\text{-}o}$]. This adequately captures the distinction between the numeration in (49) and the undesirable numeration in (58).

The Principle of Economy of Feature Projection is distinct from the constraint expressed by Giorgi and Pianesi in the passage quoted in (41) above, and distinct also from the Principle of Economy of Projection of Infl-Categories. The Economy of Feature Projection constrains the duplication of features entered into a numeration for projection onto functional categories and is therefore a constraint on what features are present in a numeration. Given the set of features to be projected onto functional categories, the Economy of Projection of Infl-Categories constrains the number of categories onto which these features are projected. The Economy of Feature Projection conspires with the Economy of Projection of Infl-Categories above to ensure that a minimal suite of functional heads, projected from a minimal numeration, is projected to meet the feature-matching needs of an initial array of lexical categories. Given an array of lexical categories, the Economy of Feature Projection regulates the introduction of matching features into the numeration, to be projected onto functional categories; the Economy of Projection of Infl-Categories ensures that these features are projected onto a minimal suite of functional categories.

2.3. Conclusion

The construction of functional categories given in section 2.2 above implicitly acknowledges points made in the following passage by van Gelderen (1993: 3); this is quoted and discussed here to illustrate the extent to which present proposals fall in line with work by other researchers, and the respects in which they are different.

> It might be argued that functional categories do not 'cost' anything: if features are present, they project automatically onto categories and maximal projections. This cannot be maintained given the evidence of languages in which e.g. tense features occur in C and not in T ... and where agreement features occur in C and not in AGR.... In these languages, there would be no automatic projection of the tense and agreement features onto a T and AGR position respectively.

This proposal and the present work agree that features should not automatically be projected onto pre-identified categories. However, in view of the construction of functional categories given in section 2.2 above, stipulated exceptions seem to be an ad hoc way to approach the matter. Features only seem to be projected onto fixed, identifiable functional categories much of the time because there is some consistency in the structure of feature matrices across languages, and across constructions within a language. Where there are exceptions, we don't want to say that the usual mapping from features to categories breaks down and alternate associations must be stipulated. Instead, we want to identify orderings of features which have the usual stock of functional categories as a predictable epiphenomenon, but which have intrinsic alternate orders encoded in them in a way which is nonexceptional, but which surfaces under particular circumstances, yielding a situation which looks like tense features occurring exceptionally in C rather than in T, agreement features occurring exceptionally in C rather than in AGR, but which in fact is just a predicted special case of feature co-occurrence which falls out from the ordering possibilities encoded regularly in the grammar. The approach to functional category acquisition in Chapters 6 and 7 will exploit this aspect of the present construction, with similar results. Developments in child language which other researchers have described as exceptional use of the C-system to represent functional elements normally represented in the I-system, for example, will be seen not to be stipulated exceptions to the normal functioning of the functional category system, but merely use of ordinary functional category resources under the exceptional circumstances of particular stages of child language acquisition.

The derivation of functional categories developed here also provides an implementation of proposals regarding the fine structure of the left periphery, particularly, multiple projections within the C-system (split CP), put forth by Rizzi (1997), and various works in Rizzi (2004), especially those by Benincá and Poletto on topic and focus in Rhaeto-Romance verb-second constructions, Giorgi and Pianesi on complementizer deletion in Italian,

Poletto and Pollock on Romance *wh*-questions, and Roberts on the C-system in Brythonic Celtic languages. The multiple functional categories at the left periphery of the clause on these proposals do not need to be stipulated within a fixed system of functional categories, but, as several of these authors are aware, should be derived from their feature contents. Rather than summarize these proposals in detail, the present work will present additional analyses along the same lines, worked out explicitly in terms of the feature-based functional categories proposed in section 2.2 above. In particular, a feature-based construction of the left-periphery of the clause is exploited in the accounts given in Chapter 3 below of variability across the Germanic languages in embedded clause verb-second (section 1) and in the occurrence of expletive subjects in existential constructions (section 2), as well as in the account of verb-second in Old and Middle English given in that chapter (section 3).

Notes

1. The displaced element is traditionally called a topic element, hence the gloss 'Top', although its actual discourse function is quite variable. The adverbial element *gestern* 'yesterday' is not included here except as a topic element.
2. The basic analysis was proposed by den Besten (1983), first published in 1977, and elaborated by Haider (1985), Vikner (1995), and others. The tree in (10) assumes a standard SOV word order for German and Dutch, not the SVO order proposed for Dutch by Zwart (1993).
3. These data are presented, as in Zepeda (1983), in the orthography developed by Albert Alvarez and Kenneth Hale, designated by the O'odham in 1974 as the official orthography of their language. In this orthography, *c* is a voiceless alveopalatal affricate and *j* its voiced counterpart, *e* is a mid central unrounded lax vowel, *d* is a voiced interdental fricative, [ʼ] is a glottal stop, and other symbols are in accord with the International Phonetic Alphabet.
4. *Wh*-questions do not exhibit the *n*- marker, but they do exhibit the *wh*-expression and auxiliary in first and second position of the clause, respectively, or in the opposite order with morphological variants. See Zepeda (1983) for details. The existence of the reversed-order variant indicates that the fronting of the *wh*-element and the auxiliary are not simply manifestations of Aux-second, but are the result of movement to a supra-Infl domain, as a reflex of question formation. Thus, *wh*-questions are syntactically similar to *yes/no*-questions, even though they lack the question particle.
5. Their framework will be discussed in more detail in Chapter 3 below, which examines some of the empirical issues which are central to their work.

6. Giorgi and Pianesi report that (37c) is grammatical for some speakers, but nearly or fully ungrammatical for others, a form of variation for which they find no obvious regional basis.
7. The relevant section of Chomsky (1995a) does not explicitly discuss economy in the number of projections, but states, more generally, that the initial array A should "fix the *reference set* for determining whether a derivation from A to [interface levels] (π, λ) is optimal, i.e., not 'blocked' by a more economical derivation." But economy in the number of functional categories projected to match features present on lexical categories in an initial array will be a major issue in the present work, and the economy constraint formulated originally by Chomsky, and directed by Giorgi and Pianesi in the passage quoted here towards the number of categories projected, will be refined further in the present work with reference to the projection of functional categories within the Infl-system.
8. Giorgi and Pianesi take a numeration to be a set of ordered sets of features, with categorial information represented in feature format. The ⟨+V, –N, ...⟩ sequence in (42) is projected as a lexical V; the other bracketed sequences are projected onto functional heads, one head for each sequence.
9. Giorgi and Pianesi leave TP out of their structure for the subjunctive complement, and therefore draw trees in which Mood/Agr takes VP as its complement. They note [p.153] that T might be present in these structures, but do not pursue the issue, presumably for expository simplicity. Adding Tense to these structures, in line with the proposals Giorgi and Pianesi make, the tense feature could be bundled with ⟨+Nom⟩ onto T in both of (42a,b); then in (42a), ⟨+φ⟩ would project independently onto Agr, and in (42b), the bundle ⟨+Mood, +φ⟩ would be projected onto a syncretic C/Agr. This would not introduce spec-TP as a possible position for the subject NP at Spell-Out (thus producing (37b)), since the subject φ-features (or the EPP feature) are strong, necessitating either a postverbal subject or overt movement of the subject to the specifier of the syncretic C/Agr, the latter option available only for some speakers. Alternatively, tense features might be bundled with ⟨+φ, +Nom⟩ in (42a) and be projected onto a syncretic Agr/T, while in (42b), tense features might be bundled with ⟨+Mood, +φ, +Nom⟩, and be projected onto a syncretic C/Agr/T.
10. If F_j^s and F_i^r bear the same orderings with respect to other features, we will write that $F_j^s = F_i^r$.
11. Of Agr_S and Agr_O, only Agr_O will play an essential role in the analyses developed in the present work. The present work could therefore accommodate Chomsky's proposal (1995b: 348–379) to eliminate $Agr_{S/O}$, and to attribute the functions of Agr_O to the light verb *v*.
12. This derivation assumes that [NOM] is checked together with subject φ-features in the specifier of "Agr_s", that is, spec-^[$F_{V\text{-}s}$, $F_{N\text{-}s}$]P, rather than in the specifier of "TP", that is; spec-^[$F_{V\text{-}T}$, NOM]P.

13. As a derivational constraint, this principle would be a special case of the economy constraint expressed by Giorgi and Pianesi (1996: 142) in the passage quoted in (41) above. Alternatively, the Economy of Projection of Infl-Categories can be regarded as a licensing condition on functional categories within the Infl-system, checked at interface levels as a requirement that Infl-categories have a V-feature or A-feature (checked or unchecked) at the interface, in which case it would function as a provision of the Economy of Representation. The constraint can be plausibly extended, with suitable adaptation, to other categories, including the nominal system, but since the present work does not deal with any phenomena that would provide the empirical motivation for this extension, the issue will not be pursued here.
14. This account is phrased procedurally in order to express a derivational theory of syntactic representations. The procedural steps described are not intended as claims about psycholinguistic processing or psycholinguistic generation. Any discovery of convergence or lack of convergence between the derivational steps posited by this theory and aspects of psycholinguistic generation or processing would be empirical discoveries, whose significance (if any) for the theory of syntactic representation would have to be determined.
15. Issues of computational complexity arise at this point. In the computationally worst case, the matching features to be projected onto functional categories might be arbitrarily chosen, and their distribution arbitrarily specified, with judicious choices subsequently ratified through convergent derivations, and injudicious choices leading to a crash. This would involve parallel computation of a potentially large – but finite – set of possible derivations of a given sentence.
16. For expository ease, the object noun phrase is presented here as preconstructed; the determiner and head noun actually would appear as separate lexical categories in the numeration. Also, tense and subject agreement features, and all case features, are left out of (58) to keep the present discussion focused on the issue at hand.
17. The Economy of Feature Projection is a feature-based counterpart to a number of category-based principles which have been formulated in the literature to constrain the projection of categories in a clause, and used more specifically to constrain the projection of functional categories to be a minimal suite sufficient to satisfy the requirements of lexical items in the clause; see Grimshaw (1991, 1997), Law (1991), Bošković (1996) and Radford (1996). Principles formulated more generally to minimize all aspects of grammatical structure include Chomsky's (1991) Economy of Representation and Safir's (1993) Structural Economy Principle.

Chapter 3
Germanic verb-second and expletive subjects

Different rankings or constraints on features across languages or language varieties can result in different matrices of features being projected as functional categories across languages. This has ramifications for verb and nominal movement, and is consequently one source of differences in verb and nominal movement across languages or dialects. The different patterns of Germanic verb-second (V2) are a prime example of the sort of cross-linguistic difference which is susceptible to analysis along these lines. In this chapter, the mechanisms for the projection of functional phrase structure described in the previous chapter will be applied to account for the different patterns of Germanic verb-second, including the pattern of Old English (West Saxon), which prevailed (in Southern dialects) through the early Middle English period.

The intent of this and subsequent chapters is to show that a framework for the construction of functional categories out of feature bundles, such as those proposed by Giorgi and Pianesi (1996, 1997) and Rambow and Santorini (1995), and that developed in Chapter 2 of the present work, can generate functional categories in a way which is less ad hoc than assuming a stock of functional categories in fixed selectional relationships to one another, and, moreover, that certain phenomena which are particularly recalcitrant to a systematic explanation on the standard view of functional categories actually fall out as expected variants on the construction of functional categories within these frameworks. The account of patterns of Germanic verb-second with which we begin, in effect, recapitulates the approach of Rambow and Santorini (1995) for modern Germanic languages, though with a substantially different implementation. We will persist nevertheless in using the construction of functional categories developed in Chapter 2 since we want a consistent formulation of the approach to the full range of problems covered in this and subsequent chapters, and, in particular, because the present construction, which refers to representational resources for functional category projection independently of the choice of lexical items, is essential for the results concerning language acquisition in Chapter 7, whereas the framework of Rambow and Santorini would not obviously serve that purpose. Nevertheless, their framework will be discussed later in this chapter for its independent merit, to highlight some contrasts with the approach developed here, and to further illuminate the mechanisms set forth in the present study.

1. Patterns of Germanic verb-second

In verb-second clauses, the finite verb occurs in second position, following an element traditionally called a topic element, although elements which appear in the first position include expletive subjects and others which are not topics in any discourse or information-theoretic sense. Recall from Chapter 2 that German main clauses are verb-second, as are subordinate clauses without overt complementizers, but subordinate clauses with complementizers exhibit SOV word order; this is illustrated in (1)–(3) below, repeated from Chapter 2.

(1)	a.	*Karl*	*hat*		*das*	*Buch*	*gelesen.*
	b.	*Das Buch*	*hat*	*Karl*			*gelesen.*
	c.	*Gestern*	*hat*	*Karl*	*das*	*Buch*	*gelesen.*
		Top	has	Karl	the	book	read

(2)	a.	*Karl*	*liest*		*das*	*Buch.*
	b.	*Das Buch*	*liest*	*Karl.*		
	c.	*Heute*	*liest*	*Karl*	*das*	*Buch.*
		Top	read	Karl	the	book

(3) a. *Sie sagt, daß Karl dieses Buch gelesen hat.*
She says that Karl this book read has
b. *Sie sagt Karl hat dieses Buch gelesen.*
c. *Sie sagt dieses Buch hat Karl gelesen.*
d. *Sie sagt gestern hat Karl dieses Buch gelesen.*
She says yesterday has Karl this book read

The V2 embedded clauses such as (3b,c,d) only occur in complements to bridge verbs such as *sagen* 'say', *glauben* 'think', *behaupten* 'claim'; they do not occur in subject clauses, adjunct clauses, interrogative clauses, or complements to negative verbs or unambiguously factive verbs.

On a standard analysis of these data, due to den Besten ([1977] 1983) and others since, the complementarity between an overt complementizer and verb-second in subordinate clauses motivates the postulation of a feature [+F], in C^{o}, associated with finite clauses (main and subordinate) in German; the feature [+F] requires lexical support, which can be provided either by a complementizer or by the finite verb. Thus, in main clauses and subordinate clauses without complementizers, the finite verb (main or auxiliary) moves to I, then to C, whereas, in subordinate clauses with a complementizer in C, the finite verb moves only to I^{o} (which is right-headed).

Mainland Scandinavian and Frisian have a somewhat different pattern. As in German, main clauses are verb-second, as illustrated by the Danish data in (4)–(5) below.[1]

(4)	a.	*Kaffe*	*drikker*	*Peter*	*ofte*		*om*	*morgenen.*
	b.	*Om morgenen*	*drikker*	*Peter*	*ofte*	*kaffe.*		
	c.	*Peter*	*drikker*		*ofte*	*kaffe*	*om*	*morgenen.*
		Top	drinks	Peter	often	coffee	in	morning-the

(5)	a.	*Kaffee*	*har*	*Peter*	*ofte drukket om morgenen.*
	b.	*Om morgenen*	*har*	*Peter*	*ofte drukket kaffe.*
	c.	*Peter*	*har*		*ofte drukket kaffe om morgenen.*
		Top	has	Peter	…

Subordinate clauses are introduced by a complementizer and are generally not verb-second, which is also in line with the German pattern.

(6) a. *...at Peter ofte drikker kaffe om morgenen.*
b. *...at Peter ofte har drukket kaffe om morgenen.*

c.	*...at*	*han*	*ikke*	*købte*	*bogen.*
	that	he	not	bought	book-the

But there is a notable exception: complement clauses to bridge verbs are optionally verb-second, with the V2 pattern following the complementizer, provided the main clause is not negated or modalized.

(7)	a.	*Vi*	*ved*	*at Peter drikker ofte kaffe om morgenen.*
	b.	*Vi*	*ved*	*at om morgenen drikker Peter ofte kaffe.*
		we	know	…

(8)	a.	*Vi*	*ved*	*at Peter har ofte drukket kaffe om morgenen.*
	b.	*Vi*	*ved*	*at om morgenen har Peter ofte drukket kaffe.*

In the presence of negation or modality in the higher clause, the bridge verb complement is non-V2 SVO, as are complements of factive and inherently negative verbs, and all subject and adjunct clauses, as illustrated by the following examples.[2]

(9) a. * *Jeg tvivler på at den film har Maria set.*
I doubt on that this film has Maria seen
b. * *Peter benægtade at den film havde Maria set.*
Peter denied that this film has Maria seen

(10) * *Johan beklager at denne bog har jeg læst.*
Johan regrets that this book have I read

(11) a. *At han ikke vil se denne film overraskede mig.*
that he not will see this film surprised me
b. * *At denne film vil han ikke se overraskede mig.*
that this film will he not see surprised me

(12) a. *Jeg går hjem hvis han ikke vil se denne film.*
I go home if he not will see this film
b. * *Jeg går hjem hvis denne film vil han ikke se.*
I go home if this film will he not see

All of this but the exceptional behavior of bridge verb complements is accounted for on the assumption that these languages, like German, have the feature [+F] in C^{o} in both main and subordinate clauses, but that, unlike German, the complementizer must be present in a subordinate clause. Then the complementizer supports [+F], and the non-V2 SVO order surfaces.

The behavior of bridge verb complements in Mainland Scandinavian poses a number of questions, including the following:
- How can a V2 pattern be accommodated in the phrase structure following a complementizer?
- Why is V2 optional in this context? And in the context of economy constraints, how can it be optional?
- Why is V2 blocked when the higher clause is negated or modalized?
- Why is V2 blocked when the higher verb is factive or intrinsically negative? Why is it not possible in adjunct clauses?

A number of researchers have addressed these questions. Iatridou and Kroch (1992) propose licensing conditions on CP-recursion, which permit a CP to be generated in complement position to a higher C just in case the first (i.e., higher) C is transparent to government by the selecting verb, thus making the lower C^{0} visible to this verb; Authier (1992) proposes a similar condition requiring the higher C to have no index marking the specialized contents of non-bridge verb complements. The structure involved is that shown in (13) below, for (7b).

(13) *Vi ved* $[_{CP}$ $[_{C}$ *at*] $[_{CP}$ *om morgenen* $[_{C}$ $[_{V\text{-}I}$ *drikker*]]
$[_{IP}$ *Peter ofte* t_V *kaffe* $t_{PP}]]]$

Only the most neutral assertive complements can be introduced by such a complementizer, lacking specialized semantic content and transparent to government. And such neutral assertive complements can occur only in complement position to an unnegated bridge verb. Factive and inherently negative verbs, as well as negation or modalization in the higher clause, are all assumed to put a burden of content on the complementizer introducing the complement clause, blocking CP-recursion and therefore blocking V2. See also Watanabe (1993a,b) for a kindred account, but with a rather different implementation.

Icelandic and Yiddish present yet another pattern, with verb-second in all subordinate clauses, following a complementizer, as well as in all main clauses. The Icelandic facts are illustrated in (14)–(17) below, with V2 in main clauses in (14), in a bridge verb complement in (15), in non-bridge verb complements in (16), and in subject clauses in (17).[3]

(14) a. *Einhver keypti bókina í gaer.*
somebody bought the-book yesterday
b. *Bókina keypti einhver í gaer.*
the-book bought somebody yesterday
c. *það keypti einhver bókina í gaer.*
there bought somebody the-book yesterday

(15) *Jón segir að þessum hring hafi Ólafur lofad Maríu.*
Jón says that this ring has Olaf promised Maríu

(16) a. *Jón efast um að á morgun fari Mária snemma á fætur.*
Jon doubts on that tomorrow will Maria get up early

b. *Jón harmar að þessa bók skuli ég hafa lesið.*
Jón regrets that this book shall I have read

c. *Jón spurði hvort þessum hring hefðu þeir lofað mér.*
Jon asked whether this ring had they promised me

(17) a. *Að Maríu hafi hann aldrei séð er kannski líklegt.*
that Maríu.ACC has he.NOM never seen is perhaps likely

b. *Að Guðmundi skuli enginn vilja hjálpa veldur mér áhyggjum.*
that Gudmund.DAT shall nobody want help.INF causes me worries

The Yiddish facts are illustrated in (18)–(22) below, with V2 in main clauses in (18), in bridge verb complements in (19), in non-bridge verb complements in (20), in an extraposed subject clause in (21), and in an adjunct clause in (22).[4]

(18) a. *Dos yingl vet oyfn veg zen a kats.*
the boy will on-the way see a cat

b. *Oyfn veg vet dos yingl zen a kats.*
on-the way will the boy see a cat

c. * *Oyfn veg dos yingl vet zen a kats.*
on-the way the boy will see a cat

(19) a. *Avrom gloybt az Max shikt avek dos bukh.*
Avrom believes that Max sends away the book

b. *Ikh meyn az haynt hot Max geleyent dos bukh.*
I think that today has Max read the book

(20) a. *Jonas bedoyert az dos bukh hob ikh geleyent.*
John regrets that this book have I read

b. *Jonas tsveyfelt az morgen vet Miriam fri oyfshteyn.*
John doubts that tomorrow will Mary early get up

(21) *Es hot undz alemen gekhidesht vos nekhtn iz*
it has us all bewildered what yesterday is
gekumen aza groyser oylem.
come such-a large audience
'It surprised all of us that such a large audience came yesterday.'

(22) *Ikh vel avekgeyn oyb morgn kumt Moyshe.*
I will away-go if tomorrow comes Moyshe

This is fundamentally different from the Mainland Scandinavian pattern since V2 in subordinate clauses following an overt complementizer is the general pattern in Yiddish and Icelandic, not an exception appearing only in a special context. One approach to this situation is to postulate provisions for V2 to occur within the IP-system (IP-V2), with [+F] in I^o instead of in C^o. The structure would be that in (23) below, for (16b). (As is clear in (23), this account must be accompanied by provisions to permit the subject to remain in spec-VP.)

(23) *Jón harmar* [$_{CP}$ [$_{C}$ *að*] [$_{IP}$ *þessa bók* [$_{I}$ *skuli*] [$_{VP}$ *ég hafa lesið* t_{DP}]]]

Assuming this is the case for all finite clauses in Yiddish and Icelandic, V2 will be uniform across finite clauses in these languages. See Diesing (1990), Santorini (1992), Iatridou and Kroch (1992), and Heycock and Santorini (1993) for development of this account for Yiddish, and see Rögnvaldsson and Thráinsson (1990) and Iatridou and Kroch (1992) for its application to Icelandic. As emphasized by Iatridou and Kroch, since this approach realizes the generalized V2 in subordinate clauses in Yiddish and Icelandic as IP-V2, it restricts CP-recursion to the special case of complements of unnegated bridge verbs in Mainland Scandinavian, where its appearance can be attributed to special licensing conditions. (See also Authier 1992.)

Alternatively, the licensing conditions for CP-recursion can be assumed to be more relaxed in Yiddish and Icelandic than in Mainland Scandinavian, permitting V2 to occur more generally through CP-recursion in Yiddish and Icelandic; see Holmberg (1986) and Platzack (1986). The structure of (16b) would then be similar to (13), rather than (23). Vikner (1995) argues that all embedded V2 under a complementizer across Germanic is due to CP-recursion. This maintains uniformity in the analysis of V2 cross-linguistically at the expense of licensing conditions on CP-recursion which might distinguish unnegated bridge verb complements from other subordinate clauses in Mainland Scandinavian.

Finally, the occurrence of embedded V2 following an overt complementizer could be accommodated without IP-V2 if [+F] is located in a functional head Z° projected between C° and I°. Then the complementizer introduces a V2 structure headed by Z°, with the rest of the clausal structure contained within IP. The head Z in proposals along these lines has been variously identified as a focus head, F° (Tsimpli 1990), or as a topic head, T° (Müller and Sternefeld 1993); see the discussion in Vikner (1995: 80–84), which surveys all three possible accounts of V2.

The above is merely a bare outline of the relevant facts and arguments pertaining to the analysis of V2 in Germanic languages. Before proceeding, some intricacies regarding V-to-I movement are worth noting. In Mainland Scandinavian, V-to-I movement does not occur independently of verb-second; in non-V2 clauses, the finite verb (auxiliary or main verb) follows negation and clause-medial adverbials, as in (6) above. This makes the contexts for V2 very clear, even in subject-initial V2 clauses, where the subject is the "topic" element of V2, since the finite verb precedes negation and clause-medial adverbials in V2 structures, as in (4)–(5) above. In Yiddish and Icelandic, in contrast, the finite verb always raises at least to I, and thus precedes negation and clause-medial adverbials. As a result, a subject-initial V2 structure (with a subject "topic") is hard to distinguish from a non-V2 SVO clause.

In the most common analyses, V2 is triggered by a finiteness feature [+F] residing in C°. The major alternative to this, first proposed in Rizzi (1996), adopts binary categorial features, {±C, ±I}, and attributes the V2-inducing properties of C° (assuming CP-V2) to its categorial feature specification, [+C, +I]. Where the complementizer of a non-V2 language is assumed to be [+C, –I], the [+C, +I] complementizer node of a V2 language attracts the finite verb to its head, and a "topic" element to its specifier. A more elaborate version of this system proposed by Rambow and Santorini (1995) is used to account for the different patterns of V2 cross-linguistically. But such an account is not readily formulated in a feature-based syntax in which the standard stock of functional heads is not available. The system developed in chapter 2 constructs functional heads, which may or may not correspond to standard functional categories, out of bundles of more primitive features. The V2 feature [+F] is an appropriate candidate member of this inventory of more primitive features, as the distinguishing property of Germanic V2 clauses. However, in the context of the theory presented here, this feature cannot be considered to be an intrinsic property of a pre-identified C or I (depending on language). In fact, it will turn out below that advantage can be gained from separating out the V2-inducing properties of this feature from its typical or common association with the complementizer feature. Specifically, the features responsible for V2 will be taken to be those in (24), where [TOP_V] is the V-feature attracting the finite verb, and [TOP_N] is a feature shared by, and attracting, the "topic" element; this is an N-feature since it is typically checked in the spec-head relation, but it may be realized on AdvPs and PPs, as well as on NPs and DPs.[5]

(24) Top = [[TOP_V], [TOP_N]]

This feature matrix is assumed to have no cross-linguistically uniform association with any particular functional head. In each language, the feature matrix Top will be ordered with respect to matrices of inflectional features, Agr_S and [Tns, [NOM]], and the matrix of mood features, M, expressed by the complementizer. For present purposes, the structure of the inflectional system will not be analyzed further, so the features in Agr_S and [Tns, [NOM]] will be assumed to be unordered with respect to one another, and denoted simply as 'I'. This amounts to positing a non-split Infl head, effectively I^o, for ease of exposition.

A typology of V2 can then be developed based on co-occurrence restrictions on the feature matrices M, Top, and I, assuming a uniform ranking of these features, namely that given in (25) below.[6]

(25) M < Top < I

Mainland Scandinavian will be addressed first since its pattern is the most intricate, and consequently, in certain respects, the most revealing.

Mainland Scandinavian lacks V2 in adjunct clauses, which typically express conditional, temporal or logical/modal relations; it also lacks V2 in complement clauses to verbs with negation or modality in the higher clause, complements to inherently negative verbs, and complements to non-bridge verbs which favor a discourse-old ("presupposed") information status of the content of the complement clause (whether through prior mention, environmental salience, or accommodation). These facts indicate that Top is incompatible with M when M contains any one (or more) of the features [NEG], [MOD/COND], [PRESUP]. The inclusion of subject clauses among the contexts which prevent V2 follows if subject clauses are introduced by a head with [PRESUP], expressing the typical topical status of subjects. Since M, with one or more of these features, is required in adjunct clauses, subject clauses, and complements to nonbridge or negated verbs, it follows that Top, which is incompatible with the features of M in all these cases, must be absent in these clauses. These clauses are thus generated with the feature structure M < I, with M expressed by an overt complementizer, and are consequently non-V2. The structure of an example of this sort is given in (26), where ^M is the functional category projected from the matrix of modal features, ^I is the functional category formed by bundling inflectional categories (or a shorthand for multiple bundles corresponding to split Infl), and ^MP and ^IP are their maximal projections. (These are not actual category labels akin to those for functional categories such as C and I on the standard conception, but rather merely labels of convenience for categories constructed from the projection of feature matrices.)

(26) *Johan* *beklager* $[_{\wedge MP}$ $[_{\wedge M[NEG,\ PRESUP]}$ *at*] $[_{\wedge IP}$ *Peter* ^I *ofte*
John regrets that Peter often
$[_{VP}$ *har* *drukket* *kaffe* *om* *morgenen*]]]
has drunk coffee in morning-the

In complement position to unnegated bridge verbs in contexts lacking modality, sometimes called "assertive" contexts, the complementizer *at* in ^M expresses none of the features mentioned in the previous paragraph, with which Top is incompatible. Assume that, in this context, there is an option for M to be interpreted as assertive by default, and, equally, an option for M to be marked as such by a feature [DECL] (for "declarative"), and assume that Top in Mainland Scandinavian is incompatible with [DECL], as with the other features of M mentioned above. Assume, furthermore, that Top is present when it is not precluded. When M is interpreted as assertive by default, then Top is present, since it is not precluded by any features of M, and then the clause is generated by functional feature matrices M < Top < I, yielding an embedded V2 structure introduced by the overt complementizer, as in (27), for (8b) above.[7]

(27) *Vi ved* $[_{\wedge MP}$ $[_{\wedge M}$ *at*] $[_{\wedge TopP}$ *om morgenen* $[_{\wedge Top}$ *har*] $[_{\wedge IP}$ *Peter* $t_{\wedge I}$
ofte $[_{VP}$ *drukket kaffe* t_{PP}]]]]

When M is labeled with [DECL], then Top is missing, and the complement clause is generated by the feature structure M < I, producing a non-V2 clause with the word order shown in (6), as in complement clauses in other environments. Since the feature content of M is optional in the assertive complement clause (and no other), these complement clauses (but not others) may surface as either V2 or non-V2.

In declarative main clauses, M is absent since these clauses are interpreted as declarative by default; thus the relevant feature structure is Top < I, yielding main clause V2 with the structures shown in (28)–(29) below, for (4a) and (5a) above.[8]

(28) $[_{\wedge TopP}$ *kaffe* $[_{\wedge Top}$ *drikker*$]$ $[_{\wedge IP}$ *Peter* $t_{\wedge I}$ *ofte* $[_{VP}$ t_V t_{NP} *om morgenen*$]]]$

(29) $[_{\wedge TopP}$ *kaffe* $[_{\wedge Top}$ *har*$]$ $[_{\wedge IP}$ *Peter* $t_{\wedge I}$ *ofte* $[_{VP}$ *drukket* t_{NP} *om morgenen*$]]]$

The structure of an interrogative main clause is determined by the feature structure M[Q] < I, which produces the "residual V2" of English interrogatives. Assuming that Top is incompatible with [Q], there is no fronting of a "topic" element in interrogative clauses; *wh*-fronting, when present, is the result of attraction by a [WH] feature in M[Q, WH] in *wh*-questions, not the Top matrix.

In Yiddish and Icelandic, declarative main clauses lack M as in Mainland Scandinavian, since they are interpreted as declarative by default, and the resulting feature structure Top < I yields V2 as in (28)–(29) above.[9] In subordinate clauses, generalized V2 will be produced by the feature structure M < Top < I, provided Top is compatible with the feature content of M in adjunct clauses, complements to factive and inherently negative verbs, and complements in negated and modal contexts and contexts in which the content of the complement clause is favored to be presupposed or discourse old. This yields subordinate clauses in Yiddish and Icelandic with the structure shown in (30) below, for (16b); this is just the structure of the Danish complement clause in (27) above, but occurring generally in Yiddish and Icelandic, not just as complements to bridge verbs.

(30) *Jón harmar* $[_{\wedge MP}$ $[_{\wedge M[\text{NEG, PRESUP}]}$ *að*$]$ $[_{\wedge TopP}$ *þessa bók* $[_{\wedge Top}$ *skuli*$]$ $[_{\wedge IP}$ *ég* $[_{VP}$ *hafa lesið* t_{DP} $]]]]$

Note that on this account, even embedded clauses in which the subject happens to be the "topic" element in Yiddish and Icelandic will have V2 structures produced by Top, outside of ^IP, that is, and so will not be IP-V2. Therefore, on this account, special theoretical provisions are not required to accommodate the subject in spec-VP, as on the IP-V2 account. In fact, these structures will be isomorphic in structure to CP-V2 structures, but without the category C labelled as such. This is in line with Vikner's (1995) conclusion that generalized V2 in Icelandic and Yiddish, and indeed, V2 throughout the Germanic languages, is CP-V2, not IP-V2. His arguments for this analysis of generalized V2 in Yiddish and Icelandic are based on subject position with respect to clause-medial sentence adverbs, which are before VP, with respect to objects which have undergone object shift, and with respect to IP-adjoined adverbials. The structure of subject-initial V2 clauses will be taken up further below.

In German, V2 in main clauses will be produced as in the languages discussed above. The complete complementarity between V2 and overt complementizers in German subordinate clauses indicates that, in German, Top is incompatible with any feature matrix M of mood features. In contexts in which M must have nondefault features (including adjunct clauses, complements to factive or inherently negative verbs, modalized or conditional contexts), the presence of M with these features will be required, and Top will be consequently missing. These clauses, produced by the feature structure M < I, are not V2, as in (31) below.

(31) *Sie bereut,* [$_{\text{^MP}}$ [$_{\text{^M[NEG, PRESUP]}}$ *daß*] [$_{\text{^IP}}$ *Karl* [$_{\text{VP}}$ *dieses Buch*
she regrets that Karl this book
gelesen] [$_{\text{^I}}$ *hat*]]]
read has

In complement clauses to unnegated bridge verbs in non-modal, non-conditional contexts, a situation similar to that of Mainland Scandinavian obtains: M can be present with feature content [DECL] and lexical content *daß*, in which case Top must be absent, and M < I yields a non-V2 structure as in (31) above; or M can be missing, with the complement clause interpreted as declarative by default, and then Top is present; in this case, the resulting feature structure, Top < I, yields a V2 clause without a complementizer, as in the structure (32) for (3c) above.

(32) *Sie sagt,* $[_{\text{^TopP}}$ *dieses Buch* $[_{\text{^Top}}$ $[_{\text{^I}}$ *hat*]] $[_{\text{^IP}}$ *Karl* $[_{\text{VP}}$ t_{NP} *gelesen* $t_{\text{Aux}}]$ $[_{\text{^I}}$ $t_{\text{Aux}}']$]]

The difference between assertive complements in German and Mainland Scandinavian is that in German, ^M is just a projection of mood features, and therefore is not projected at all when there are no mood features (whether [COND], [PRESUPP], or [DECL]), whereas in Mainland Scandinavian, ^M is projected as a lexical category with *at*, even when it has no mood features. That is why Mainland Scandinavian can have V2 under a complementizer in the complement of a bridge verb, whereas in German, V2 in complement clauses alternates with the overt complementizer, and is only possible in bridge verb complements when the complementizer is absent.[10]

As is well known, English has a very restricted form of V2 with the fronting of "affective" elements (see Klima 1964), as illustrated in (33); this will be called affective inversion, or, when it involves explicitly negative elements, Neg-inversion.

(33) a. *Not a single person did I see there.*
b. *Never have I seen such a mess.*
c. *Under no circumstances should you go there.*
d. *Under no circumstances will he arrive early.*

These are produced by the feature structure, Top < I, with Top = $[\text{TOP}_{\text{V}}, \text{TOP}_{\text{Aff}}]$. Inversion can occur as well in complements to unnegated bridge verbs, but not in adjunct clauses, subject clauses, or complements to factive or inherently negative verbs, as shown below. (See Emonds 1976: 29, Authier 1992, Iatridou 1993/94.)

(34) a. *She has often said that under no circumstances should you go there.*
b. *I thought that never in my life had I seen such a mess.*
c. *She claims that under no circumstances will he arrive early.*

(35) a. ??*If under no circumstances should you go there, then we will send the packages by mail.*
b. * *Because never had they seen such a mess, they returned home immediately.*

c. * *While never have you seen such a mess, you won't understand how awful it is.*
d. * *You lost the clients that only on workdays would you see.*

(36) a. * *That under no circumstances should you go there was strongly recommended.*
b. * *That never had they seen such a mess was clear.*

(37) a. ??*I doubt that never have they seen such a mess.*
b. ??*She regrets that under no circumstances should you go there.*
c. ??*She didn't say that under no circumstances should you go there.*

The instances of embedded Neg-inversion in (34) will be produced by the feature structure, M < Top < I, with M optionally lexicalized by the complementizer, as in (38) for (34c).

(38) *She claims* [$_{\wedge\text{MP}}$ [$_{\wedge\text{M}}$ *that*] [$_{\wedge\text{TopP}}$ *under no circumstances* [$_{\wedge\text{Top}}$ *will*] [$_{\wedge\text{IP}}$ *he* [$_{\text{VP}}$ *arrive early*]]]]

But the failure of Neg-inversion in (35)–(37) indicates that [TOP_{Aff}] in English is incompatible with M when M contains negative, temporal, modality/conditional, or presuppositional features. By making co-occurrence conditions on features central to the explanation of the facts, this account obviates the need for conditions on CP-recursion of the sort proposed by Iatridou and Kroch (1992), Authier (1992), Iatridou (1993/94), Watanabe (1993a), and Watanabe (1993b).

Finally, this approach accounts for the pattern of V2 in non-Germanic V2 languages. In Kashmiri, main clauses are V2, as well as complement clauses introduced by the complementizer *ki*. Adjunct clauses, which are introduced by complementizers other than *ki*, are not V2. This pattern is produced by the feature structure, M < Top < I, as above, provided that Top is compatible with *ki*, but not with any other complementizers. See Rambow and Santorini (1995) for relevant data, and their analysis of Kashmiri.

On this account, the distinguishing feature of the Germanic languages is the feature matrix Top, with features ordered between mood or clausal subordination features and inflectional features, M < Top < I. The source of cross-linguistic variation lies not in licensing conditions for CP-recursion structures, nor in the major phrase structure difference between IP-V2 and CP-V2, but rather, in feature co-occurrence restrictions: Top has varying degrees of compatibility with the featural content of M across languages, ranging from total incompatibility with any features of M in German, to compatibility with virtually all features expressed by M in Icelandic and Yiddish. The features which occur in M in different clauses on this account, including [DECL], [Q], [MOD], [COND], [PRESUP], [AFF] (the last of these for negative complementizers), and in other examples, subjunctive and imperative features, [SUBJ] and [IMP], constitute a natural class insofar as they have scope over the rest of the clause and can serve as points at which syntactic structure interfaces with pragmatics in situating the content of the clause with respect to a wider semantic-pragmatic context. Finally, English is assimilated to the other Germanic languages in having exactly the same mechanisms for verb-second, but realizing them only for a highly restricted featural content of Top, containing [TOP_{Aff}].

The account of verb-second given above amounts to a feature-based construction of the topic field of Benincá and Poletto (2004), which itself extended proposals of Rizzi (1997). In section 3 below, it will be seen that Old and Middle English made similar, but even more extensive, use of such a topic field under a feature-based construction.

In essential respects, the present account is directly parallel to that proposed by Rambow and Santorini (1995), though the implementation is significantly different in its notation, motivations, and conceptual foundation. They separate out the functions of clausal subordination and mood expression for complementizers by positing separate features, M for mood, and C for the subordinating function. Thus, their inventory of features is {C, M, Top, I}, and they impose a superficially similar (if reversed) ordering, C > M > Top > I, which they construe as expressing selectional properties, rather than as being part of a general (partial linear) ordering of morpho-syntactic features. They conceive of these as categorial features rather than as matrices of morpho-syntactic features, but they construct functional heads through order-preserving conglomerations of these features, which they call multi-functional heads, in a way that is parallel in some respects to that proposed here. The main difference in implementation is that Rambow and Santorini do not distribute functional features into feature matrices and project the matrices as functional heads. Instead, on their account, multi-functional heads are created when lexical items bearing the appropriate features are introduced into a derivation, or when a verb bearing the appropriate features moves out of VP. For example, a German verb with feature content [+M, +Top] in their notation, to appear in a (non-subject initial) V2 structure, moves out of IP, creating a functional head with feature content M/Top, which projects to M/TopP, the functional projection hosting the topic element. Functional phrase structure is thus generated upon movement of verbs with particular feature complexes on their account, rather than to host matching features which attract the lexical items.

The major theoretical difference between the accounts is that the present account achieves different distributions of the feature matrices {M, Top, I} on functional heads cross-linguistically through feature co-occurrence restrictions, whereas Rambow and Santorini specify differing complexes of their features {+C, +M, +Top, +I} cross-linguistically on verbs and complementizers, resulting in the creation of functional heads with different multi-functional feature specifications produced as these lexical items are inserted or move out of VP. A significant difference in implementation between the two accounts is that Rambow and Santorini must endow a V2 verb with different feature contents in subject-initial V2 clauses and V2 clauses with a non-subject topic element. On the present account, to capture the facts noted above, there is no difference in the feature matrices on either verbs or functional categories in subject-initial V2 and other V2 clauses; subject-initial V2 clauses and ones with non-subject topics are produced identically, except that different elements host the TOP_N feature. (In discussion of coordination below, a difference will be proposed in the derivation of subject-initial V2 and non-subject topic V2 clauses which, in effect, mirrors Rambow and Santorini's account. But it will exploit available options for ordering features, rather than positing verbs with different feature matrices in subject-initial V2 and other V2 clauses.)

Finally, as Rambow and Santorini note, the flexibility in construction of the feature content of functional heads provides a straightforward account of the phenomenon of Subjektlücke in Finiten Sätzen (SLF), otherwise known as Subject Gap Clauses (SGC), in German coordination structures such as the following (from Heycock and Kroch).

(39) *Das Gepäck ließ er fallen und rannte zum Ausgang.*
the pack let he fall and ran to-the exit

Putting aside the second conjunct, the sentence in (39) is a main clause V2 structure in which the "topic" element is the direct object, *das Gepäck*, of the verb *fallen*. It therefore has the structure shown in (40), in standard phrase structure.

(40) [$_{CP}$ *das Gepäck*$_3$ [$_{C'}$ [$_C$ [$_I$ *ließ*]$_2$] [$_{IP}$ *er* [$_{I'}$ [$_{VP}$ [$_{VP}$ t$_3$ *fallen*] t$_2$] [$_I$ t$_2$']]]]]

But, as much discussed in the literature (Höhle 1983, 1990; Heycock and Kroch 1993; Rambow and Santorini 1995), the occurrence of the second conjunct in the context of the structure in (40) is paradoxical. Since the second conjunct is not verb-final, it must be derived from a V2 structure, which means that it is a C′ (or a CP with an empty initial element). To obtain the correct interpretation of (39), the "topic" element of the second conjunct should be the subject *er*, which is missing, and the only way for *er* to be missing in the second conjunct is for the first occurrence of *er* to be shared under coordination of I′ and I′ (or for the second instance of *er* to be elided under identity with the subject of the first conjunct). But, by the parallelism required for a shared subject, or for ellipsis, this entails that the second conjunct is an I′ coordinated with the first clause I′, with the shared subject *er* in the first clause spec-IP, or else the second conjunct is an IP, with elided subject *er* in spec-IP, coordinated with the first clause IP. So V2 considerations require the second clause to be a C′ (or CP), as in (41a) below, while shared subject considerations require it to be an I′ (or IP), as in (41b), with ellipsis of the subject indicated by the strikethrough in both cases.

(41) [$_{CP}$ *das Gepäck*$_3$ [$_{C'}$ [$_C$ [$_I$ *ließ*]$_2$] [$_{IP}$ *er* [$_{I'}$ [$_{VP}$ [$_{VP}$ t$_3$ *fallen*] t$_2$] [$_I$ t$_2$']] (])(])(])

a. *und*([$_{CP}$ ~~*er*~~) [$_{C'}$ [$_C$ [$_I$ *rannte*]$_2$] [$_{IP}$ … *zum Ausgang*]]]

b. *und* ([$_{IP}$ ~~*er*~~) [$_{I'}$ [$_{VP}$ *zum Ausgang* t$_2$] [$_I$ *rannte*$_2$]]]]]

But neither of these can be correct. CP or C′ coordination in (41a) would not put the subject *er* of the second clause in a position to be elided under parallelism with the subject of the first clause. IP or I′ coordination in (41b) would not permit the second clause to be V2, and thus would leave the verb in final position, contrary to fact.

Heycock and Kroch address this problem by looking at the derivation of the second clause more closely. It is a subject-initial V2 structure with subject-topic, in which both the subject and the verb vacate the I-system for the C-system, under V2.

(42) $[_{CP}$ *er*$_3$ $[_{C'}$ $[_{C}$ $[_{I}$ *rannte*$]_2]$ $[_{IP}$ t_3 $[_{I'}$ $[_{VP}$ *zum Ausgang* $t_2]$ $[_{I}$ $t_2']$ $]]]]$

In this structure, the verb and its subject enter into a configuration of spec-head agreement within the I-system satisfying licensing relations for nominative case and subject-verb agreement. Heycock and Kroch point out that this configuration is then repeated in the C-system. But Heycock and Kroch assume a plausible Principle of Minimal Satisfaction for the projection of phrase structure, which requires that "[t]he structure projected from syntactic heads is the minimum in which all the licensing relations in which they participate can be satisfied." [p.263] Heycock and Kroch claim that (42) violates this principle and propose that, in order to rectify the situation, the traces of the verb and subject in the I-system delete, leaving the I-system bereft of syntactic content and function. The licensing relations that would normally be established within the I-system are established within the C-system instead, effectively combining the licensing functions of the I- and C-systems, resulting in the structure shown in (43).

(43) $[_{CP/IP}$ *er*$_3$ $[_{C'/I'}$ $[_{C/I}$ *rannte*$]_2]$ $[_{VP}$ t_3 *zum Ausgang* $t_2]$ $]]$

In this structure, the 'IP' part of the label on the highest node, with the subject *er* in spec-IP, in a sisterhood relation to a node with 'I′' as part of its label, is presumed to establish parallelism between (43) and the IP of the first clause in (41), permitting ellipsis of the subject in (43) and coordination of the two IP nodes (or of the two I′ nodes).

The point is not that the C-system in (42) duplicates the function of the I-system: it doesn't. The I-system in (42) licenses relations of nominative case and subject-verb agreement, while the C-system licenses relations pertinent to V2 – the checking of Top features on the implementation given above. But by the Principle of Minimal Satisfaction, if the spec-head relation is established within the C-system for V2 requirements, then the structure in (43), with all the relations associated with spec-head agreement within the C- and I-systems established together, is more minimal than that in (42). Rambow and Santorini embrace this conclusion, and obtain the result not through derivational deletion of traces, but by positing the feature matrix [+Top, +I] on the finite verb in subject-initial V2 clauses; on their formulation of the grammar, the movement of such a verb creates a

Top/I multi-functional head, and in the projection of Top/I, V2 relations are satisfied in the same structural configuration as nominative case and subject-verb agreement relations. The resulting structure, essentially that in (43), permits shared subject coordination of its C′/I′ with the I′ of the first clause in (41).[11]

On the formulation developed here, the insight about subject-initial V2 clauses from Heycock and Kroch can be captured by revising (25) above as shown in (44).

(44) $M < Top \leq I$

The derivation of V2 clauses with non-subject topics, marked XP[TOP_N], proceeds as described above, from the choice of Top < I. When the subject is marked [TOP_N], on the other hand, a more economical derivation can be obtained by taking advantage of the possibility Top = I, which bundles the features in the Top feature matrix, [[TOP_V], [TOP_N]], together with the I-features, [Agr_S, [Tns, [NOM]]], and projects them all together onto a single functional head. This head attracts the finite verb and the subject, resulting in a spec-head configuration in which all Top-features and all I-features can be checked at once. This results in (45), which realizes (43) within the framework developed here; as usual, Top = [[TOP_V], [TOP_N]] and I = [Agr_S, [Tns, [NOM]]], and furthermore, Tns = [$F_{V\text{-}T}$] and Agr_S = [$F_{V\text{-}s}$, $F_{N\text{-}s}$].

(45)

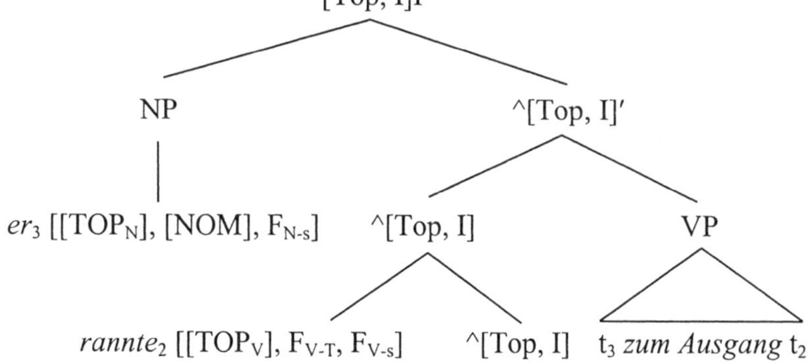

Suppressing the adjunction structure of the verb to ^[Top, I] and suppressing the feature matrices of lexical items, this result can be represented more simply as in (46).

(46) $[_{\wedge[\text{Top, I}]\text{P}}$ *er*$_3$ $[_{\wedge[\text{Top, I}]'}$ $[_{\wedge[\text{Top, I}]}$ *rannte*$_2$] $[_{\text{VP}}$ t_3 *zum Ausgang* t_2]]]

The ^[Top, I]P in (45)–(46) can undergo shared subject coordination with the IP *er fallen* in (41), yielding a structure for (39). (Or, alternatively, the ^[Top, I]′ in (45)–(46) can undergo shared subject coordination with the I′ in (41), yielding a structure for (39).)

This explanation is almost parallel to that offered by Rambow and Santorini, but is crucially different in that the subject-initial V2 structure does not need to be an independently stipulated case. They propose that the V2 verb in a subject-initial V2 clause introduces the features [+M, +Top, +I], resulting in the projection of a functional category with these features when the verb moves out of VP. The subject, in moving to the specifier of this functional category, serves the purposes of V2 and the checking of inflectional features under spec-head agreement. In a non-subject-initial V2 clause, the V2 verb introduces the features [+M, +Top], and the features [+I] must be introduced by a separate, non-V2 verb, thus distinguishing the "topic" element, which moves to the specifier of the [+M, +Top] category, and the subject, which moves to spec-IP. The theoretical drawback of this method of generating functional categories is that the V2 verb must effectively be marked as "subject-initial V2" or as "non-subject-initial V2". An empirical drawback of this approach is that it requires a separate verb with Infl-features in a non-subject-initial V2 clause, and consequently does not seem suited to generate a non-subject-initial V2 clause in which the main verb is the V2 verb, as in the German example in (2b) above, *Das Buch liest Karl*. Rambow and Santorini (1995: 381, ex. (17)), in discussion of a comparable Yiddish example, handle this by positing a verb with features [+M, +Top] in this case, and assuming that it creates a functional category with feature content [+I] when it moves out of VP, creating the I projection (which will be right-headed in German), and then that it creates a [+M, +Top] left-headed category when it moves out of IP. But in permitting a verb with features [+M, +Top] to create a functional head with feature content [+I] upon initially moving out of VP, they give up the construction of I out of the feature content of the moved verb in this instance and effectively embrace a primitive head I. This defeats the program of constructing functional categories purely on the basis of the feature content of lexical heads.

In contrast, constructing functional categories directly out of feature matrices consisting of features introduced to match features on lexical items, ordered as in (44), the sentence *Das Buch liest Karl* is declarative by default, so that M is missing; the sentence can then be derived from the Top < I provision of (44). This allows for projection of a (right-headed) ^I, distinct from the (left-headed) ^Top. The resulting structure is shown in (47).

(47) $[_{\text{^TopP}}$ *das Buch*$_3$ $[_{\text{^Top}}$ $[_{\text{^I}}$ *liest*$_2$-^I]-^Top] $[_{\text{^IP}}$ *Karl* $[_{\text{VP}}$ t_3 t_2] $t_{\text{^I}}$]]

Furthermore, the option Top < I must be chosen in deriving phrase structure from the numeration for *Das Buch liest Karl*, since the object *das Buch* is marked with [TOP_N] in this numeration. If the option Top = I were chosen with this numeration, then the subject and the object would both need to merge with ^Top′, which is not possible in German since German does not permit multiple specifiers of functional categories. (Old English did permit multiple specifiers of ^Top′, as will be seen in section 3 below, and therefore does permit structures with multiple elements in the Top domain.) Thus, in German, the Top = I option is compatible only with a subject marked [TOP_N]. Conversely, the option Top < I is compatible only with a non-subject topic: with a subject topic, the option Top < I would produce a structure with more functional heads and more derivational steps than the option Top = I, and is therefore barred by principles of the economy of derivation and representation.

Subject-initial versus non-subject-initial V2 patterns thus result directly from the occurrence of [TOP_N] on a subject or a non-subject; this in turn determines which of the options Top = I and Top < I in (44) must be chosen. Choice of the wrong derivational option either leaves some N-features unchecked, rendering the result illicit, or leads to a structure violating economy principles, as described above. Thus, the linear ordering of features in (44) makes provision for subject-initial and non-subject-initial V2 alike, with no further stipulation.

2. Expletive subjects

In this section, it will be observed that the feature-based account of verb-second given above, along with the construction of the topic field as ^Top, has implications for the analysis of certain facts about variation in expletive constructions across the Germanic languages and across construction types within these languages. This discussion relies extensively on Vikner

(1995), as did the discussion of verb-second above; it also relies on Holmberg and Platzack (1995) and a central idea of Ward and Birner (1995).

Where verb-second is produced through the action of Top = [[TOP_V], [TOP_N]] in Germanic languages, a wide range of constructions with expletive subjects are in evidence, with the expletive in the "topic" position. These contexts include main clauses, as in (48a–d), from Vikner (1995: 185).[12]

(48)	a.	*Es*	*ist*		*ein*	*Junge*	*gekommen.*	(German)
	b.	*Es*	*iz*	*gekumen*	*a*	*yingl.*		(Yiddish)
	c.	*það*	*hefur*	*komið*		*strákur.*		(Icelandic)
	d.	*Der*	*er*	*kommet*	*en*	*dreng.*		(Danish)
		there	is	(come)	a	boy	(come)	

However, subordinate clause data suggest that expletive constructions in Mainland Scandinavian are of a different nature from those in German, Yiddish and Icelandic. We will focus comparison on the differences between Mainland Scandinavian versus Icelandic and Yiddish since the latter have ubiquitous V2, including in subordinate clauses, although German patterns with Icelandic and Yiddish in most respects examined here. In Icelandic and Yiddish, expletive subjects occur with active transitives (49), passivized transitives (50), unaccusatives (51), unergatives (52), and with passivized unergatives (impersonal passives) (53); these are illustrated by subordinate clause data from Vikner (1995: 189, 202, 197, 209).

(49)	a.	…	*az*	*es*	*hot*	*imitser*	*gegesn*	*an*	*epli.* (Yiddish)
	b.	…	*að*	*það*	*hefur*	*einhver*	*borðað*		*epli.* (Icelandic)
			that	there	has	someone	eaten	an	apple

(50)	a.	…	*az*	*es*	*vert*	*gegesn*	*an*	*epl.*
	b.	…	*að*	*það*	*var*	*borðað*	*eitthvert*	*epli.*
			that	there	was	eaten	an	apple

(51)	a.	…	*az*	*es*	*iz*	*gekumen*	*a*	*yingl.*
	b.	…	*að*	*það*	*hefur*	*komið*		*strákur.*
			that	there	is/has	come	a	boy

(52) a. … *az es hot imitser getantst in gortn.*
b. … *að það hefur einhver dansað í garðinum.*
that there has someone danced in garden

(53) a. … *az es iz getantst gevorn.*
that there is danced been
b. … *að það hefur verið dansað.*
that there has been danced

In Mainland Scandinavian, expletive constructions are much more restricted, as illustrated by the Danish examples in (54)–(58), from the same source.

(54) * … *at der har nogen spist et able.*
that there has someone eaten an apple

(55) … *at der blev spist en able.*
that there was eaten an apple

(56) … *at der er kommet en dreng.*
that there is come a boy

(57) * … *at der har nogen danset i haven.*
that there has someone danced in garden-the

(58) … *at der er blevet danset.*
that there is been danced

Furthermore, the expletive subject must be the V2 topic element in Icelandic and Yiddish, but need not be in a Danish V2 clause, as in the following examples from Vikner (1995: 185).

(59) a. * *Nekhtn iz es gekumen a yingl.* (Yiddish)
b. * *I gær hefur bað komið strákur.* (Icelandic)
c. *Igår er der kommet en dreng.* (Danish)
yesterday is/has there come a boy

Thus, expletive constructions in Yiddish and Icelandic are tied to conditions which underlie verb-second in a way which requires the expletive to be the topic element of a verb-second clause. To see why this might be so, note that the associate nominal is indefinite and the interpretation of the structure exhibits distinct information structural properties. These merit detailed investigation in their own right, but some relevant points can be made to get on with. For English existentials such as *There is a boy in the garden*, Ward and Birner (1995) argue that the associate must be hearer-new in a sense derived from (and expanding upon) Prince (1992). (They argue, correspondingly, that the associate in English existentials need not be indefinite.) This seems to be an appropriate characterization of the informational status of the associate in (48)–(53). In any event, it is clear that the associate introduces an entity which is new to an extent which is sufficient to produce an informational contour in these examples. Taking this to be the interpretive point of introducing the expletive, the syntactic form can be seen as a reflex of keeping the hearer-new subject out of the topic domain created by the projection of Top = [[TOP_V], [TOP_N]]. For these reasons, expletive constructions in Icelandic and Yiddish should be expected to be possible in any V2 clause in which basic conditions on the expletive-associate pair are met. (These conditions will be discussed below.)

The expletive constructions in Danish subordinate clauses, where we generally don't have verb-second, as in (54)–(58), seem to serve a different purpose. These examples are grammatical just in case the external argument of the verb is not projected in a subject position, whether because the verb has no external argument, or because the external argument was demoted by passivization. This suggests that the purpose of the expletive construction in Danish subordinate clauses is to project a grammatical subject in the absence of an external argument.[13] As a result, expletive constructions in Danish are not intrinsically tied to the conditions for V2, and can occur in non-V2 clauses, and in V2 clauses in which the topic element is something other than the expletive subject, as in (59c) above.

This recapitulates a long-standing generalization regarding the availability of expletive subjects in existentials across Germanic languages (Platzack 1983; Maling 1987, 1988; Christensen 1991; and others): the expletive in Insular Scandinavian and Yiddish has the characteristics of a V2 topic, while in Mainland Scandinavian, the expletive has the characteristics of a subject.

The basic mechanisms for the projection of an expletive-associate pair can be formulated as follows on the present account. If an expletive subject is needed solely to serve as a subject in the absence of an external argument, then it is introduced into the numeration with a copy of the feature matrix F_{NP} of the associate nominal. If an expletive subject is needed to keep the associate out of the ^Top domain, then it is introduced into the numeration with the feature matrix [F_{NP}, [TOP_N]]. In either case, the associate is merged into phrase structure in the construction of the lexical VP (or AP) core of the clause, and the expletive is merged to create the specifier of a higher, functional, projection. The expletive checks features at its point of merger and all higher positions (if any) at which N-features of the subject need to be checked. The associate then moves and adjoins to the expletive at LF, which serves to check any features on the associate which were checked by the expletive. The only aspect of the derivation of an expletive construction which remains to be specified is the exact point of the derivation at which the expletive is merged into phrase structure; this is linked directly to the question of how much checking of subject N-features the associate performs before the expletive is merged into phrase structure. This issue has been investigated at length in Chomsky (1995a, 1995b, 2000, 2001), Frampton (1997), and others. Some issues to which we now turn suggest that the merge point of the expletive, and the exact way in which the task of checking subject N-features is divided up between the expletive and the associate nominals, varies across the Germanic languages in ways which depend on feature-checking needs in conjunction with the purpose of the expletive-associate chain in a language.

In Icelandic and Yiddish, there is an interesting difference in movement properties between an internal argument associate and an external argument associate. An internal argument associate can either remain in place, as in (50)–(51) above, or it can raise to a position checking Infl-features, as in (60)–(61) below; what it cannot do is raise to a position where it does not check Infl-features, as in (62)–(63). (These data are from Vikner 1995: 191, 194–195.)

(60) a. … *az es volt a yingl gevolt kumen.* (Yiddish)
that there will a boy would come
'That a boy would want to come.'

b. … *að það mundi einhver strákur hafa komið.* (Ice.)
that there would some boy have come

(61) a. … *az es iz an epl gegesn gevorn / gevorn gegesn.*
that there is an apple eaten been / been eaten

b. … *að það hefur eitthvert epli verið borðað.*
that there has an apple been eaten

(62) a. * … *az es volt gevolt a yingl kumen.*
that there will would a boy come
b. * … *að það mundi hafa einhver strákur komið.*
that there would have some boy come

(63) a. * … *az es iz gevorn an epl gegesn.*
b. * … *að það hefur verið eitthvert epli borðað.*
that there is/has been an apple eaten

In all of (60)–(63), the associate is an internal argument generated as the complement of the verb, and has raised to a higher position in the clause. In (60)–(61), the expletive is in spec-^TopP, and the highest auxiliary is in ^Top; the associate DP, which immediately follows the auxiliary, then appears in the specifier of an Infl head, either ^Agr_S or ^[Tns, [NOM]]. In (62)–(63), in contrast, the associate has raised to spec-VP, where it checks no Infl-features. Similarly, in examples with a single auxiliary, the auxiliary is in ^Top, and the associate can immediately follow it in a high Infl head, as in (64) (Vikner 1995: 192).

(64) a. … *az es vert an epl gegesn.*
b. … *að það var eitthvert epli borðað.*
that there was an apple eaten

The following data show that when the associate is an external argument, its options are more restricted: the associate must raise to a high Infl head, as in (65)–(66); it does not have the option of remaining in-situ, as shown by (67)–(68). (From Vikner 1995: 191–192.)

(65) a. … *az es volt imitser gevolt esn der epl.*
that there will someone would eat the apple
b. … *að það mundi einhver hafa borðað þetta epli.*
that there would someone have eaten this apple

(66) a. … *az es volt imitser gevolt getantst in gortn.*
that there will someone would danced in garden

b. … *að það mundi einhver hafa dansað í garðinum.*
that there would someone have danced in garden

(67) a. * … *az es volt gevolt imitser esn der epl.*
b. * … *að það mundi hafa einhver borðað petta epli.*

(68) a. * … *az es volt gevolt imitser getantst in gortn.*
b. * … *að það mundi hafa einhver dansað í garðinum.*

On the present account, why should there be such a difference in raising requirements between an internal argument associate and an external argument associate in Icelandic and Yiddish? In both cases, we have proposed above that the expletive is introduced to keep the new-information associate out of the Top domain of the V2 clause. But the obligatory movement of the external argument associate indicates that it nevertheless needs to behave more like an ordinary subject than the internal argument associate; in fact, we could entertain the supposition that it needs to behave as much as possible like an ordinary subject, consistent with its participation in the expletive-associate construction. This would mean that the external argument associate nominal raises through the inflectional category system, creating a specifier with each movement step, to the highest inflectional level (^Agr_S′), and that the merger of the expletive is delayed until the latest possible derivational step, when it is merged to ^Top′. The feature-checking performed by the associate is thereby maximized, and feature-checking by the expletive is minimized. The internal argument associate, in contrast, is free to raise to the highest inflectional head, as in (60)–(61), or not do so, as in (50)–(51). To explain this, assume that the introduction of the expletive with an internal argument associate in Yiddish and Icelandic has a dual purpose: to keep the associate out of the Top domain (as we have so far supposed for Icelandic and Yiddish), and to provide a subject in the absence of an external argument (as was assumed above for Danish). By virtue of this latter function, the expletive can take over all the feature-checking functions of the subject, leaving the internal argument associate in-situ; there is, consequently, no constraint that the subject N-feature checking by the expletive must be minimized, as there is when the associate is an external argument.

On this proposal, the constraints on expletive-associate pairs in Icelandic and Yiddish are structurally expressed constraints which follow from the function of the expletive construction. When the associate is an external argument, the expletive is introduced solely to keep the associate out of the Top domain, and the associate correspondingly behaves like a normal subject, and must raise to the highest Infl head, as in (66), with the structure in (69).[14]

(69) … [$_{\wedge\text{MP}}$ *að* [$_{\wedge\text{TopP}}$ *það mundi* [$_{\wedge\text{IP}}$ *einhver*$_i$ [$_{\wedge\text{AspP}}$ *hafa* [$_{\text{VP}}$ t$_i$ *dansað í garðinum*]]]]]

When the associate is an internal argument, the expletive is introduced to keep the associate out of the Top domain and to provide a subject in the absence of an external argument projected as a subject; in this case, the expletive is free to take over feature-matching functions of the subject, leaving the associate nominal in-situ. Thus, alongside examples in which an internal argument associate raises, such as (60)–(61), we also have ones in which the expletive is merged into spec-^IP and raises, while the associate stays within the VP, as in (51), with the structure in (70).

(70) … [$_{\wedge\text{MP}}$ *að* [$_{\wedge\text{TopP}}$ *það*$_i$ *hefur* [$_{\wedge\text{IP}}$ t$_i$ [$_{\text{VP}}$ *komið strákur*]]]]

In Danish, there are no external argument associates since the expletive construction is used only in the absence of a syntactically projected external argument. The expletive in this case is effectively a grammatical substitute for the subject, and it would therefore be expected that the expletive should check all subject N-features, and that the associate, correspondingly, should stay in place. This is, in fact, what happens, as shown by the following Danish counterparts to (61) and (64), from Vikner (1995: 194–195, 202).

(71) a. … *at der blev spist et æble.*
that there was eaten an apple
b. * … *at der et æble er blevet spist.*
that there an apple is been eaten
c. * … *at der er et æble blevet spist.*
d. ??… *at der er blevet et æble spist.*

Although (71d) is unexpectedly better than (71b,c), it does not appear that the associate has raised high enough to check any subject N-features, which must therefore be checked by the expletive in this example, as in (71a).

To summarize, in Yiddish and Icelandic, an expletive with an external argument associate is introduced solely to keep the hearer-new associate out of the Top domain of the V2 clause; the expletive is not a substitute subject to any degree, and the associate therefore raises through the Infl system to perform checking of all subject N-features. An expletive in a Danish clause is possible only with an internal argument associate and is introduced solely to provide a subject in the absence of an external argument; the expletive therefore performs checking of all subject N-features. An expletive in Yiddish or Icelandic with an internal argument associate has dual motivation: it is introduced in part to keep the associate out of the Top domain, and in part to provide a subject in the absence of an external argument. As a result, it exhibits a dual nature: it can perform the checking of all subject N-features, or remain in place and leave this task to the expletive subject.

Vikner's (1995: 167–213) account of expletive subject constructions across the Germanic languages gets some of its greatest leverage in its explanation of the facts reproduced above regarding the different positions of the associate nominal depending on the construction type. Vikner assumes that the subordinate clause Icelandic and Yiddish expletive constructions discussed here are V2 clauses in which the finite verb has moved through I to C, and the expletive is generated in spec-IP, where it receives nominative case under government by the [+F] C^o, before it moves to spec-CP. Vikner proposes (p.183) that the associate nominal, not being a direct recipient of case, is alternatively licensed by being either governed by a thematic role assigner (in complement position of V^o), or by being governed by the [–F] I^o of a V2 language (where [+F] is in C^o), specifically, by being in the specifier of the complement of I^o. In Icelandic and Yiddish, therefore, the internal argument associate, which is generated in a theta-governed position (complement of V^o) is thereby subject to alternative licensing whether or not it moves, and so is free to move or not; the external argument associate, generated in the lowest spec-VP, is not the beneficiary of theta-government, and must therefore appear (by moving, if necessary) in the specifier of the highest VP, where it is alternatively licensed under government by I^o. In Danish, I^o is barred from alternative licensing since it performs the normal case-licensing by assigning nominative case to spec-IP; consequently, external argument associates in an expletive construction in Danish have no opportunity for alternative licensing, and are therefore impossible. Vikner's account is quite elegant and comprehensive; it is therefore significant if, as argued here, equivalent coverage can be obtained as described above, expressed not in terms of licensing under government, but in terms of the feature-matching properties of the expletive and its associate, coupled with consideration of the different functions of the expletive-associate pair in each construction in each language.

Copular expletive constructions, such as those in (72) below, pose a particular challenge for Vikner's account since the copular verb *BE* does not assign a thematic role to its complement; thus the indefinite DP, the associate of the expletive, is not theta-governed in these examples, and since it is not governed by I° either (which would only count in the languages with pervasive subordinate clause V2 anyway), it would not be alternatively licensed. The data in (72)–(74) are from Vikner (1995: 212), where the English example essentially provides a gloss for the others.

(72) a. … *az es hot gemuzt zayn a guter film in televizye.* (Yi.)
b. … *að það mun hafa verið góð mynd i sjónvarpinu.* (Ic.)
c. … *at der må have været en god film i TV.* (Da.)
d. … *that there must have been a good film on TV.* (En.)

In accounting for these, Vikner appeals to the fact that copular *BE* does not assign any thematic roles, and proposes that it would therefore be unreasonable to hold an associate in complement position to *BE* to the alternative licensing requirement; an associate in this position therefore automatically (or vacuously) counts as satisfying the alternative licensing requirement. If the associate raises to a higher position in the clause, it will appear in an unlicensed position, unless it surfaces in a position governed by a [–F] I°, which is an alternative licenser. This accounts for the failure of the associate to be licensed in any of the examples in (73), and it accounts for the mixed results in (74), where the associate is governed by I°, which counts as a licenser only in the languages with pervasive subordinate clause V2.

(73) a. * … *az es hot gemuzt a guter film zayn in televizye.*
b. * … *að það mun hafa góð mynd verið i sjónvarpinu.*
c. * … *at der må have en god film været i TV.*
d. * … *that there must have a good film been on TV.*

(74) a. … *az es hot a guter film gemuzt zayn in televizye.*
b. ? … *að það mun góð mynd hafa verið i sjónvarpinu.*
c. * … *at der må en god film have været i TV.*

d. * … *that there must a good film have been on TV.*

However, the notion that the associate in the complement position of *BE* should vacuously satisfy the alternative licensing requirement seems strained. Among other things, it raises the question why the associate nominals in (73) should not likewise vacuously satisfy the alternative licensing requirement since the auxiliary verbs which govern them also do not assign thematic roles. Vikner attempts to answer this question by providing a principled distinction between, on the one hand, main verb *BE* and passive *BE*, which both license an associate of an expletive, and on the other hand, the other auxiliaries. The distinction is that main verb *BE* and passive *BE* can both be inflected for aspect by taking an aspectual verb, while other auxiliaries can't. But this appeal is undermined by the fact that the other auxiliaries examined seem to be aspectual verbs themselves, which would suggest that their failure to take an aspectual verb may not be truly correlated in any meaningful way with their failure to license the associate of an expletive.

Thus, the case Vikner makes for his account of these data is rather vexed. On the approach to expletive-associate chains developed here, the results follow directly from the proposals made above. In Icelandic and Yiddish, since *BE* has no external argument, the expletive is introduced in part to keep the associate out of the Top domain and in part to provide a subject in the absence of an external argument projected as a subject. Thus, the expletive is free to take over feature-matching functions of the subject, leaving the associate nominal in-situ; but the associate is also free to raise, provided it thereby checks subject N-features. In (72a,b), the associate remains in-situ, while in (74a,b), it raises to the highest inflectional head, checking all inflectional N-features for the subject. In (73a,b), the associate has raised, but not to a position allowing it to check all subject N-features; this example will therefore not be derived. In Danish, the expletive is introduced solely to provide a subject in the absence of an external argument, and the expletive must therefore perform matching of all N-features for the subject, while the associate stays in place. This in itself rules out (73c) and (74c). But since the finite verb does not raise in (73c) or (74c), it is clear that the associate in these examples has raised only partly, and is not in a position to check subject N-features anyway; therefore the leftward shift of the associate in these examples is doubly unmotivated, and these examples will not be derived. In English, as in Danish, the expletive is introduced solely to provide a subject in the absence of an external argument and therefore checks all subject N-features, while the associate remains in-situ, as in (72d). The raising of the associate in (73d) and (74d) is therefore unmotivated. As in Danish, movement of the associate in English is doubly unmotivated since the expletive is in the specifier of the highest inflectional head (in the absence of subordinate clause V2), which would prevent the associate from checking all subject N-features anyway, even if the associate were to raise.

In summary, since the licensing of the associate does not depend on thematic properties of the verb at all on the feature-based account developed here, the copular constructions do not pose any special problem for the account.[15]

Other influential approaches to the variation in existential constructions across the Germanic languages include that of Platzack and Holmberg (1989) and Holmberg and Platzack (1995), who posit an Agr element in I^{0} in Icelandic, but not in Mainland Scandinavian. On their account, Agr in I^{0} licenses the occurrence of the associate of a transitive expletive construction in spec-VP in Icelandic, but not in Mainland Scandinavian. Arguments of Jonas and Bobaljik (1993) and Bobaljik and Jonas (1996) count against this and other accounts which accommodate Icelandic transitive expletive constructions by assuming that the associate remains within the VP.

3. Verb-second and the Top domain in Old English and Middle English

3.1. Early English verb-second

The approach to verb-second developed in section 1 above sheds new light on the verb-second pattern of Old English, which is different from the patterns in the modern Germanic languages surveyed above. The Old English facts are discussed by Pintzuk (1993), Kroch and Taylor (1997), van Kemenade (1997), Fischer et al. (2000), among others. The verb-second pattern of the West Saxon texts, which comprise the bulk of the surviving Old English texts, holds as well in early southern texts of Middle English, which dominate available texts of early Middle English.

Old English exhibits general verb-subject inversion in *wh*-interrogative clauses, and clauses introduced by the negation morpheme *ne*, by the adverbial *þa* 'then', and, less consistently, by some other adverbials, including *nu* 'now', in all such cases producing a verb-second word order. This happens in both root and embedded clauses. Furthermore, it happens with both pronominal and nominal (that is, nonpronominal) subjects; the significance of this will become clear in a moment. These facts are schematized in (75) and (77), accompanied by some illustrative data in (76) and (78), respectively.[16]

(75) *wh/ne/þa* V_{fin} NP_{sub} …

(76) a. *hwi wolde God swa lytles þinges him forwyrnan?*
why would God so small thing him deny
b. *ne sende se deofol ða fyr of heofenum, …*
not sent the devil then fire from heavens
'The devil did not send fire from heaven then, …'
c. *þa com God and axode hwi he his bebod tobræce*
then came God and asked why he his commandment broke

(77) *wh/ne/þa* V_{fin} Spron …

(78) a. *Hwæt tacnað us ðonne Saul buton yfle hlafurdas?*
what betokens us then Saul except evil lords
b. *Ne sceal he naht unaliefedes don.*
not shall he nothing unlawful do
'He shall not do anything unlawful.'
c. *þa foron hie mid þrim scipum ut.*
then sailed they with three ships out

The appearance of genuine verb-second "topic" constructions, featuring a non-subject first element and inversion of the finite verb with the subject, is more restricted in Old English. It occurs almost exclusively in root clauses, and then only in the presence of a nonpronominal subject. With a pronominal subject, the construction is actually realized as verb-third since the subject must precede the finite verb. These two possibilities are schematized in (79) and (81), accompanied by some illustrative data in (80) and (82), respectively.[17]

(79) XP_{top} V_{fin} NP_{sub} …

(80) *On twam þingum hæfde God þæs mannes sawle*
in two things had God the man's soul
gegodod.
endowed
'With two things God had endowed man's soul.'

(81) XP_{top} Spron V_{fin} ...

(82) *Forðon we sceolan mid ealle mod & mægene*
therefore we must with all mind and power
to Gode gecyrran.
to God turn

In a variant of (81), noted by Pintzuk (1993: 24), the subject pronoun can appear before the initial "topic" element, as shown in (83).

(83) Spron XP_{top} V_{fin} NP_{sub} ...

And, as would be expected, Old English had subject-initial V2, shown in (84).

(84) NP_{sub}/Spron V_{fin} ...

Researchers have tended to analyze the V2 patterns with initial *wh*, negative, or adverbial elements in (75) and (77), as different from those with an initial "topic" element in (79), (81), and (84). Nevertheless, there is some strain involved in trying to account for the pattern in (75)–(84) using a fixed stock of functional categories. Some prominent accounts will be reviewed briefly in order to highlight the issues these data present to an attempt to posit a functional category system for Old English.

For Pintzuk (1993), *wh*-questions, *þa*-initial clauses, and *ne*-initial clauses are CP-V2 structures, as in (85). Van Kemenade (1997: 352, fn.22) suggests that *ne* is an independent topic element in Old English, which would justify its placement in spec-CP in (85); alternatively, if *ne* is a proclitic of the finite verb, the structure of these clauses would be as shown in (86).

(85) $[_{CP}$ *wh* / *þa* / *ne* $[_{C}$ $[_{I}$ $V_{fin}]]$ $[_{IP}$ NP_{sub} t_{I} $[_{VP}$ t_{NP} $[_{V'}$ ...

(86) $[_{CP}\ [_{C}\ [_{I}\ ne\text{-}V_{fin}]]\ [_{IP}\ NP_{sub}\ t_{I}\ [_{VP}\ t_{NP}\ [_{V'} \ldots$

Pintzuk's approach to the "topic initial" clauses in (81) and (83) is taken in the context of her double base hypothesis, according to which Old English exhibits head-final IPs, with rightward $V_{fin} \rightarrow$ I movement in non-V2 clauses, in alternation with head-medial IP, with leftward $V_{fin} \rightarrow$ I movement in V2 clauses. This establishes a foundation of uniform $V_{fin} \rightarrow$ I movement from which to analyze the alternation between V2 and non-V2 finite clauses in Old English. Pintzuk notes that there is leftward movement of the finite verb in adverbial adjunct clauses, relative clauses, and interrogative subordinate clauses, which suggests that they are IP-V2, assuming that CP-recursion is restricted to bridge verb complements. On this approach, the "topic-initial" clauses in (81) and (83) are IP-V2 with clause-medial I and XP_{top} in spec-IP, and a full nominal subject in spec-VP, as in (87a) below; a pronominal subject is a clitic to the left or right periphery of the initial or "topic" element (following Pintzuk 1991), as in (87b,c).

(87) a. $[_{IP}\ XP_{top}\ [_{I}\ V_{fin}]\ [_{VP}\ NP_{sub}\ [_{V'} \ldots$
b. $[_{IP}\ XP_{top}\ \text{Spron}\ [_{I}\ V_{fin}]\ [_{VP}\ t_{Spron}\ [_{V'} \ldots$
c. $[_{IP}\ \text{Spron}\ XP_{top}\ [_{I}\ V_{fin}]\ [_{VP}\ t_{Spron}\ [_{V'} \ldots$

Fischer et al. (2000) note that Pintzuk's account would seem to predict that embedded topicalization (with XP_{top}) should be as free as root topicalization, as is the case in Modern Icelandic and Yiddish, whereas, in fact, (as Pintzuk herself notes), topicalization of non-subjects in embedded clauses is systematic but limited in Old English (embedded topicalization only happens in passive clauses and clauses with unaccusative verbs). They therefore charge that Pintzuk's account of V2 is too symmetric between root and embedded clauses. They also point out that if V2 is IP-V2, then loss of V2 should correspond to the loss of $V_{fin} \rightarrow$ I movement. But loss of $V_{fin} \rightarrow$ I correlates with the rise of *do*-support (Kroch 1989) at the end of the fifteenth century, whereas V2 decline was well underway by the mid fourteenth century, and had proceeded by the end of the fifteenth century to a point that left verb-second as an occasional stylistic option. So Pintzuk's account does not correctly predict the chronology of the loss of verb-second.

Kroch and Taylor (1997) follow Pintzuk in the placement of the finite verb in the various types of V2 constructions, but capture the variant orders of V_{fin} and the subject in (79) and (81) by assuming that Spron adjoins to

IP, yielding (89) below for (81), while the full nominal subject in (79) remains inside VP, yielding (88) for this clause type.

(88) [$_{CP}$ XP$_{top}$ C [$_{IP}$ ø [$_{I}$ V$_{fin}$] [$_{VP}$ NP$_{sub}$ [$_{V'}$ …

(89) [$_{CP}$ XP$_{top}$ C [$_{IP}$ Spron [$_{IP}$ ø [$_{I}$ V$_{fin}$] [$_{VP}$ t$_{Spron}$ [$_{V'}$ …

But Kroch and Taylor assume that *wh/þa/ne*-clauses involve V$_{fin}$ → C, so they constitute a special case of CP-V2. With full nominal subjects, this yields the structures in (85)–(86) above, as assumed by Pintzuk; for pronominal subjects, it yields the structure in (90) below.[18]

(90) [$_{CP}$ *wh* / *þa* [$_{C}$ [$_{I}$ V$_{fin}$]] [$_{IP}$ Spron [$_{IP}$ ø t$_{I}$ [$_{VP}$ t$_{Spron}$ [$_{V'}$ …

According to Kroch and Taylor, the distinction between the structures in (88)–(89) for topic-initial V2, and the structures in (85)–(86) and (90) for V2 in clauses with *wh*, *þa* or *ne* as initial element provides a structural foundation for the subsequent historical developments concerning these constructions. V → I → C remained in *wh*-questions, subjunctives, and (some) negative clauses as "residual V2" after the regular V2 in (79)–(82), which Kroch and Taylor analyze as IP-V2, was lost with the decline of independent V → I movement. However, while this account gets the overall difference in loss between (75)–(78) and (79)–(82) correct, it seems vulnerable to Fischer et al.'s (2000) objection that this sort of account does not capture the timing of the loss of V2 correctly since V2 declined significantly in the late fourteenth century and throughout the fifteenth century, while independent V → I declined with the rise of *do*-support, which did not become well established until the end of the fifteenth century.

Fischer et al. (2000) posit a special functional head, F, projected above TP, specifically to serve as a host for subject pronouns, which appear in spec-FP; the functional structure of the clause they adopt (with all relevant categories represented) is given in (91).

(91) [$_{CP}$ C [$_{FP}$ F [$_{NegP}$ Neg [$_{TP}$ T [$_{VP}$ …

In the "topic-initial" constructions in (79) and (81), the finite verb raises to F, not to C, thus appearing after a subject pronoun in spec-FP, but before a full nominal subject, which surfaces in spec-TP.

(92) $[_{CP}\ XP_{top}\ C\ [_{FP}\ [_{F}\ [_{T}\ V_{fin}]]\ [_{TP}\ NP_{sub}\ t_{T}\ [_{VP}\ t_{NP}\ [_{V'}\ \ldots$

(93) $[_{CP}\ XP_{top}\ C\ [_{FP}\ Spron\ [_{F}\ [_{T}\ V_{fin}]]\ [_{TP}\ t_{Spron}\ t_{T}\ [_{VP}\ t_{Spron}\ [_{V'}\ \ldots$

In wh-clauses, negative clauses, and clauses introduced by *þa* (and certain other adverbials), the finite verb moves to C, with the results shown in (94)–(95).

(94) a. $[_{CP}\ \textit{wh / þa}\ [_{C}\ [_{T}\ V_{fin}]]\ [_{TP}\ NP_{sub}\ t_{T}\ [_{VP}\ t_{NP}\ [_{V'}\ \ldots$
b. $[_{CP}\ \textit{wh / þa}\ [_{C}\ [_{F}\ [_{T}\ V_{fin}]]]\ [_{FP}\ Spron\ t_{F}\ [_{TP}\ t_{Spron}\ t_{T}$
$[_{VP}\ t_{pron}\ [_{V'}\ \ldots$

(95) a. $[_{CP}\ [_{C}\ [_{Neg}\ \textit{ne-}[_{T}\ V_{fin}]]]\ [_{NegP}\ \textit{na}\ t_{Neg}\ [_{TP}\ NP_{sub}\ t_{T}\ [_{VP}\ t_{NP}\ \ldots$
b. $[_{CP}\ [_{C}\ [_{F}\ [_{Neg}\ \textit{ne-}[_{T}\ V_{fin}]]]]\ [_{FP}\ Spron\ t_{F}\ [_{NegP}\ \textit{na}\ t_{Neg}$
$[_{TP}\ t_{Spron}\ t_{T}\ [_{VP}\ t_{Spron}\ \ldots$

This distinguishes the forms of V2 which will become "residual" V2 in (94)–(95) from the "topic" V2 forms in (92)–(93), thus permitting an account by which the "residual V2" forms remain after the decline (and eventual disappearance) of "topic V2". Furthermore, the "topic" V2 forms in (92)–(93) involve V → I movement only as an intermediate step to achieve V → F; to the extent that this decouples "topic" V2 from independent V → I movement, it makes it more explicable that "topic" V2 should decline for more than a century before the loss of independent V → I movement. However, the postulation of the functional head F just in order to capture the relative orders of the finite verb, subject pronoun, and full nominal subject seems to be a rather ad hoc device in this account.

3.2. A feature-based account of Old and Middle English verb-second

The pattern for *wh*-interrogatives, negative clauses and *þa*-clauses (along with some clauses introduced by other adverbials) is repeated in (96a,b). As Kroch and Taylor (1997) note, this is essentially the pattern of subjunctive clauses as well, indicated in (96c).

(96) a. *wh/ne/þa* V_{fin} NP_{sub} …
b. *wh/ne/þa* V_{fin} Spron …
c. $V_{fin/subj}$ NP_{sub} / Spron …

In the interrogatives, [Q] and [WH] features will attract the finite verb and a *wh*-expression. There is no need to endow a fixed C^o with these features; it is enough that they be ranked lower than inflectional features as in (97), bundled together in a feature matrix and projected onto a functional head merged above the inflectional projections at the appropriate point in the derivation. The inflectional features can, of course, be distributed into multiple feature matrices, effecting split Infl, but with each of the component features within each inflectional feature matrix subject to the ordering condition in (97).

(97) [Q, WH] < F_I for all Infl-features F_I.

Subjunctive and negative clauses will be generated similarly by projecting [SUBJ] and [NEG] onto a functional head merged above the inflectional projections. The *þa*-clauses and similarly behaving adverbial clauses will follow suit if they have conditional or modal force. Thus, the implementation of a feature-based approach to the pattern in (96) is a fairly straightforward matter of translating over to the present notation.

To address the "topic V2" constructions, first note that object pronouns typically occur in the same position as subject pronouns in these constructions. A fuller paradigm for these is therefore as given in (98) below (which all obtain almost exclusively in root clauses).

(98)	a.	XP_{top}		V_{fin}	NP_{sub} …
	b.	XP_{top}	Spron/Opron	V_{fin}	NP_{sub} …
	c.	Spron/Opron	XP_{top}	V_{fin}	NP_{sub} …

This fuller paradigm suggests a new generalization: in these structures, the inflectional systems are preceded by a TOPIC domain. That, is, the fronting of the finite verb is associated with the fronting of elements which can fulfill the role of "topics," in a sense which is comprehensive of standard V2 topic elements and elements having the discourse topic status of pronouns. We unite these somewhat disparate elements here, not just because they have been put under the same rubric (whose denotation has thereby lost some conceptual unity), but because of parallelism in their grammatical effects, coupled with whatever V2 "topics" have in common with subject and object pronouns as discourse topics. This is, in fact, an idea with a long history; see the discussion by Bean (1983: 18–40), who traces the idea from Weil (1844) and McKnight (1897), cited therein, and places it within the context of the functional sentence perspective of the Prague School of Linguistics and more recent work by Li and Thompson (1976). However, this TOPIC domain need not be conceived of as a vague region of the clause; it can be precisely constructed through the projection of appropriate features onto functional heads. Assume that XP_{top}, Spron, and Opron are all attracted to a N-feature TOP_N, and that TOP_N is accompanied by a corresponding V-feature, TOP_V, which attracts the finite verb. Then $[TOP_V, TOP_N] < F_I$ for all Infl-features F_I. So the matrix $[TOP_V, TOP_N]$ is projected as a supra-Infl head, $\hat{}[TOP_V, TOP_N]$. TOP_V attracts V_{fin}, producing inversion with a nominal subject in spec-^IP (except when NP_{sub} is the topic element). TOP_N attracts XP_{top}, as well as Spron and Opron, so the functional projection $\hat{}[TOP_V, TOP_N]$ is an all-purpose TOPIC domain, whose effects are evident in (98), producing a topic-comment bifurcation in information structure. When multiple TOPIC elements move to the $\hat{}[TOP_V, TOP_N]$-system, they merge to the left of the target phrase structure as multiple specifiers. (See Koizumi 1994 for multiple specifiers of – essentially – CP for various processes, including multiple *wh*-movement in Slavic languages and Romanian, English topicalization, and embedded V2 in Germanic; Ura 1996 for multiple specifiers of Agr; and Sabel 2002 for the role of multiple specifiers of CP in *wh*-movement.) On this account, the TOP_N feature can be successively checked by a "topic" element, XP_{top}, and by a pronoun in either order; thus these two fronted constituents can be merged with a projection of $\hat{}[TOP_V, TOP_N]$ in either order, producing structures with the order in (98c) as well as those with (98b).

The option of ranking $\{TOP_V, TOP_N\} = F_I$ for the highest ranked Infl-features should also be available, producing subject-initial V2 clauses. Thus, in general, $\{TOP_V, TOP_N\} \leq F_I$. The option $\{TOP_V, TOP_N\} = F_I$ permits $\{TOP_V, TOP_N\}$ to be projected with inflectional features on a highly syncretic functional category, so that subject φ-features and TOP features can be checked in the same position, yielding subject-initial V2.[19]

Evidently, TOPIC elements, in the sense introduced above, do not appear with *wh*-interrogative structures. This follows since $\{TOP_V, TOP_N\}$ are incompatible with {Q, WH}. It is clear that they should not be compatible to the extent of being capable of being ranked equally and projected together, since the *wh*-element has a focal status, and therefore cannot be topical. TOPIC elements also do not occur in negative clauses or *þa*-clauses with verb raising, such as (99a,b); these have non-TOPIC negative and conditional V-features attracting the verb.[20]

(99) a. *Ne het he us na leornian heofonas to wyrcenne.*
not ordered he us not learn heavens to make
'He did not bid us learn to make the heavens.'

b. *þa foron hie mid þrim scipum ut.*
then sailed they with three ships out

In Old English, "topic V2" structures typically do not occur in embedded clauses except in bridge verb complements, as in (100) below.[21]

(100) *Gregorius se trahtnere cwæð þæt forði wolde*
Gregorius the interpreter said that therefore wanted
drihten getrahtnian þurh hine sylfne þæt bigspel ðe …
God interpret through himself the parable that

This restriction follows if {TOP_V, TOP_N} are incompatible with all non-default features which would introduce a subordinate clause. The declarative features in a bridge verb complement are default features, compatible with {TOP_V, TOP_N}, as in Modern Mainland Scandinavian. However, this simple proposal stands in need of refinement in light of a systematic exception to the restriction of embedded verb-second to bridge verb complements. As noted in the literature (cf. van Kemenade 1997, Fischer et al. 2000: 116) verb-second occurs in contexts other than bridge verb complements when the clause is passivized or the verb is unaccusative, as in the following examples.[22]

(101) *for þan þe on me is afunden ætforan Gode rihtwisnyss*
because that in me is found before God justice
'because justice before God is found in me'

(102) *þonne ælce dæge beoð manega acennede þurh*
when each day are many.NOM given-birth through
hys mihte on worulde
his power on world

This type of example is also obtained when the first element (between the complementizer and the finite verb) is a pronoun, moved to the topic domain.[23]

(103) *forðam þe him burston ut butu his eagan*
because that him.DAT burst out both his eyes.NOM
'because both his eyes burst out'

(104) *gif we wyllað secgan be þam ðe us secgað béc,*
if we want declare.INF by that us.DAT declares book
of þam ðe us becymð se widsom and
from that.DAT that us.DAT results the wisdom and
seo wissung,
the guidance

These sometimes exhibit the subject clause-finally, as (101) and (103) do. Another example with a full nominal subject is given in (105) below, from *The West Saxon Gospels* (Grünberg, ed., 1967: 38, line 54).

(105) *of þe forð gæð se heretoga se ðe recð*
from which forth goes the chieftain who that rules
min folc israhel
my people israel

Fischer et al. (2000: 185–201) show that particles such as *forð* are distinct from separable prefixes, and that Old English particles exhibit syntactic independence of the verb in various respects (such as that verb raising strands the particle). Assuming that the verb raises by itself in V2, *forð* is placed before the verb as a V2 topic element in (105). Furthermore, as noted by Fischer et al. (2000: 116), OE *gan*, 'go' (of which *gæð* is 3.SG.PRES) behaves as unaccusative.

What can we make of this? Within standard approaches to verb-second, it certainly seems odd that the passive syntax of the clause or the unaccusativity of the verb should have any effect on the circumstances higher in the clause which pertain to the contexts in which subordinate clause verb-second can appear. Van Kemenade (1997) approaches this problem under the assumption that V2 in Old English is asymmetric between root and subordinate clauses, with embedded V2 restricted to complements of bridge verbs. It follows that the examples in (101)–(105) are not a product of normal verb-second processes which move the finite verb to C and a topic element to spec-CP. Van Kemenade notes that the distinguishing property of these constructions is that the main verb lacks an external argument, either through passivization or inherent unaccusativity, a context in which Old English permits expletive *pro*-drop, and links her account of this exceptional construction to this distinguishing fact. Focusing on cases in which the subject occurs within VP, and spec-IP is empty or filled by a dative element, van Kemenade proposes that these examples involve movement of the finite verb to a clause-medial I, and licensing of the nominative subject within VP by chain government by C, transmitted from spec-IP to spec-VP by virtue of the lack of a nominative subject in spec-IP. On this analysis, the subject in (102) is in spec-VP since *beoð* 'are' is in I^o.

On the feature-based approach, we are not confined to accommodate V2 within the standard stock of functional categories, and there are plausible mechanisms available for a link between the projection of the TOPIC domain and some well known properties of passivized and unaccusative structures. Turning to the structures in (101)–(105), the clause-final position of the subject (the lone argument of the verb) in some of these examples seems to be a focalizing device to give this argument greater prominence. Now the unique properties of passive and unaccusative structures in relation to focus projection come into play. As discussed by Selkirk (1984) and others, focus can project from the object of a verb, but not generally from its subject; as a result, passivized and unaccusative verbs uniquely have the property of projecting focus from their subjects since their subjects are underlying objects.[24] That is, focus registered on the subject of a transitive structure such as that in (106) below, or the subject of an unergative verb as in (107), does not permit an interpretation in which the entire clause is the focus, as would be favored by the contexts indicated.

(106) A: *What's new about the children these days?*
B: *SAM likes brussels sprouts.*
#[$_{\text{Foc}}$ *Sam likes brussels sprouts*]

(107) A: *What happened here?* [surveying a mess]
B: *SAM swam across the bathtub.*
#[$_{\text{Foc}}$ *Sam swam across the bathtub*]

But focus on an object does project, as in (108)–(109) below, with the focal domains of B's responses as indicated, in which focus associated with nuclear stress on the object NP can project to the VP, as in (108), and from thence to the entire IP, as in (109).

(108) A: *What did Bill do most recently?*
B: *Bill attacked SAM.*
Bill [$_{Foc}$ *attacked Sam*]

(109) A: *What happened here?*
B: *Bill attacked SAM.*
[$_{Foc}$ *Bill attacked Sam*]

Correspondingly, focus on the subject of a passivized clause, or the lone argument of an unaccusative verb, whether it is in subject position or not, does project since this argument originates in object position, as in (110)–(111).[25]

(110) A: *What's going on here?*
B: *SAM is being attacked.*
[$_{Foc}$ *Sam*$_i$ *is being attacked* t_i]

(111) A: *What's going on here?*
B: *SAM is arriving.*
[$_{Foc}$ *Sam*$_i$ *is arriving* t_i]

The conjecture regarding (101)–(105) is now straightforward on the assumption that the TOP features are averse to information-theoretic focus. These structures come about when the subject is focal and when this focus projects to the entire ^IP of which it is the subject. In this instance, if TOP features are projected, they cannot be projected together with the lowest ranked (and highest projected) I-features, F_I, since this would put them within the focal domain. In this circumstance, the constraint against TOP being projected in the same clause as non-default subordinating features seems to be a soft constraint which can be violated in order to permit projection of TOP features when they are effectively flushed out of ^IP by projection of focus from the subject. The resulting projection of Top = [[TOP_V], [TOP_N]] as a head ^Top, merged just above ^IP, will yield the structures in (101)–(105). This solution to the problem of how the unaccusative nature of the clause influences possibilities for embedded topicalization in non-bridge-verb complements appeals solely to effects of feature projection and not (as with van Kemenade's account) to non-local relationships of case licensing across the clause. On this account, the frequent sentence-final position of nominative subjects in these examples is explicable as a focalizing device, but by no means necessary, so examples such as (102) and (105) can be accommodated with nominative subjects in spec-^IP.

The constraints on feature projection given in Chapter 2, repeated below, can play a role in formulating other aspects of the account of Old and Middle English verb-second developed here.

> *Economy of Feature Projection*
> Given the lexical categories in a numeration, a minimal suite of matching features is entered into the numeration to be projected onto functional categories.
>
> *Economy of Projection of Infl-Categories*
> If features F_1, F_2, ..., F_n are elements of a feature matrix M projected as a functional head ^M within the Infl-system of a clause, then one of F_1, F_2, ..., F_n must be a clausal feature (V/A-feature matching some $F_{V/A}$ on a verb/adjective within that clause).

The Economy of Projection of Infl-Categories narrows the range of possible accounts. In particular, the Kroch and Taylor structure given in (112) below, repeated from (89) above, would be ruled out by the condition that CP would not be projected if there is no V-feature in C.

(112) $[_{CP}$ XP_{top} C $[_{IP}$ Spron $[_{IP}$ ø $[_{I}$ $V_{fin}]$ $[_{VP}$ t_{Spron} $[_{V'}$ …

The Economy of Projection of Infl-Categories also gives us a purchase on the following examples in ways which will anticipate the analysis of clitic climbing of object clitics in Modern Italian in the next chapter.[26]

(113) … *ðæt he wisdom mæge wið ifernetta æfre gemengan*
that he wisdom may with pride ever mingle

(114) *ðæt he Saul ne dorste ofslean*
that he Saul not dared murder

Fischer et al. (2000: 123) call attention to these, but their account of Old English clause structure, summarized above, does not readily account for them, nor do any of the others summarized above. Their account of (113) illustrates the difficulties they face. Fischer et al. propose that (113) results from the movement of the object NP to the specifier of an Agr_O node associated with the modal verb; this is the exercise of an option they accord to the object NP to freely move or not to move to the local Agr_O.

In the present framework, these structures are an indirect result of the lack of NP-verb agreement with the uninflected main verb. The object has N-features (φ-features and case features) which need to be checked. Therefore, matching N-features are entered into the numeration. However, since there is no NP-verb agreement with the main verb, there are, correspondingly, no V-features on the main verb, and thus no matching V-features entered into the numeration with which the N-features of the object could be bundled and projected as a functional head (in what would be, in effect, a construction of Agr_O). By the Economy of Projection of Infl-Features, the matrix of N-features of the object cannot be projected as a functional head by themselves; therefore, they must associate with lower ranked V-features and be projected higher in the clause. The object must therefore raise to the specifier of this higher position.

3.3. Middle English dialects and language change

Verb-second in English was the dominant pattern in root clauses in Old English, but declined in the late Middle English period, through the fourteenth and fifteenth centuries, to become merely a diminishing stylistic variant in Early Modern English. On the present account, the phrase structure of English need not have undergone any major adjustment to effect this change; the loss of V2 is at heart just the diminishing use and ultimate loss of the $\{TOP_V, TOP_N\}$ features.

We can address the difference between the southern dialects of Middle English, which had the verb-second pattern of Old English, and the northern (central west Yorkshire) dialect of Middle English represented in the *Prose Rule of St. Benet.* As argued by Kroch and Taylor (1997), the northern dialect had generalized V2 with finite verb inversion over pronominal as well as nominal subjects in ordinary V2 topic constructions with a preverbal topic element. Kroch and Taylor analyze all of these as CP-V2. On the present account, one main difference between these two dialects is that TOP_N in the northern dialect is restricted to formal V2 "topic" elements, and does not act on pronominals, whereas in the southern dialects of Middle English and in Old English, TOP_N acts on pronominals and V2 "topics" alike. Another main difference is that $\{TOP_V, TOP_N\}$ in the northern dialect determines the structure of all adjunct-initial V2 clauses, including *þa-*

clauses, so *þa*-initial clauses are assimilated to the normal V2 pattern. Both of these differences can be attributed to the employment of {TOP_V, TOP_N} in the northern dialect as more akin to its employment in Scandinavian languages. This acknowledges Kroch and Taylor's (1997) observation that the differences between northern and southern dialects are not merely due to the behavior of subject pronouns, but furthermore it provides a single, and minimal locus for these two differences.

The fact that TOP_N in the northern dialect is not active on subject pronouns is illustrated by the following "doubly-filled comp" example from *The Prose Rule of St. Benet*, cited by Kroch and Taylor (1997: 315).

(115) *I sal yu lere þe dute of god, his wille þat ye may do*
I shall you teach the duty of God, his will that you may do

The V-feature TOP_V is not present in this structure, but TOP_N is projected on the category lexically filled by *þat*, attracting XP_{top} to spec-^[TOP_N]P. But the subject pronoun remains in spec-^IP.

3.4. Streamlining accounts of Old English word order below the TOPIC domain

The variety of word orders below the TOPIC domain in Old English poses issues for the system of inflectional features, I. These issues will be explored in the remainder of this section, to determine what conclusions can be drawn regarding the nature of the system of inflectional features in Old English.

When not in verb-second position, Old English main verbs exhibit both OV and VO orders with respect to an object. OV order can be seen in the non-V2 subordinate clauses in (116)–(118) below.[27]

(116) *þa he ða þas andsware onfeng*
when he then that answer received

(117) … *ond þurh Godes gife þone songcræft onfeng.*
And through God's gift that songskill received

(118) *ðæt he hwelc gerisenlic wundor wyrcean mæge*
that he some suitable miracle perform can

The position of the auxiliary in (118) might result from the same processes that produce OV order with the main verb (such as base generation of right-headed VPs), or it might reflect movement of the auxiliary to a right-headed $^\wedge I^o$. Examples of VO order can be seen in (119)–(120) (from *Ælfric's Catholic Homilies, the First Series*, cited by Fischer et al. 2000: 140, 142).

(119) *þæt he nolde niman mancyn neadunga of ðam deofle*
that he not-would take mankind forcibly from the devil

(120) *We willað secgan eow sum bigspell.*
we want tell you a parable

These can be produced from an OV base, assuming movement operations to produce structures which do not surface as OV, or from a VO base, assuming a rather different set of movements to produce non-VO orders. Alternatively, as Pintzuk (1991, 1993) has argued, Old English might have had a dual base, with separate OV and VO grammars co-existing, competing to produce an alternation of OV/VO forms even within a single manuscript by a single writer. As Pintzuk points out, if Old English underwent a change from an OV grammar to a VO grammar, with competing OV and VO in the interim, then the number of VO structures should exhibit the S-shaped curve of the sort which Kroch (1989) argues is associated with a grammatical characteristic when it is introduced to a speech community, spreads through the community, and gradually attains dominance across speakers. Pintzuk argues that the spread of VO in Old English exhibits just such a curve.

But even on the dual base hypothesis, most structures cannot be derived without some further movement. Consider the example in (121).[28]

(121) *for-þon he gewunade gerisenlice leoð wyrcan,*
for that he was-accustomed fittingly songs make.INF
þa ðe to æfestnisse ond to arfæstnisse belumpon
DEM REL to religion and to virtue pertained

From an OV base, this would be generated as (122) below, and derived from movement of the finite verb to check TOP_V, together with extraposition of the relative clause.

(122) *for-þon he gerisenlice [leoð [þa ðe to æfestnisse*
for that he fittingly songs DEM REL to religion
ond to arfæstnisse belumpon]] wyrcan gewunade
and to virtue pertained make.INF was-accustomed

From a VO base, (121) would be generated as (123) below, and derived by movement of the finite verb to check TOP_V, combined with object shift of the relativized object to a position before the infinitival verb, followed by extraposition of the relative clause; object shift would also have to apply within the relative clause.

(123) *for-þon he gerisenlice gewunade wyrcan [leoð*
for-that he fittingly was-accustomed make.INF songs
[þa ðe belumpon to æfestnisse ond to arfæstnisse]]
DEM REL pertained to religion and to virtue

But the required combinations of operations tend to be much more elaborate on a single base hypothesis, and, assuming feature-driven movement, this complexity of hypothesized movement operations is relevant to the system of functional features.[29] For example, Fischer et al. (2000: 151–160) propose a uniform VO base for Old English, with alternate orders produced through feature-driven leftward movements. On this approach, OV order is typically produced by V → Agr_O movement, accompanied by object shift to spec-Agr_OP. By making both of these optional (thereby suspending Holmberg's Generalization – which predicates object shift upon verb raising – for Old English), Fischer et al. account for various orders of the verb and object with respect to one another and with respect to other nearby elements, such as adverbs and particles. These possible combinations of movement and nonmovement are accounted for under the assumption that the relevant features attracting the verb and object are optionally strong or weak features, thus active in the overt syntax or not, as the case may be. In more complex examples, such as (124) below, Fischer et al. (2000: 155) appeal to further possibilities of movement. (Example from *Ælfric's Catholic Homilies, the First Series*.)

(124) *þæt he ure sawle fram synna fagnyssum gehælen mæge*
that he our soul from sins' ulcers heal can

From a VO base such as that given in (125) below, the derivation of (124) proceeds through object shift of *ure sawle* to spec-Agr_OP.[30]

(125) *þæt he mæge* [$_{VP}$ *fram synna fagnyssum* [$_{VP}$ *gehælen*
that he can from sins' ulcers heal
ure sawle]]
our soul

To obtain *mæge* in clause-final position, Fischer et al. assume that the entire lower Agr_OP thereupon moves to the specifier of an Agr_O node associated with the modal; they suggest that the existence of such a higher Agr_O is plausible in light of the fact that Old English modals were fully thematic verbs, unlike their Modern English descendants.

But across a broad range of cases, this strategy leads to derivations which are more complex than can be comfortably sustained. As applied to the clauses in (126)–(127), for example (from Bede, Book IV, Ch.24), it would require movement of a lower Agr_OP, following object shift as in the derivation of (124), to the specifier of an Agr_O associated with the auxiliary BE (*wæron/wæs*); the existence of such a higher Agr_O in these examples is considerably less plausible than in (124) since auxiliary *BE* does not have the main verb characteristics of Old English modals.

(126) *Ond for his leoþsongum monigra mona*
and on-account-of his poemsongs many men's
mod oft to worulde forhogdnisse ond to geþeodnisse
minds often to [of] world disdain and to service
þæs heofonlice lifes onbærnde wæron.
[of] the heavenly life kindled were

(127) *for-þon he nalæs from monnum ne þurh mon*
for that he not-at all from men not through man
gelæred wæs
taught was

Furthermore, as illustrated by examples (121), (124), and (126) above, this strategy would require object shift of object PPs and infinitival complements. Fischer et al. appeal to the nominal character of Old English infinitival verbs as justification for the latter, but it isn't clear why the nominal character of an infinitive verb would be reflected in object shift of an entire infinitival clause (with attendant arguments and adjuncts of the infinitive). Fischer et al. assume that adjunct PPs are freely generated left-adjoined or right-adjoined to the VP; a more constrained treatment of these will be suggested below.

In short, a uniform VO base with leftward verb raising and object shift would put a strain on the system of functional features driving such movement. This strain is considerably reduced if the dual base hypothesis is adopted, with OV and VO base orders both available. The strain can be further reduced if we note that PPs often appear left-stacked according to their semantic scope. In (128) below, for example (Bede, Book IV, Ch.24), in the subordinate clause beginning with the topicalized demonstrative pronoun *þæt* (in bold face, extracted across-the-board from the object positions of *geglængde* 'adorned' and *forþ brohte* 'forth brought'), *þæt* is generated directly before or after the verb, depending on the order in the base, but the adjunct PPs appear with their appropriate semantic scopes, provided they are left-stacked, that is, left-adjoined to the VP, merged in succession from bottom to top in the structure, and from right to left in linear order.

(128) *swa ðætte swa hwæt swa he of godcundum stafum*
so that so what so he of divine letters
*þurh boceras geleornode, **þæt** he æfter medmiclum*
through scholars learned that he after medium
fæce in scopgereorde mid þa mæstan swetnisse ond
time in poetic speech with the greatest sweetness and
inbryrdnisse geglængde ond in Engliscgereorde wel
inspiration adorned and in Englishspeech well
geworht forþ brohte.
worked forth brought

Note that (129), a subordinate *þæt*-clause, and (130), both from the same source, follow suit.

(129) *þæt heo ealle sceoldon þurh endebyrdnesse be*
that they all should through succession with
hearpan singan
harp sing.INF

(130) *þonne aras he for scome from þæm symble ond*
then arose he from shame from that banquet and
ham eode to his huse
home went to his house

Assuming that early Old English left-stacked PPs above the object, before the verb, and that VO order was introduced and gradually spread, and that PP placement was subsequently loosened up allowing right or left adjunction, the amount of ad hoc allowance of optionality in feature strength is minimized. The appeal to optional and ad hoc movements is thus also minimized.

Notes

1. Examples (4)–(8) are from Vikner (1995: 47).
2. Examples (9), (11), and (12) are from Iatridou and Kroch (1992: 6–7); example (10) is from Vikner (1995: 72).
3. The examples in (14) are from Thráinsson (1985: 192), and (15) and (16c) from Thráinsson (1985: 179). Examples (16a,b) are from Vikner (1995: 72), and (17a,b) are from Iatridou and Kroch (1992).
4. The examples in (18) are from Santorini (1992: 597). Examples (19a,b) are from Diesing (1990: 42, 58). Examples (20a,b) are from Vikner (1995: 72). Examples (21)–(22) are from Iatridou and Kroch (1992).
5. Rambow and Santorini (1995) likewise adopt a feature [+Top] in the context of a construction of functional heads building on the categorial features in Rizzi (1996). Some remarks on the adoption of Top in (24) are in order. As noted in Chapter 2, the "topic" element, attracted to check [TOP_N] on the present account, tends to have, but need not have, the informational status of a topic. Despite the imperfect correlation, there might be a temptation to reify Top as an expression of information-theoretic topichood. But the feature matrix Top = [[TOP_V], [TOP_N]] is internal to the syntactic system, driving movements to produce a verb-second structure, whether or not the element attracted to check [TOP_N] is an information-theoretic topic. A substantive interface between the syntactic system and information structure, considerably more complex and subtle than a one-to-one correlation between syntactic fea-

tures and informational statuses, is implicated by this relationship. Mulkern (2003), drawing on a wide range of constructions in disparate languages, argues that informational status is not directly expressed by syntactic features, and provides grounds for a substantive interface between syntax and information structure, realized as a nontrivial, parameterized mapping between distinct modules of the grammar. See also Clamons, Mulkern, Sanders, and Stenson (1999) for a version of one of these arguments, based on the information status and subject-verb agreement properties of subjects in the Cushitic language Oromo.

6. Rambow and Santorini propose a similar, but reversed, ordering, interpreted as an order of categorial selection rather than as a checking order for primitive morpho-syntactic and semantic features. Their formulation will be compared with the present one below.
7. The inventory of bridge verbs varies somewhat cross-linguistically. In Danish, *vide* 'know' behaves as a bridge verb, as Vikner (1995) shows. Its counterpart in English, *know*, on the other hand, is typically used as factive and behaves in many respects as a non-bridge verb, although not as uniformly as some members of that class.
8. The central role of declarative marking is a point of rough analogy between this account and Brandner's (2004) account of verb-second as resulting from the need to establish declarative force marking. Brandner's account is otherwise very different, however, in that it dispenses with feature attraction as the basic determinant of movement in the analysis of verb-second effects.
9. As in English and Mainland Scandinavian, interrogative main clauses have verb fronting by attraction to [Q], not to [TOP_V], and *wh*-questions have *wh*-fronting by attraction to [WH], not [TOP_N].
10. See Chapter 7, section 7.2, below for discussion of a stage of Swiss German child language in which Top is compatible with nondeclarative M features, producing embedded clause verb-second constructions which the adult language lacks. This discussion is based on the results presented by Schönenberger (2001).
11. Because Rambow and Santorini separate out mood from complementizer features, they actually posit the feature structure [+M, +Top, +I] in finite verbs in subject-topic V2 clauses.
12. Following much of the literature, expletives in existential constructions will be uniformly glossed as *there*, regardless of their pronominal affiliations.
13. Vikner (1995: 203) also cites the following, which might seem at odds with the claim that the expletive is introduced to project a grammatical subject in the absence of an external argument.

    (i) … *at der har danset nogen i haven.*
    that there has danced someone in garden-the

But Vikner (1995: 202–207) gives a variety of arguments that the indefinite subject in (i) appears in the complement position to the unergative verb *danset*, so it is not clear that the associate DP *nogen* counts as a projected external argument in this example.

14. This is basically in line with Jonas and Bobaljik (1993) and Bobaljik and Jonas (1996), who argue that the associate of a transitive expletive construction in Icelandic does not remain in spec-VP, or (as argued by Christensen 1991) adjoined to VP, but that it raises to an Infl-spec. They identify the position of the associate as spec-TP, assuming that the expletive is in spec-Agr_SP; but, making due allowance for their claims regarding the role of spec-TP, the specification of these positions can be reinterpreted in light of the assumption that the expletive is in spec-^TopP, adopted here.
15. English was included in the discussion of copular expletive constructions above since the English data cited were parallel to the Danish data, and the explanations offered for these data were parallel in the two languages. English was not included in discussion of the other expletive constructions since the English data don't quite parallel the Danish data, or that for any of the other Germanic languages, and the reasons for this divergence are not clear. Like Danish, English cannot introduce an expletive for an external argument associate. This suggests that English introduces an expletive solely to project a subject in the absence of an external argument. As a result, as in Danish, we expect the expletive to perform checking of all subject N-features, and for the associate to remain in-situ. But the English counterpart to (71d), *There was an apple eaten*, which was already unexpectedly good in Danish, is quite perfect in English; in fact, it is much better than *??There was eaten an apple*, the English counterpart of (55) and (71a). Furthermore, the English counterpart of (48d) and (56) is notoriously fickle, varying across speakers, and varying from quite colloquial to quite formal or awkward, depending on lexical choices, tense and aspect, and other properties of the clause, as illustrated below. ((iia,b) are adapted from Vikner 1995: 197.)

    (i) a. *Finally, there have arrived some people I can talk to.*
    b. ?? *There has arrived a boy.*
    (ii) a. *There will come a time when you will be sorry.*
    b. ?? *There will come a letter from your mother.*
16. Examples in (76) and (78) are cited by Fischer et al. (2000: 106, 115, 118–119, 124). The examples in (76) are from *Ælfric's Catholic Homilies, the First Series*; (78a,b) are from *King Alfred's West Saxon Version of Gregory's Pastoral Care*; and (78c) is from *The Anglo-Saxon Chronicles*, Parker Chronicle, MS A.
17. Examples in (80) and (82) are cited by Fischer et al. (2000: 107, 114). Example (80) is from *Ælfric's Catholic Homilies, the First Series*; (82) is from the *Blickling Homilies* (Homily 8).

18. Kroch and Taylor add subjunctive clauses to the list of contexts for finite verb inversion with a subject pronoun, as in (i) below, from *The Anglo-Saxon Chronicle*, cited by Kroch and Taylor (1997: 303). Compare with Modern English, *Had they received the books, ...*
    (i) *hæfdon hi hiora onfangen ær Hæsten to Beamfleote come*
    had they them received before Hæsten to Beamfleote came
19. If {TOP_V, TOP_N} = F_I is chosen when a non-subject is marked with [TOP_N], this will produce a verb-third structure in which the subject and topic element both move to spec-^[Top, F_I]P. In this case, Old English evidently requires one or both of the subject and topic element to be pronominal.
20. Example (99a) is from *Ælfric's Lives of the Saints*, cited by Fischer et al. (2000: 125); example (99b) is repeated from (78c) above.
21. From *Ælfric's Catholic Homilies, the Second Series*, cited by van Kemenade (1997: 333), and by Fischer et al. (2000: 116).
22. These examples are from *Homilies of Ælfric: A Supplementary Collection*, J. C. Pope, ed.; they are cited by van Kemenade (1997: 335) and by Fischer et al. (2000: 116–117).
23. Example (103) is from *Ælfric's Lives of the Saints*, cited in van Kemenade (1997: 337), and (104) is from *Homlies of Ælfric: A Supplementary Collection*, John C. Pope, ed., Vol.II, XXII, lines 80–84. Oxford University Press, 1968.
24. Diesing (1991) claims that focus can project from any argument which originates within the VP, and claims thereby a distinction between projection of focus from subjects of stage-level predicates and subjects of individual-level predicates, because, following Kratzer (1995), she takes the former to be generated in spec-VP, and the latter to be generated outside the VP.
25. These facts, particularly (110) have been variously advanced and denied in the literature; see Selkirk (1984) for discussion and sources. (Selkirk is among those who deny the possibility of focus projecting in examples such as (110).) In fact, (110)–(111) are best obtained with the focus structure indicated when the idea of Sam (or someone) being subject to attack in (110), or of Sam (or someone) arriving in (111), has a certain degree of prior salience in the discourse; if it had no prior salience whatsoever, the intended interpretation in (110)–(111) would be best conveyed by (ia,b) below.
    (i.) a. *SAM is being ATTACKED.*
    b. *SAM is ARRIVING.*

    But the idea of someone being attacked, or someone arriving, should not be too salient when A's utterance is made, since otherwise the most favored interpretation would be with contrastive focus on the subject, rather than focus projecting to the entire clause. The indicated interpretations of B's responses, with focus projecting, are obtained exactly when the idea of Sam (or someone) being attacked or arriving has a nonzero but fairly low degree of prior salience.

26. Cited by Fischer et al. (2000: 123). Example (113) is from *The Meters of Boethius*, and (114) is from *King Alfred's West Saxon Version of Gregory's Pastoral Care.*
27. Examples (116) and (117) are from the Old English version of Bede's *Ecclesiastical History of the English People*, Book IV, Ch.24, glosses by Lisi Oliver. Example (118), cited by Fischer et al. (2000: 140), is from *King Alfred's West Saxon Version of Gregory's Pastoral Care.*
28. From the Old English version of Bede's *Ecclesiastical History of the English People*, Book IV, Ch.24, glosses by Lisi Oliver. This holds for all sources hereafter referenced as Bede, Book IV, Ch.24.
29. In a feature-based syntax, at least leftward movements to head and specifier positions are driven by feature-checking requirements. Rightward movements such as the extraposition of relative clauses seen in (121) above must either be analyzed as leftward movement of other material, a tall order in most such examples, or as a different kind of movement, motivated by prosodic requirements rather than checking of morpho-syntactic features.
30. In (125), the PP *fram synna fagnyssum* is assumed to be adjoined to VP to minimize the complexity of the derivation. This serves the argument that the derivation in question is too complex on other grounds.

Chapter 4
Aspects of clitic placement and clitic climbing

In a Minimalist formulation of syntax of the sort presented in Chapter 2, the derivation of a sentence is directed by features on functional and lexical categories in a numeration. Chomsky (1995a, 1995b) explores the derivational options across a range of examples in which features on lexical categories are attracted to matching features projected onto functional categories. Giorgi and Pianesi (1996, 1997) and the discussion in Chapter 2 above articulate some principles by which functional features are distributed onto functional categories, and argue that there is a limited and constrained range of derivational options for a numeration, generated by different possible distributions of features onto functional categories. The present chapter seeks to apply these principles to account for some well known facts regarding clitic placement and clitic climbing in certain Romance languages, focusing on the role played in the explanation of these phenomena by the organization of features on functional categories in a numeration.

1. Head movement accounts of clitic placement

In much generative syntactic work on clitic placement in Romance languages, the relative orders of the verb and an object clitic are analyzed as results of the interaction of verb and clitic movement, essentially following Kayne (1989a, 1991a), assuming association of the clitic with a particular functional category. In European Portuguese (extendible to Galician), Madeira (1993) and Manzini (1994) assume that the clitic must move to C^o, and subsequent left-adjunction of the verb to C yields enclisis, [V-cl]; when movement of the clitic to C is blocked by a complementizer or [+wh] feature in C, or by an intervening Neg or Focus element, the clitic must left-adjoin to the verbal complex, yielding proclisis, [cl-V]. Martins (1994) assumes that the clitic is oriented towards the highest Infl-head, Agr_S, while the verb moves to Laka's (1990) Σ node above Agr_S in [V-cl] cases; when V-to-Σ is precluded, V moves to Agr_S, and subsequent left-adjunction of the clitic to Agr_S yields [cl-V]. Uriagereka (1995a, 1995b) assumes that the clitic moves to a supra-Infl head F (posited with the semantic function of expressing a notion of point of view), with verb movement yielding different orders of verb and clitic, depending on the nature of the clause. The facts of clitic placement in these languages thus fall out on various accounts from facts of verb movement together with the C/F-orientation or $Agr_{(S)}$-orientation of the clitic.

In nonimperative forms in (most varieties of) Italian and Spanish, the orders [V-cl] and [cl-V] within a clause do not depend on the presence of a complementizer or [+wh] feature or Negation or Focus, or other factors which could be attributed to the contents of C or Σ or which would influence clitic or verb movement to C or Σ, but only on finiteness, hence the contents of Infl.[1] The facts of proclisis in finite clauses are illustrated by the Italian data in (1) and (2) below.[2]

(1) a. *Gianni la incontrò.*
Gianni her met
b. *Sarebbe assurdo che tu gli parlassi.*
it-would-be absurd that you him.DAT spoke

(2) *l'ha sempre fatto.*
it-has-3.SG always done
'He has always done it.'

Enclisis is exhibited in nonfinite forms, including infinitivals and gerunds, as illustrated in (3)–(6) below.[3]

(3) a. *Parlargli sarebbe un errore.*
to-speak- him.DAT would-be an error
b. *Gianni tentò di incontrarla.*
Gianni tried meet-her

(4) *Gianni sostiene di averlo letto.*
Gianni claims have-it read

(5) *dicendoglielo.*
saying-him.DAT-it.ACC

(6) *dopo averti detto ...*
after having-you told

On most accounts, proclisis in finite clauses in these languages results from the convergence of the verb and clitic on an Infl head. Enclisis in nonfinite clauses in these languages has been given more varied treatments. Kayne (1991a) resorted to adjunction of V to T′ in infinitivals in these languages to protect PRO from government by the complementizer *se* ('if'); the clitic, in T°, is consequently an enclitic on the verb. This recourse is obviated by Martin's (1996) analysis of infinitives in these languages and the licensing conditions on PRO. Rooryck (1992) relies on excorporation of V from the complex $[_T$ [cl-V]-T] formed by movement of the verb to T; excorporation of the verb from this complex strands the clitic, as V moves to Agr_S, resulting in an enclitic structure.

For Madeira (1993), Manzini (1994), and Belletti (1999), the relative ordering of verb and clitic in Spanish and Italian type languages depends on the exact sequencing of movement operations. Madeira assumes that clitics must move to the highest nonoperator functional head in the clause. In Italian and Spanish, Madeira assumes that C is an operator head, and the highest nonoperator head is the highest Infl head, which Madeira takes to be Agr (adopting the phrase structure of Belletti 1990, in which Agr takes TP as its complement).[4] In finite clauses, the verb moves to Agr for its own morphological reasons, and the clitic subsequently left-adjoins to [V-Agr] due to its morphological requirements as a clitic, yielding proclisis. This derivation is outlined in (7a,b) below, which shows successive representations derived by the movement steps described above.[5]

(7) a.

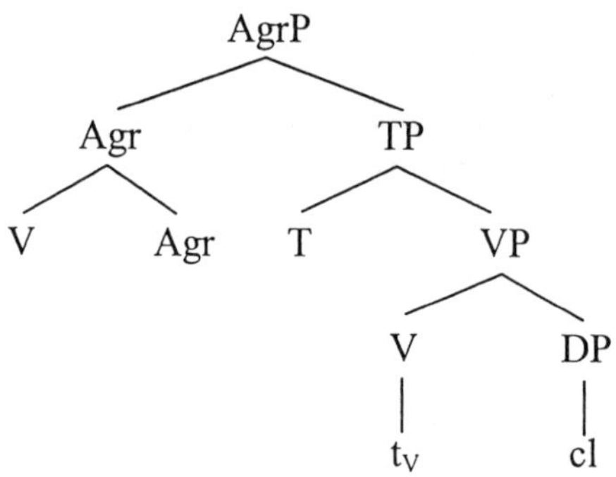

b.

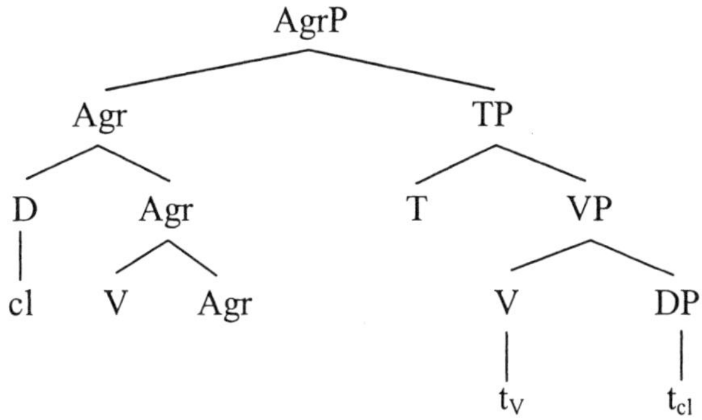

In nonfinite forms, the verb does not have a morphological relationship with Agr, and consequently the clitic moves and left-adjoins to an empty Agr; the verb subsequently left-adjoins to [cl-Agr] in order to satisfy morphological requirements of the clitic, yielding enclisis; the relevant representations are given in (8a,b).

(8) a.

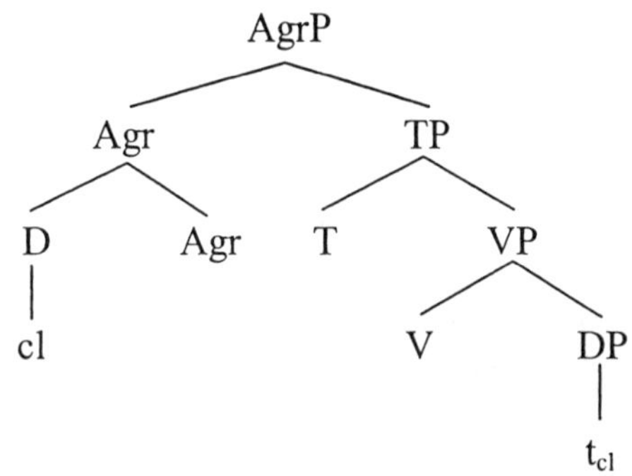

b.

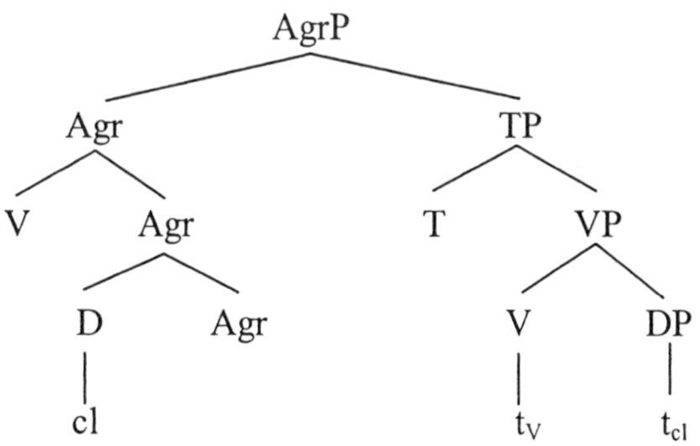

Manzini adopts the outlines of Madeira's account, but reduces the Infl-orientation of object clitics in Modern Italian and Spanish to the supposition that "clitics overtly behave like agreement elements [p.312]" in these languages (as opposed to European Portuguese), and Manzini casts the motivation for movement in explicitly Minimalist terms as feature-checking.

These accounts seem right in assuming an Infl-orientation of the object clitic, but they posit non-uniform motivations for clitic movement. According to Madeira, the clitic adjoins to [V-Agr] in finite clauses on account of its phonologically dependent nature, which requires it to be adjacent to a host for cliticization at the PF interface, whereas in nonfinite clauses, the clitic moves to Agr on account of its independent attraction to the highest non-operator functional head. Furthermore, the attraction to Agr (when that is what drives clitic movement), understood as a subject agreement category, is not motivated by an identifiable instance of feature checking and particularly, not one which stems from the status of the clitic as an object clitic.

Summarizing and simplifying slightly, the Madeira/Manzini approach to clitic placement in Italian proposes that in finite clauses, V moves to Agr to check Infl-features; then the clitic left adjoins to [V-Agr] for morphological reasons (or to check a clitic feature against Agr), yielding proclisis. In nonfinite clauses, the clitic moves to Agr first (to check the clitic feature), and the verb subsequently left-adjoins to [cl-Agr] to satisfy morphological requirements of the clitic, yielding enclisis. The main problem with this approach is that V moves to the highest Infl head anyway in Italian infinitives (as shown by Belletti 1990 and Zanuttini 1991), so it is unclear what determines that in finite clauses, V moves first, and then the clitic, while in nonfinite clauses, the clitic moves first, and then V.

Belletti (1999) proposes that the object clitic moves to check a case feature against Agr_O. In finite clauses, with the clitic in Agr_O, the verb moves to T, skipping Agr_O; the clitic then left-adjoins to the [V-T] complex, producing proclisis. This derivation is illustrated in (9) below.

(9) a.

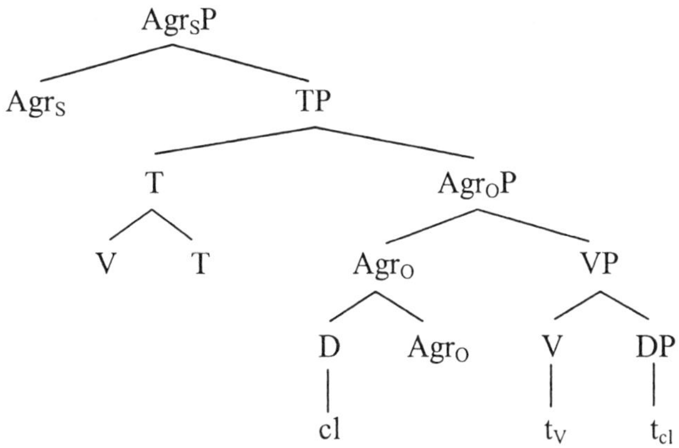

b.

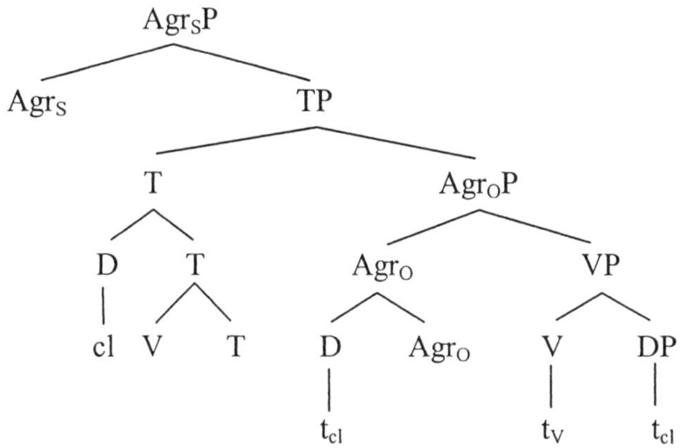

By not moving the verb through Agr_O, this account removes the verb from a role in case feature checking for the clitic in Agr_O (and likewise, for a full NP or DP direct object in spec-Agr_OP). Belletti claims that it is crucial that the verb not move through Agr_O, picking up the clitic, since the presence of the clitic in the verbal complex would prevent further checking of verbal morphology features on V as V moves to higher functional heads. But it's not clear why this should be so: passing through a lower head X and checking features on X does not ordinarily prevent the verb from subsequently moving to a higher functional head Y and checking further morphological features against Y.

In nonfinite clauses, Belletti assumes that the object clitic moves to Agr_O, thus maintaining a uniform motivation for clitic movement. The verb checks verbal morphology against a head Inf below Agr_O (as proposed by

Kayne 1991a); the verb then moves to Agr_O, T, and Agr_S, in succession, but does not check further verbal morphology features after Inf. In this derivation, the verb can move through Agr_O, picking up the clitic by left-adjunction, since the clitic will not interfere with checking of any verbal morphology features above Agr_O. The derivation is illustrated in (10).

(10) a.

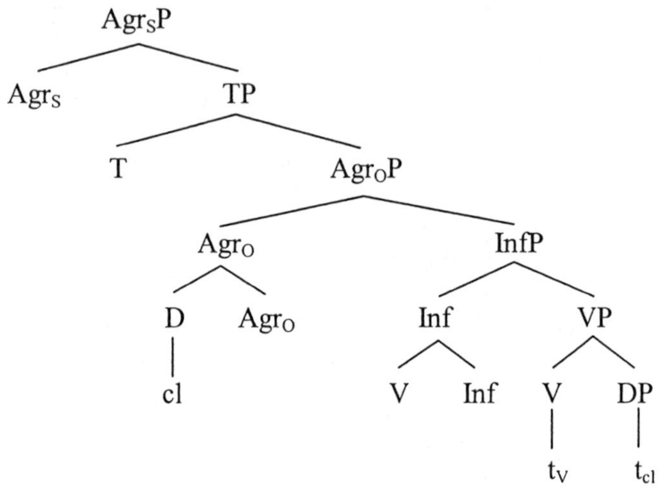

b.

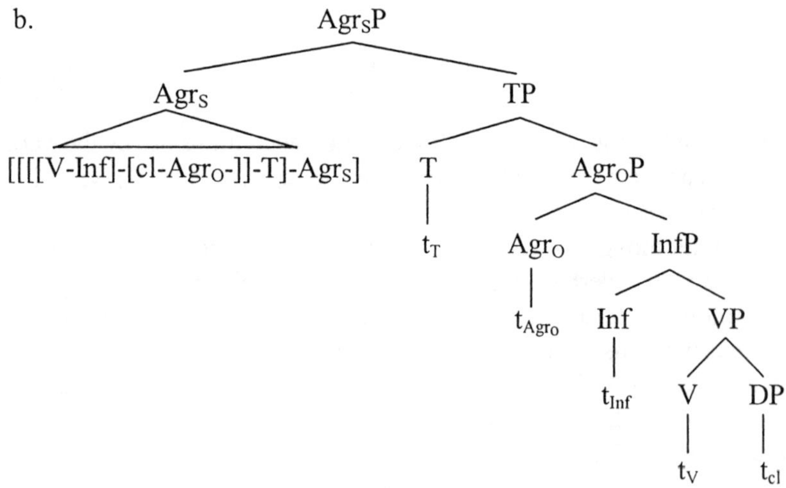

But in this derivation, it is unclear why the verb should move out of Inf if it has no further features to check. While the sequences of verb and clitic movement proposed by Belletti do not seem to be as well motivated as those proposed by Madeira and Manzini, the Agr_O-orientation of the object clitic, and the uniform movement of the object clitic to Agr_O, are desirable qualities of this analysis which will be adopted here.

The present chapter provides an implementation of an analysis of the sort given for Spanish/Italian type languages by Madeira and Manzini, but with more detail regarding the organization of the relevant features on functional categories within the numeration, how these features are entered into the numeration, and how they are distributed onto functional heads. The Infl-orientation of object clitics in the overt syntax in these languages is due to the fact that N-features matching those on the clitic are projected onto an Infl-category. Assuming the derivation of functional categories proposed in Chapter 2, the category in question does not have an absolute categorial label, and depends on the suite of V-features for the local clause available in the numeration, constrained by an Economy principle that limits functional categories within the Infl-system to ones which support V-features. The sequencing of movements required by Madeira and Manzini then falls out from the ordering of features in a numeration. On this implementation, the features relevant to clitic placement are morphological (agreement) features, following Manzini (1994), but ones associated with the object, yielding the equivalent of an Agr_O-orientation of the object clitic, along the lines assumed by Belletti. Furthermore, the account adheres throughout to the strict left-adjunction of verbs and clitics upon movement, following Madeira, Manzini, Kayne (1991a, 1994), and Belletti (1999). On the basic approach, Modern French falls into line as a language with Infl-oriented clitics, but with differences from Italian and Spanish in the distribution of V-features onto functional heads in infinitival clauses, as revealed by its different pattern of verb movement in infinitivals.

Such an implementation of clitic placement, developing proposals along the lines of those of Giorgi and Pianesi (1996) and Chapter 2 above for the projection of features in a numeration onto functional categories, yields an account of clitic climbing in Modern Italian varieties and Modern Spanish that follows from the constraints on the projection of Infl-related features onto functional categories. A variety of recent accounts of clitic placement and clitic climbing are cast nominally or explicitly in Minimalist terms. On some of these accounts, clitic climbing would violate basic principles of syntactic movement, including the "shallowness" provision of Attract-F, by which matching features projected onto a functional category attract the nearest matching features on lexical items already merged into phrase structure. Furthermore, these accounts do not handle the optionality of clitic climbing in consistent Minimalist terms. The problem that the optionality of clitic climbing presents to Minimalist syntax is acknowledged and addressed in Rooryck (1994); however, Rooryck's exact solution, based on excorporation of the clitic out of a verbal complex within the infinitival clause under government by the matrix [V-T-Agr_S], is not available under a formulation of the grammar which motivates movement by feature checking requirements. Another possible type of account assumes that N-features of the clitic are not checked off upon matching, opening up the possibility that the clitic is attracted successively to N-features on a local Infl-head, and then by N-features on an Infl-head in a higher clause. Consideration of this possibility raises the issue, considered in Chapter 2, of how functional categories come to be within a numeration and why they have the features they do. The principle of Economy of Feature Projection from Chapter 2 restricts features projected onto functional categories in a numeration to be limited to a minimal suite required for matching features present on lexical categories in the numeration. This principle rules out an analysis of clitic climbing relying on the duplication of N-features matching those of the clitic on local and higher Infl-heads. Instead, it is proposed that clitic climbing results from the status of object N-features within restructuring infinitives, which, due to a lack of associated V-features within the infinitive, must be associated with V-features of the higher verb. This produces a transference of clitic-attracting features in restructuring contexts, in a way that is reminiscent of LaPolla's (1988) proposal.

The intent is to provide a feature-based formulation of clitic placement appealing to general principles regarding the distribution of features in a numeration and their projection onto functional heads. Certain issues cannot be resolved within the scope of this investigation, and require detailed empirical study in their own right, in terms of the present, or other, mechanisms. Among these are complex issues concerning the placement of subject clitics in Northern Italian dialects, a matter which seems to involve more than simply head movement; see Rizzi (1986), Brandi and Cordin (1989), Poletto (1993), Poletto (1996), and Poletto (1999). Furthermore, there is a wealth of variation across dialects which will not be addressed here; see Zanuttini (1997), Manzini and Savoia (2004), and the works concerned with subject clitics just cited.

2. Verb and clitic movement

2.1. Mechanics of clitic placement in Italian and Spanish

An account of clitic placement in terms of verb and clitic movement to functional categories depends on the exact architecture of functional projections within the clause. The present account will adopt the merge-order of heads given in (11a) below (with V merged first, then Asp, etc.) for finite nonparticipial (simple tense) clauses, and the merge-order of heads given in (11b) for finite participial (complex tense) clauses.[6]

(11) a. $Agr_S < T < Agr_O < Asp(ect) < V$
b. $Agr_S < T < Agr_O < Aux < Agr_{prt} < Asp < V_{prt}$

In accordance with the construction of functional categories outlined in Chapter 2, these node labels are not primitives of the syntactic system, but merely convenient labels for matrices of features, where a familiar node label X (such as T or Agr_O) is used for ^M when the feature matrix M contains exactly or approximately the features that would standardly be associated with X. These node labels will be used initially below in setting forth the overall structure of the clause, but they will have to give way to the underlying features for the discussion of clitic placement.

In the derivation of a participial structure from the categories in (11b), the participle V_{prt} moves to Aspect, and Aux raises through successive head movement of Aux to Agr_O, Agr_O to T, and T to Agr_S. A crucial property of these structures is that Agr_O is clustered together with T and Agr_S, above the site at which an auxiliary verb is entered into phrase structure in a participial clause. This is crucial since both V and Aux are entered into phrase structure below Agr_O in (11a,b), from which the parallel behavior of V and Aux in clitic placement will follow on the hypothesis that object clitics are Agr_O-oriented. If Agr_O were placed directly above the main VP in (11b), below the auxiliary verb, then the auxiliary could not raise through Agr_O, and therefore, on an account of clitic placement that depends on verb movement through Agr_O (which is essentially what happens in the account given below for finite clauses), the auxiliary would diverge in behavior from a main verb, contrary to fact.

This property of the order in (11b), though appropriate for clitic placement, raises questions about the checking of an accusative case feature against an ordinary object DP: since Aux, not the main verb, is in a position to raise to Agr_O in (11b), it follows that accusative case cannot be checked at Agr_O in the presence of the main verb. This, in turn, casts doubt on the joint role of Agr_O and the participle in accusative case checking. The present account will disassociate accusative case from Agr_O, and will assume instead that accusative case is checked off against a "light verb" *v* (Chomsky 1995b), or a Voice node (Kratzer 1994), projected directly above the main VP; this structure will not be depicted or discussed further here.

Features in a numeration are ranked according to their checking order. The merge-orders of functional heads in (11a,b) indicate that the subject N-features and V-features, Tense V-features, and object N-features and V-features are ordered as shown in (12) below, where the strong features among those in (12) are ordered as indicated in the overt syntax, and the weak features among those in (12) are ordered in the covert syntax, after Spell-Out, in the mapping to LF.

(12) $[F_{V\text{-s}}, F_{N\text{-s}}] < F_{V\text{-T}} < [F_{V\text{-o}}, F_{N\text{-o}}]$

This ordering of features will be refined below.

Overt clitic movement will be driven, under Chomsky's (1995b) Attract-F conception of movement, by attraction of strong features of the clitic to a functional category. This requires that the clitic be generated in a low position in clausal phrase structure. Following Uriagereka (1995b) and Belletti (1999), it will be assumed that the object clitic is generated as head of a complex DP, which itself appears in the thematic object position.[7] The nature of clitic movement will be derived from the view from Chomsky (1995a) that clitics are both minimal and maximal projections, minimal because they are selected from the lexicon as bare heads, and maximal, on the relational conception of this notion as the highest projection of a category, since clitics do not project to any higher category. As a result, clitic movement proceeds as proposed by Sportiche (1990), specifically, the initial steps of clitic movement are XP-movement, thus not subject to the constraints of head movement, and the last step is X^o-movement, involving adjunction to another head. Finally, all instances of head movement will be assumed to be by left-adjunction, in accord with Kayne's (1994) theory of adjunction structures.

Consider first the proclitic order [cl-V] in finite clauses, illustrated by (1a), repeated below in (13).

(13) *Gianni la incontrò.*
Gianni her met

Following Madeira (1993) and Manzini (1994), these will be produced by a proper sequencing of verb and clitic movement to Infl-heads. Adopting the formulation of movement as Attract-F, the sequence of movements is determined by the organization of features on functional heads attracting matching features on the verb and clitic. The relevant feature matrices are given in (14) below, where for clarity, subject N-features and V-features have been suppressed, and 'V' and 'cl' denote the feature matrices for the verb and clitic.

(14)
$$\begin{array}{llll} & & \mathrm{V} & \mathrm{cl} \\ F_{\mathrm{V\text{-}T}} & \mathbf{F_{V\text{-}o}} & F_{\mathrm{V\text{-}o}} & F_{\mathrm{N\text{-}o}} \\ & \mathbf{F_{N\text{-}o}} & F_{\mathrm{V\text{-}T}} & \end{array}$$

The finite verb is attracted by features on Infl-heads,[8] and the clitic, in the languages under consideration here, is attracted by the N-features $F_{N\text{-}o}$. Since all movements are by left-adjunction, if the clitic moves to ^[$F_{V\text{-}o}$, $F_{N\text{-}o}$] first, and the verb subsequently moves to this head, an enclitic ordering will be derived. In contrast, if the verb moves to ^[$F_{V\text{-}o}$, $F_{N\text{-}o}$] first, and then the clitic, proclisis will be derived. Movement is precipitated by features on the target, ^[$F_{V\text{-}o}$, $F_{N\text{-}o}$], attracting corresponding features on the moved item, clitic or verb. The order of movement operations is determined by the ranking of the corresponding features on ^[$F_{V\text{-}o}$, $F_{N\text{-}o}$]. The proclisis facts indicate that the V-features on ^[$F_{V\text{-}o}$, $F_{N\text{-}o}$] that must be checked off by the verb are ranked above the N-features that must be checked off by the clitic; thus $F_{V\text{-}o}$ are operative first, attracting the verb to ^[$F_{V\text{-}o}$, $F_{N\text{-}o}$], at which point $F_{N\text{-}o}$ are operative, attracting the clitic. The required organization of features in the matrix [$F_{V\text{-}o}$, $F_{N\text{-}o}$] is recorded in (15) below, indicating that $F_{V\text{-}o}$ are superior to $F_{N\text{-}o}$ and must be checked off first (if they are of the same strength).[9]

(15) $F_{N\text{-}o} < F_{V\text{-}o}$

This will be taken to be indicative of a general pattern: when object N-features and V-features are both strong on a functional category F, the V-features are ranked higher and must be checked before the N-features; likewise for subject N-features and V-features.

Now consider enclisis, as in (3), repeated below as (16).

(16) a. *Parlargli* *sarebbe* *un* *errore.*
to-speak-him.DAT would-be an error
b. *Gianni* *tentò* *di* *incontrarla.*
Gianni tried meet-her

On the approach adopted here, derived from Madeira and Manzini, enclisis results from movement of the clitic to a functional category X, followed by movement and left-adjunction of the verb to [cl-X]. The movements required for enclisis would not be produced by the feature ordering given in (15) since then ^[$F_{V\text{-}o}$, $F_{N\text{-}o}$] would attract the verb to check off $F_{V\text{-}o}$ before it would attract the clitic. However, the lack of subject agreement in nonfinite forms is an overt indication that there are no V-features $F_{V\text{-}s}$ and $F_{V\text{-}o}$ in nonfinite forms. The question that then arises is whether the feature matrices $F_{N\text{-}s}$ and $F_{N\text{-}o}$ are projected as functional heads in these circumstances. Focusing on the object, the question is whether the grammar will project a functional head ^[$F_{N\text{-}o}$] in order to support $F_{N\text{-}o}$, matching the N-features on the object (clitic or NP) in a nonfinite clause, when there are no corresponding V-features, $F_{V\text{-}o}$. If so, then the sequence of steps required by the Madeira and Manzini approach would be straightforwardly obtained. Considering an infinitival clause for discussion, at the appropriate point in the derivation, ^[$F_{N\text{-}o}$] would be merged into the syntactic structure, carrying N-features, $F_{N\text{-}o}$, which would attract those of the clitic; the clitic would then move to ^[$F_{N\text{-}o}$], producing [cl-^[$F_{N\text{-}o}$]], as in (17).

(17) a. $[_{\text{^}[F_{N\text{-}o}]P}$ [cl-^[$F_{N\text{-}o}$]] $[_{VP}$ PRO V t_{cl}]]
b. $[_{\text{^}[F_{N\text{-}o}]P}$ [cl-^[$F_{N\text{-}o}$]] $[_{VP}$ Aux $[_{AspP}$ [V_{prt} -Asp]
$[_{VP}$ PRO $[_V\ t_v]$ t_{cl}]]]]

A functional head ^[$F_{V\text{-}T}$], with V-features for infinitival tense, would be subsequently merged into phrase structure, attracting the highest verb. If verb raising proceeds through left-adjunction to the intervening head complex [cl-^[$F_{N\text{-}o}$]], then the complex [V-[cl-^[$F_{N\text{-}o}$]]] will be produced, which would then move to ^[$F_{V\text{-}T}$]. The derivation for the participial case would be similar, with Aux the highest verb, producing [Aux-[cl-^[$F_{N\text{-}o}$]]]. In either case, the rest of the derivation of the nonfinite clause, involving the merging of ^[$F_{N\text{-}s}$, EPP] and the movement of ^[$F_{V\text{-}T}$] to ^[$F_{N\text{-}s}$, EPP], would preserve enclisis.

However, economy constraints rule out this derivation. To begin with, it requires the movement of the verb through ^[$F_{N\text{-}o}$], which lacks V-features; this move is not motivated by feature-matching requirements, and if an alternate derivation is possible in which the projection of such a functional head can be dispensed with, it should be preferred by the principle that Giorgi and Pianesi state in the passage quoted in (41) of Chapter 2, on which "the actual number of projections is defined according to economy considerations, that is, the shortest derivation compatible with the initial array is selected." Furthermore, the projection of a functional head X within the Infl-system should be blocked in principle when X carries no V-features. The requirement that functional heads within the Infl-system should carry V-features blocks the projection of extraneous functional categories within the Infl-system, as a plausible implication of the Economy of Representation. The substance of this implication is the content of the Economy of Projection of Infl-Categories from Chapter 2 above, reproduced in (18) below, which trims the derivation in line with the derivational economy considerations brought up by Giorgi and Pianesi.

(18) *Economy of Projection of Infl-Categories*
If features F_1, F_2, ..., F_n are elements of a feature matrix M projected as a functional head ^M within the Infl-system of a clause, then one of F_1, F_2, ..., F_n must be a clausal feature (such as a V/A-feature matching some $F_{V/A}$ on a verb or adjective within that clause).

The projection of ^[$F_{N\text{-}o}$], without $F_{V\text{-}o}$, would violate the Economy of Representation; furthermore, if there exists a shorter derivation that would not require movement of the verb through ^[$F_{N\text{-}o}$], the derivation based on the projection of ^[$F_{N\text{-}o}$] would violate the Economy of Derivation as well, assuming that the conception of the Economy of Derivation proposed in Chapter 2, as favoring the shortest derivation relative to the features present in the numeration.

If (18) holds, the $F_{N\text{-}o}$ features cannot be projected onto a functional head on their own. How, then, are the $F_{N\text{-}o}$ features projected onto a functional category in a nonfinite clause? In order to answer this question, compare the situation in an infinitival clause with that in a finite clause, considered above. In a finite clause, by the Economy of Projection of Infl-Categories, the $F_{N\text{-}o}$ are dependent on $F_{V\text{-}o}$ for their projection onto a functional head; the resulting feature matrices are those given in (14) above, subject to the additional ordering constraint in (15). In an infinitival, the associated $F_{V\text{-}o}$ are not present, and the $F_{N\text{-}o}$ are consequently floating features, which cannot be projected by themselves onto a functional category on account of the Economy of Projection of Infl-Categories. In these circumstances, the $F_{N\text{-}o}$ can be bundled with their neighboring V-features, $F_{V\text{-}T}$, with the resulting feature matrix projected as a functional head. This yields the set of feature matrices given in (19), in which, crucially, the $F_{N\text{-}o}$ retain their order above $F_{V\text{-}T}$ in the numeration; the complete numeration for the sentence in (16b) is given in (20), where the top line gives the lexical items and the traditional functional category labels in their merge order, and where features of the higher clause are suppressed. (In an infinitive, there are no $F_{V\text{-}s}$ or $F_{N\text{-}s}$ features projected. But the Extended Projection Principle feature, EPP, is projected as a head ^[EPP]. This is identified as "Agr$_S$" for the infinitival clause in (20).)[10]

(19)		V	cl
	$F_{V\text{-}T}$	$F_{V\text{-}T}$	$F_{N\text{-}o}$
	$\mathbf{F_{N\text{-}o}}$		

(20)	"*Gianni tentò* [*di*	Agr$_S$	T	PRO	*incontrar*	***la***]"
		EPP	$F_{V\text{-}T}$		$F_{V\text{-}T}$	$F_{N\text{-}o}$
			$\mathbf{F_{N\text{-}o}}$			

Since $F_{V\text{-}T} < F_{N\text{-}o}$, the clitic is the first element attracted to the infinitival ^[$F_{V\text{-}T}$, $F_{N\text{-}o}$], checking $F_{N\text{-}o}$; then the infinitival verb is attracted to ^[$F_{V\text{-}T}$, ~~$F_{N\text{-}o}$~~], checking $F_{V\text{-}T}$ and producing enclisis. This yields a second account of enclisis in Italian and Spanish infinitival clauses within the broad assumptions of the present work.

This second account of enclisis in Italian and Spanish, on which ^[$F_{N\text{-}o}$] is not projected as an independent functional head in an infinitival clause, is to be preferred since it imposes tighter constraints on feature-driven movement and on the projection of functional categories. This account applies to clitic placement in gerunds, as in (5)–(6), as well as infinitival clauses. Gerunds also lack $F_{N\text{-}s/o}$, and assuming that the gerund has V-features $F_{V\text{-}T}$ that are analogous to infinitival tense features, but appropriate to the gerund, the results in (5)–(6) are obtained exactly as in infinitival clauses.[11]

In Standard Italian and other varieties in which a single negation marker serves as clausal negation, the negation element appears above the projection site of $F_{V\text{-}T}$ (above TP, in more standard terms; see Belletti 1990 who proposes that Neg takes TP as its complement, and Zanuttini 1997, who proposes that this negation element is projected above all tense and agreement heads), unlike in French and English, where negation (the position of which is marked by *pas* in French) is below the projection site of $F_{V\text{-}T}$. As a result of the high position of this negation element in clausal phrase structure in Italian, Neg does not interfere with the bundling of N-features matching those on the clitic with the $F_{V\text{-}T}$ features attracting the verb. As a result, enclisis is obtained in Italian infinitives with negation, such as (21) below, exactly as in ones without it, discussed above.

(21) *Sapevo cosa non dirgli.*
knew-1.SG what NEG say-him.DAT
'I knew what not to say to him.'

The interactions between multiple negation elements and clitic placement in various dialects of Italian are too complex to be addressed here; see Zanuttini (1997) for an extensive investigation of these interactions.

On the present analysis, structures of enclisis as well as structures of proclisis in languages with Infl-oriented clitics have the verb and clitic together in a complex head; on this point it falls into line with Madeira (1993), Manzini (1994), and Belletti (1999), contrary to Kayne (1991a) and Rooryck (1992). Madeira (1993) offers explicit arguments against splitting up the verb and clitic in enclisis, in general, and also with special attention to the structures of enclisis in Modern European Portuguese. To Madeira's arguments may be added one specific to Modern Italian with Infl-oriented object clitics, based on the movement of verb and enclitic together in Aux-to-Comp structures in gerunds, such as the following (from Roberts 1994a).

(22) a. *Avendolo Gianni fatto, ...*
having-it Gianni done, ...
b. * *Avendo Gianni lo fatto, ...*

If structures of enclisis are produced by left-adjunction of the gerundive auxiliary to [cl-^[$F_{V\text{-}T}$, $F_{N\text{-}o}$]], as proposed here, producing [Aux-[cl-^[$F_{V\text{-}T}$, $F_{N\text{-}o}$]]], then further movement of this verbal complex to C^o in Aux-to-Comp (however the motivation for this last movement step is analyzed) will keep the Aux and clitic together with enclitic order, yielding exactly the results in (22).

2.2. Clitic placement in French

In Modern French, proclisis obtains in finite and infinitival clauses, as illustrated in (23)–(24).[12]

(23) a. *Marie le connait.*
Marie him knows
b. *Marie nous a parlé.*
Marie us.DAT has spoken

(24) a. *Lui parler serait une erreur.*
him.DAT to-speak would-be an error
b. *l'avoir donné serait une erreur.*
it-have given would-be an error

Proclisis in finite clauses follows directly as in Italian, assuming that $F_{N\text{-}o} < F_{V\text{-}o}$ in the context of the numeration given in (14) (subject features suppressed for clarity). Then the finite verb V_{fin} moves first to ^[$F_{V\text{-}o}$, $F_{N\text{-}o}$], checking $F_{V\text{-}o}$, followed by left-adjunction of the clitic to [V_{fin}-^[$F_{V\text{-}o}$, $F_{N\text{-}o}$]].

In French infinitival clauses, other processes need to be taken into account before clitic placement is addressed. The infinitive verb can optionally appear before a clause-medial adverb in French, as in (25a,b). (Examples (25)–(27) are from Pollock 1989.)

(25) a. *A peine parler l'italien après cinq ans d'étude…*
hardly to-speak Italian after five years of-study…
b. *Parler à peine l'italien après cinq ans d'étude…*

An infinitive main verb, however, remains below the position of negation, as shown by (26), while an auxiliary can optionally move to a position higher in the clause, above Neg, as shown in (27).

(26) a. *Ne pas posséder de voiture en banlieue rend*
NEG not own of-a car in suburbs makes
la vie difficile.
the life difficult
b. * *Ne posséder pas de voiture en banlieue rend la vie difficile.*

(27) a. *Ne pas avoir eu d'enfance herueuse est une*
NEG not have had childhood happy is a
condition pour écrire de romans.
prerequisite for writing novels
b. *N'avoir pas eu d'enfance herueuse est …*

An object clitic is a proclitic on the auxiliary, and when Aux undergoes movement above negation, the proclitic order is preserved, as shown in (28) (from Sportiche 1996: 218).

(28) a. *ne pas l'avoir donné …*
NEG not it-have given
b. *ne l'avoir pas donné*

A standard interpretation of these facts is that the infinitive verb either remains in place, or it undergoes Pollock's (1989) optional short verb movement to a position preceding clause-medial adverbs, but following negation; an infinitive main verb stops in this position, while an auxiliary may optionally move to a position above negation. On the assumption that French has a merge order of heads along the lines of that given in (29), with clause-medial adverbials adjoined to VP, this would mean that the infinitive verb moves to an Agr head below Neg (Agr_O in (29)), and that if it is an auxiliary, it may optionally move on to T.[13]

(29) $Agr_S < T < Neg < Agr_O < V$

Turning to a feature-based account, the absence of verbal agreement means that $F_{V\text{-}o}$ features are missing, and therefore that $F_{N\text{-}o}$ features matching those on the clitic will have to be projected with other V-features. But it is clear from (28b) that the $F_{N\text{-}o}$ features cannot project with the infinitival tense features on a head $^\wedge[F_{V\text{-}T}, F_{N\text{-}o}]$, for if they did, then, since $F_{N\text{-}o}$ has a higher checking order than $F_{V\text{-}T}$, the head $^\wedge[F_{V\text{-}T}, F_{N\text{-}o}]$ would attract the clitic first, then the infinitival auxiliary, producing enclisis. Instead, there seems to be something about the structure of the French infinitive below negation which is different from Italian. We'll begin with the least well understood part of the standard account of French infinitives, the optional short verb movement of the infinitive verb, V_{inf}. The evidence for this is the optional [V_{inf} AdvP] order, alongside [AdvP V_{inf}] in (25a,b). But these options would be produced as a special case of a much more general process if an Asp(ect) node is merged just above the projection of the highest verb (main or auxiliary) in both finite and infinitival clauses, and if the highest verb invariably undergoes movement to Asp, provided the clause-medial adverbial can be adjoined equally well to the highest VP, or to AspP. The resulting possible structures are shown in (30), given on the next page. The movement of the verb to Asp on this account is formulated as a basic and obligatory operation in both finite and nonfinite clauses, rather than as an optional and unmotivated movement which only takes place in infinitives, and it is essential to see why circumstances conspire to give it the appearance of an optional and ad hoc operation. To begin with, in finite clauses, the effect of movement to Asp is masked by subsequent movement of the finite verb to higher heads. The movement of the finite verb to Asp is therefore posited here with no theoretical cost: if there is an Asp head projected, the finite verb will move through it as it does through all inflectional heads in a finite clause. Only in an infinitival clause is the surface position of an infinitive verb low enough to (sometimes) reveal the effects of movement. Furthermore, the multiple adjunction sites of the adverbial assumed by this account are also not much of an ad hoc assumption if we accept the results of Travis (1988) and others that adverbials do not have rigidly specified positions in clause structure, but rather loci within clause structure determined by their interpretive effects which specify a range of (generally contiguous) syntactic adjunction sites. The adverbials participating in the alternation in (25a,b) include ones such as *à peine* 'hardly', *complètement* 'completely', *presque* 'almost', and *souvent* 'often', which can be identified as qualifying the extent, degree of completion, or repetition of the event. As such, they are appropriate for adjunction to sites low in the clause at which the event and its aspect are introduced. These are just the sites posited for these adverbs in (30).

(30) a.

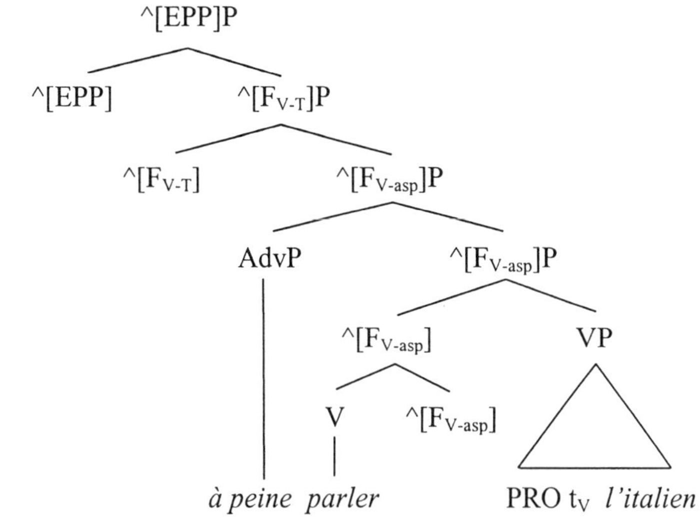

b.

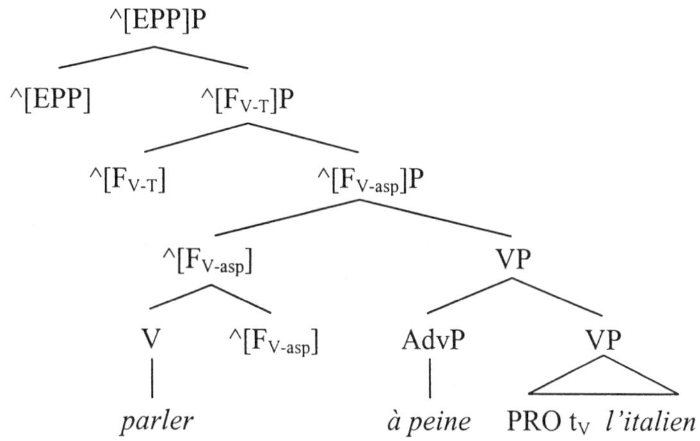

The optional short verb movement in French infinitives is thus merely the obligatory movement of the infinitive verb to Aspect observed against the backdrop of the appropriate attachment sites for a particular class of adverbials.[14] The relationship between aspect and the adverb class involved in the alternations in short verb movement in French infinitives also counts against replacing Asp with the empty verbal head *v* in the account above, since *v* is not as plausible a candidate for being the loci of these adverbs as Asp.

On the basis of these considerations, we posit the set of feature matrices shown in (31) below for a French infinitive with no auxiliaries, and (32) for a perfective form, with a main verb participle. The $F_{N\text{-}o}$ feature matrix introduced to check the $F_{N\text{-}o}$ features on the clitic is depicted here as a floating feature matrix (in bold typeface) since, by the Economy of Projection of Infl-Categories, it cannot be projected as a functional head on its own. The copy of aspectual V-features introduced to check the aspectual V-features on the verb have a high checking order, and are projected on a functional head directly above the highest VP; these are strong features which cause obligatory overt short verb movement. As before, the top line, in quotation marks, is not part of the representation, and is provided merely for expository clarity; the functional category labels on this line are merely familiar labels for projections of particular feature matrices, which in some cases merely approximate the feature matrices standardly associated with the functional category label.

(31)	“Agr_S	T	Neg		Asp	V	cl”
		$F_{V\text{-}T}$	[Neg]		$F_{V\text{-}asp}$	$F_{V\text{-}asp}$	$F_{N\text{-}o}$
	EPP			$\mathbf{F_{N\text{-}o}}$		$F_{V\text{-}T}$	

(32)	“Agr_S	T	Neg		Asp	Aux	Agr_{prt}	V_{prt}	cl”
		$F_{V\text{-}T}$	[Neg]		$F_{V\text{-}asp}$	$F_{V\text{-}asp}$	$F_{V\text{-}prt}$	$F_{V\text{-}prt}$	$F_{N\text{-}o}$
	EPP			$\mathbf{F_{N\text{-}o}}$		$F_{V\text{-}T}$			

At this point, the question is whether the floating $F_{N\text{-}o}$ feature matrix will associate with the higher ranked $F_{V\text{-}asp}$ features, to be projected on a lower functional head, or with the lower ranked tense features $F_{V\text{-}T}$, to be projected on a higher functional head. The basic requirement imposed by the Economy of Projection of Infl-Categories, that the $F_{N\text{-}o}$ matrix cannot be projected unless accompanied by V-features, does not favor either option. But other considerations resolve the issue. The $F_{N\text{-}o}$ and $F_{N\text{-}s}$ features are strong in both finite and infinitive clauses in French, the main difference between French infinitives and finite clauses being the strength of the tense feature in $F_{V\text{-}T}$, which is weak in infinitives. Given this fact, together with the possible intrusion of [NEG] between the floating $F_{N\text{-}o}$ and $F_{V\text{-}T}$, it is explicable that the floating $F_{N\text{-}o}$ feature matrix will associate with the strong, and higher ranked features $F_{V\text{-}asp}$, projecting a functional head ^[$F_{V\text{-}asp}$, $F_{N\text{-}o}$], rather than associating with the weak feature matrix $F_{V\text{-}T}$. Since $F_{N\text{-}o} < F_{V\text{-}asp}$, the infinitive verb (main verb or auxiliary) is attracted and left-adjoins to ^[$F_{V\text{-asp}}$, $F_{N\text{-o}}$] first, after which the clitic is attracted and left-adjoins to [V/Aux-^[$F_{V\text{-asp}}$, $F_{N\text{-o}}$]], producing proclisis.[15]

It is crucial on this account that the basis for the difference between proclisis in French infinitives and enclisis in Italian infinitives lies in the feature matrices driving movement rather than on how high in the clause the infinitive verb raises, since, in the case of an auxiliary which undertakes optional movement to the site of $F_{V\text{-T}}$, as in (28b), there is no obvious difference in the extent of verb movement.

On the present approach, the (optional) agreement of an object clitic with a past participle, illustrated in (33b) below (from Kayne 1989b), cannot be the result of participle movement to Agr_O since the auxiliary, not the participle, moves through the major Infl-heads Agr_O, T, and Agr_S.

(33) a. *Paul a repeint les chaises.*
Paul has repainted the chairs
b. *Paul les a repeintes.*
Paul them has repainted-PL

However, as Kayne (1989b) suggests, participle agreement might be mediated by a local Agr above the maximal projection of the participle, and, as Uriagereka (1995b) argues, distinct from Agr_O.[16] Arguments for such a phrase structure for a participial clause are given by Friedemann and Siloni (1993); Laenzlinger (1993) and Belletti (1999) also adopt this structure. If the object clitic moves through the specifier of this Agr in its XP-movement phase, then agreement with the participle will be obtained.[17]

2.3. Imperatives

There are imperatives in Romance languages which exhibit a morphological paradigm which is unique to imperatives; these are called true imperatives. In addition, there are forms which have the morphological marking of indicatives, subjunctives, infinitives or gerunds, which are nevertheless used as imperatives, and which have properties distinguishing them from the non-imperatives to which they bear morphological similarity; these are called surrogate or suppletive imperatives. See Rivero (1994), Rivero and Terzi (1995), and Zanuttini (1997). Typically, there is morphological marking for second person singular and second person plural, but in many languages (e.g. Italian, Catalan), the second person singular form is a true imperative, while the second person plural form is suppletive; in other languages (e.g. Spanish), there are true imperatives for both singular and plural, but there are in addition suppletive forms for the plural.

In certain sub-paradigms, such as Italian second person singular and plural formal or polite imperatives, which take suppletive forms consisting of present tense third person singular and third person plural subjunctives, the inflectional paradigm is full enough to support the inflectional features of a finite declarative clause; see Zanuttini (1997: 106). In these cases, agreement V-features can reasonably be expected to be present, and by the account given in section 2.1 above, we predict a proclitic ordering of an object clitic and the verb: the feature matrix $F_{N\text{-}o}$ of inflectional features matching those on the object clitic are projected with corresponding V-features, $F_{V\text{-}o}$, on a head ^[$F_{V\text{-}o}$, $F_{N\text{-}o}$], which, due to the constraint in (15), attracts the verb before it attracts the object clitic. And proclisis is, in fact, exhibited in these cases, as in (34); see Zanuttini (1997: 106).

(34) *Lo dica pure!* (Ital. suppletive imp., 3sg subjunctive)
it say indeed
'Go ahead and say it!'

But most positive imperatives, whether true imperatives or suppletive, exhibit an enclitic ordering of verb and clitic, as in (35)–(38) below. The exception is subjunctive suppletive imperatives with a complementizer, as in (39)–(40).[18]

(35) *Fallo di sicuro!* (Ital. true imperative, 2sg)
do-it of sure
'Definitely do it!'

(36) *Fate-lo di sicuro!* (Ital. suppletive imp., 2pl indicative)
do-it of sure

(37) a. *Envía lo!* (Span. true imperative, 2sg)
send it
b. *Dí-me-lo!* (Span. true imperative, 2sg)
tell-me-it

(38) a. *Den-me el libro!* (Span. suppl. imp., polite, 2pl subj.)
give-me the book
'Give me the book!'

b. * *Me den el libro.* (Span. suppletive imp., polite, 2pl subj.)

(39) *Le ordino che lo faccia subito!* (Ital. suppl. imp., 3sg subj.)
her order that it do immediately
'I order you (sg) to do it right away!'

(40) a. *Que me den el libro!* (Span. suppletive imp., 2pl subj.)
that me give the book
'Give me the book!'

b. *Ordeno que me deis el libro!* (Span. suppl. imp., subj.)
order that me give the book
'I order that you give me the book.'

In true imperatives, the verb raises to a high (supra-Infl) head, an analysis which is widely agreed upon in the literature (Laka 1990, Rivero 1994, Zanuttini 1997). Within the present framework, this requirement can be implemented by a low-ranked imperative feature, [IMP], projected above all Infl heads. Agreement in true imperatives is very limited: in languages which use a true imperative for the second person singular and a suppletive for the second person plural, there are no contrasts in subject agreement for true imperatives, and in languages which have a second person singular and plural in the true imperative, there exists a suppletive option in the plural nevertheless. With little or no alternation in the agreement paradigm, there is reason to assume that there are no agreement V-features in true imperatives. In the absence of object V-features, $F_{V\text{-}o}$, the matrix of features for the clitic, $F_{N\text{-}o}$, will be left floating, free to associate with whatever V-features are available. In the absence of tense and other Infl-features, $F_{N\text{-}o}$ will associate with [IMP], and be projected as a head ^[[IMP], $F_{N\text{-}o}$]. Since [IMP] is lower ranked than all Infl-features, the clitic will be attracted to this head before the verb, producing enclisis, as in (35).

True imperatives do not occur with preverbal negation elements (those which Zanuttini characterizes as ones which can negate a clause by themselves). But suppletive imperatives do; the next paragraph deals with their positive forms; then we turn to their negative forms.

In indicative suppletive imperatives, and subjunctive suppletive imperatives without a complementizer, Zanuttini (1997) notes that the highest verb appears before the same classes of adverbs as in true imperatives, and concludes thereby that the extent of verb movement to a supra-Infl head in these forms is the same as in true imperatives. This suggests that [IMP] is present in these forms and that it attracts the verb, as in true imperatives. Where evidence of verb movement is lacking, in subjunctive suppletive imperatives with a complementizer, the complementizer evidently checks [IMP], rendering overt verb movement unnecessary. The morphological difference between indicative and subjunctive suppletive imperatives is in the marking for tense versus subjunctive mood. Although the morphological paradigms are extremely sparse, the need to distinguish the two types of suppletive imperative is grounds for positing tense features in the indicative, and subjunctive mood features in the subjunctive. In indicative suppletive imperatives, the tense features are ranked lower than $F_{N\text{-}o}$, assuming the usual ordering in (12); thus, [IMP] < $F_{V\text{-}T}$ < $F_{N\text{-}o}$. As a result, ^[$F_{V\text{-}T}$, $F_{N\text{-}o}$] is projected in indicative suppletive imperatives, attracting first the clitic, and then the verb, and the resulting enclitic structure is preserved upon movement of [V-[cl-^[$F_{V\text{-}T}$, $F_{N\text{-}o}$]]] to ^[IMP]. In subjunctive suppletive imperatives, subjunctive mood features are present along with the object agreement features matching those of the clitic. According to Zanuttini (1997) and Cinque (1999), the functional head Mood is projected below tense and other high inflectional heads in Italian and other Romance languages at issue. Accordingly, subjunctive features $F_{V\text{-}M}$ are higher ranked than $F_{N\text{-}o}$. Assuming that the complementizer in (39) checks [IMP] (essentially following Zanuttini (1997: 144), the only V-feature matrix with which $F_{N\text{-}o}$ can associate is $F_{V\text{-}M}$. Since $F_{N\text{-}o}$ < $F_{V\text{-}M}$, the verb is attracted first to ^[$F_{V\text{-}M}$, $F_{N\text{-}o}$], then the clitic, producing the proclisis ordering. In (38), where [IMP] is not checked by the complementizer, the V-features available include [IMP], ranked lower than $F_{N\text{-}o}$, and $F_{V\text{-}M}$, ranked higher than $F_{N\text{-}o}$. In some constructions in some languages (which will be explored below), this situation leads to optionality in verb and clitic order, but in the positive subjunctive suppletive imperatives, only an enclitic ordering is possible, indicating a preference for $F_{N\text{-}o}$ to associate with [IMP] rather than $F_{V\text{-}M}$. Possible sources for this preference will be considered when other instances of its type are discussed below.[19]

Negative imperatives are a quite different story. As is well known, true imperatives do not occur with preverbal negation. We will assume that the feature [NEG], expressing this form of negation, is simply incompatible with [IMP]. This means that negated suppletive imperatives lack [IMP]; this, in fact, seems to be the right supposition since the highest verb appears within the Infl system in negated suppletive imperatives, as described by Zanuttini (1997).[20] Our account at this point will "merely" implement proposals by Zanuttini (1997: 126–149), but "merely" is in quotes since Zanuttini mainly accounts for the large scale co-occurrences in negative imperatives, but is rather vague on the issue of clitic placement with respect to the verb, which is precisely the issue which can be made more precise with the theoretical apparatus developed here. The present account is thus offered as an emendation of existing accounts, transcribing their major points straightforwardly into the notation of the framework developed here, while providing refined precision on the fine points.

Zanuttini (1997: 126–149) posits a determinative relationship between preverbal negation elements and mood in negative imperatives. Comparing suppletive forms of negative imperatives in Standard Italian and northern and central varieties with their counterparts in southern varieties, which have subjunctive particles akin to Greek *na*, Zanuttini argues that preverbal negation requires that mood be syntactically represented in the imperative clause (both indicative and subjunctive), where the mode of syntactic representation (subjunctive particle versus verbal morphology) varies with the type of suppletive imperative and the language. Accordingly, on the present implementation, mood V-features, $F_{V\text{-}M}$, are present in negative suppletive imperatives (both indicative and subjunctive), and the matrix $F_{V\text{-}M}$ is ranked higher than agreement and tense features. The relevant features in negative subjunctive suppletive imperatives is thus $F_{N\text{-}o} < F_{V\text{-}M}$. Associating the floating $F_{N\text{-}o}$ with $F_{V\text{-}M}$, and projecting them as a head ^[$F_{V\text{-}M}$, $F_{N\text{-}o}$], the higher rank of $F_{V\text{-}M}$ will produce proclisis, as in the following Spanish example, from Zanuttini (1997: 148).

(41) *No me den el libro!* (Span. suppletive imp., 2pl subjunctive)
NEG me give the book
'Don't give me the book!'

In negative indicative suppletive imperatives, the tense V-features are present as well, and the complete ordering of relevant features is $F_{V\text{-}T} < F_{N\text{-}o} < F_{V\text{-}M}$. Since $F_{V\text{-}T}$ and $F_{V\text{-}M}$ are both strong feature matrices, there are no grounds for $F_{N\text{-}o}$ to necessarily associate with one or the other of them. This creates multiple possibilities for association of the $F_{N\text{-}o}$ matrix, and it seems that some languages realize these possibilities as true optionality, while others impose a preference. Negative indicative suppletive imperatives in Standard Italian show both proclitic and enclitic orderings of the verb and clitic, as in (42a,b) (Zanuttini 1997: 149), whereas northern varieties show only the enclitic ordering in (42a).

(42) a. *Non datemi il libro!* (suppletive imperative, indicative)
NEG give-me the book
'Don't give me the book!'
b. *Non mi date il libro!*
NEG me give the book

On the present account, this reflects free association of $F_{N\text{-}o}$ in Standard Italian with either of the linearly adjacent feature matrices in the ordering $F_{V\text{-}T} < F_{N\text{-}o} < F_{V\text{-}M}$, while in northern varieties, $F_{N\text{-}o}$ is more strongly oriented to its local tense features. (Note that, among negative suppletive imperatives, the enclisis order in (42a) is obtained only in the indicative, for only in indicative suppletives are there V-features ranked lower than $F_{N\text{-}o}$, along with the higher ranked mood features.) As in Zanuttini's (1997: 184, footnote 68) account, the present account can relate the preference for enclisis in (42a) to the preference for local association of the clitic over clitic climbing in northern varieties. But Zanuttini accomplishes this by supposing (in an admittedly speculative suggestion) that negation licenses a phonologically empty auxiliary in negative indicative suppletive imperatives, and that the clitic raises to this empty Aux, producing the proclitic ordering with the phonologically overt main verb. On the present account, invoking the account of clitic climbing developed in section 4 below, nothing special is needed to tie the preference of northern varieties for (42b) with a preference for local placement of the object clitic over clitic climbing: both reflect a preference to associate the floating $F_{N\text{-}o}$ feature matrix with local tense features over other available alternatives.

We have met two cases where there are both higher and lower ranked V-features than $F_{N\text{-}o}$ and where the language in question exhibits a preference for one over the other: Spanish subjunctive suppletive imperatives without a complementizer, and negative suppletive imperatives in northern Italian varieties. In both cases, the preference is for associating $F_{N\text{-}o}$ with V-features with immediately lower rank, projected on the next higher functional head within the clause, resulting in enclisis. Whether or not this is a general tendency cannot be inferred from just two cases. However, the cases of optionality, such as (42) for central and southern Italian varieties, emerge as the simpler type of case since the optionality reflects a lack of any preference for direction of association of the floating $F_{N\text{-}o}$ feature matrix.

2.4. The orders of multiple object clitics in Modern Greek

When both direct and indirect objects are expressed as pronominal clitics in a clause, it does not always seem possible to give a purely syntactic explanation of the relative order of the multiple clitics, since phonological factors at the PF interface seem to be a factor in the spell-out of multiple clitics and their relative ordering in many cases; see Bonet (1991) for extensive discussion of such effects. But a language in which the spell-out and ordering of pronominal clitics does not seem to be primarily morphophonological should present an opportunity to find independent evidence of the mechanisms of pronominal clitic placement proposed here. In such a language, in a clause with a ditransitive verb in which both the direct and indirect objects are expressed by pronominal clitics, we would expect $F_{N\text{-}DO}$ and $F_{N\text{-}IO}$ matrices of features matching features on the object clitics to have corresponding V-features with which they are projected, resulting in functional heads ^[$F_{V\text{-}DO}$, $F_{N\text{-}DO}$] and ^[$F_{V\text{-}IO}$, $F_{N\text{-}IO}$]. The ordering of these two heads with respect to one another would depend on the relative order of the V-features. The N-features are lower ranked than the corresponding V-features, so in finite clauses, in which all these features are present, we expect the finite verb to raise through the lower of these two heads, attract the corresponding clitic cl_1, and then we expect the lower head, with [cl_1-V], to raise to the higher head, subsequently attracting the other clitic, cl_2, producing a complex [cl_2-cl_1-V] with a determinate order of object proclitics, which is preserved as the verb moves to higher heads. For example, if $F_{V\text{-}IO} < F_{V\text{-}DO}$, then the derivation proceeds through the steps shown in (43a,b), where (43a) results from the merging of direct object features, and subsequent verb and direct object clitic movement, and (43b) results from the merging of indirect object features, and subsequent movement of the lower functional head, with [cl_{DO}-V], to the higher functional head, capped by movement of the indirect object clitic. All left-adjunctions are executed in accord with the cycle on head movement, that is, as adjunction to all previously derived material in the target head; the previously derived material retains its structure.

(43) a.

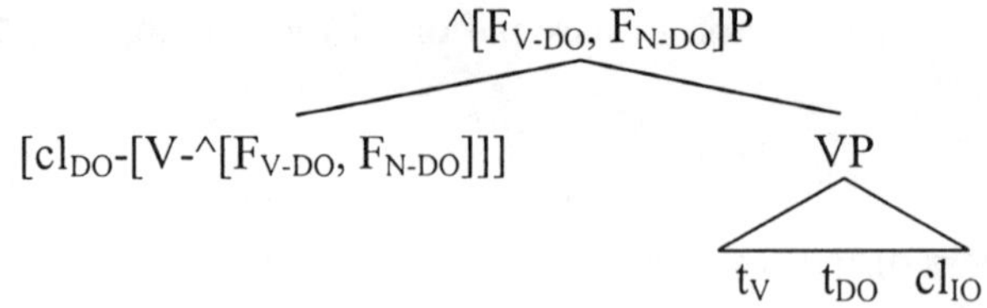

b.

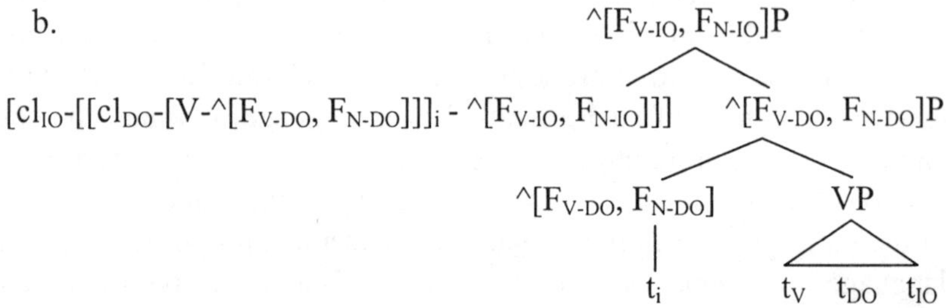

But this raises a question: Are the N-feature matrices $F_{N\text{-}DO}$ and $F_{N\text{-}IO}$ ordered with respect to one another in the partial linear ordering of features in the numeration? Note that they wouldn't have to be in the finite clause case just described since the N-features associate with the corresponding V-features, and the V-features are ordered with respect to one another. If we assume that the partial linear ordering on features in a numeration is a minimal specification of ordering relationships required to drive the derivation, then the N-features will, in fact, not be ordered with respect to one another. Such a principle, formulated in (44) below, would be a natural concomitant to the Economy of Projection of Infl-Categories, which asserts that N-features cannot be projected by themselves in the clausal functional category system, but must accompany a matrix of V-features; (44) asserts that the N-features are not ordered amongst themselves, but have their checking order determined derivatively from the associated V-features. This principle of minimal feature ordering is stated in a narrow form pertaining to the ordering of N-features in (44a), and in a more general form in (44b). (In accord with our usual practice, a feature matrix in (44) can consist of a single feature, or a set whose elements are any mix of individual features and hierarchically structured feature matrices.)

(44) *Minimal Feature Ordering*

a. The partial linear order defining the checking order of features in a numeration does not specify the checking order of N-features with respect to one another, but only with respect to V-features.

b. The partial linear order defining the checking order of features in a numeration is minimal to determine a convergent derivation of a syntactic structure from the numeration.

Now we return to consideration of a language in which the spell-out and ordering of multiple object clitics is not determined by morpho-phonological factors. In corresponding nonfinite forms in such a language, the object V-features will not be present, and the N-feature matrices $F_{N\text{-}DO}$ and $F_{N\text{-}IO}$ will have to "float" and associate with other V-features, F_V, to project a head ^[F_V, $F_{N\text{-}DO}$, $F_{N\text{-}IO}$]. The V-feature matrix on this head will have a determinate ranking with respect to the N-features, but the N-feature matrices are not ordered with respect to one another. The expectation, therefore, is that both possible orderings of the two object clitics should be possible, either as proclitics on the verb, or as enclitics, depending on whether F_V is higher ranked or lower ranked than the N-feature matrices.

Modern Greek is a suitable language to test these predictions. Multiple object clitics do not seem to interact with one another morpho-phonologically in Modern Greek, that is, they do not alternate in phonological form depending on the presence of other pronominal clitics, and the ordering of multiple clitics does not seem to be determined by phonological factors. Greek lacks infinitives, but the behavior of nonfinite forms can be observed in gerunds. The functional structure of the Greek clause will be taken to be that proposed by Rivero (1994), in which tense and agreement heads are projected below a higher inflectional head. Rivero identifies the higher head as Mood, where the subjunctive particle *na* appears, but also identifies it as the landing site of movement of the gerundive verb; this suggests that, in fact, the higher head should be identified as Mood/Asp, or that there are separate mood and aspect heads projected above tense and agreement. On the present account, the functional structure of the Greek clause is projected from the feature matrices given in (45), with the usual constraint that V-features are ordered higher than the corresponding N-features. The two lowest ranked feature matrices are separated by a slash to indicate that they alternate with one another, depending on the nature of the clause.

(45) $[F_{V\text{-}M} / F_{V\text{-}ger}] < [F_{V\text{-}s}, F_{N\text{-}s}] < F_{V\text{-}T} < [F_{V\text{-}o}, F_{N\text{-}o}]$

Modern Greek exhibits the Italian pattern of proclisis in finite clauses and enclisis in gerunds and true imperatives, as in (46)–(48) below.

(46) a. *Ton sinandisa.*
him met-1.SG
'I met him.'
b. *To eho fai.*
it have-1.SG eaten

(47) a. *troghondas to*
eating it
b. *ehondas to fai*
having it eaten

(48) a. *Dhjavase to!*
read-2.SG it
b. *Dhjavaste to!*
read-2.PL it

These are obtained as in Italian. With multiple object clitics of a ditransitive verb in a finite clause, proclisis is obtained on the finite verb, as in (49)–(50), with the indirect object clitic preceding the direct object clitic; the reverse order of clitics is ungrammatical.

(49) a. *Tu to edhosa.*
him.GEN it.ACC gave
'I gave it to him.'
b. * *To tu edhosa.*

(50) a. *Tu to eho dhosi.*
him.GEN it.ACC have given
'I have given it to him.'
b. * *To tu eho dhosi.*

These show that $F_{V\text{-}IO} < F_{V\text{-}DO}$, so that the head $\hat{}[F_{V\text{-}DO}, F_{N\text{-}DO}]$ is projected first, attracting the verb and direct object clitic, yielding $[cl_{ACC}\text{-}[V_{fin}\text{-}\hat{}[F_{V\text{-}DO}, F_{N\text{-}DO}]]]$. The head $\hat{}[F_{V\text{-}IO}, F_{N\text{-}IO}]$ is then merged with $\hat{}[F_{V\text{-}DO}, F_{N\text{-}DO}]P$, and V_{fin} is attracted to the newly merged head. It moves, pied-piping the entire $[cl_{ACC}\text{-}[V_{fin}\text{-}\hat{}[F_{V\text{-}DO}, F_{N\text{-}DO}]]]$ complex with it. Finally, $F_{N\text{-}IO}$ attracts the indirect object clitic, which, in accordance with the cycle in head movement, left-adjoins to the entire $[[cl_{ACC}\text{-}[V_{fin}\text{-}\hat{}[F_{V\text{-}DO}, F_{N\text{-}DO}]]]\text{-}\hat{}[F_{V\text{-}IO}, F_{N\text{-}IO}]]$ complex, yielding a proclitic structure with the indirect object clitic preceding the direct object clitic. This is the structure diagrammed in (43b) above, and it is preserved upon further movement of the finite verb to check tense features.

Now turn to gerunds with multiple object clitics. In the absence of corresponding agreement V-features, the N-feature matrices $F_{N\text{-}DO}$ and $F_{N\text{-}IO}$ are floating matrices in this case, and will associate with the lower ranked gerundive V-features $F_{V\text{-}ger}$ and be projected onto a head $\hat{}[F_{V\text{-}ger}, F_{N\text{-}DO}, F_{N\text{-}IO}]$. Since the N-features on this head are ranked higher than the V-feature matrix, the object clitics will be attracted to this head first, after which the verb will be attracted, producing enclisis. But by the Minimal Feature Ordering principle, $F_{N\text{-}DO}$ and $F_{N\text{-}IO}$ will not be ordered with respect to one another. Thus, the object clitics can be attracted to the head $\hat{}[F_{V\text{-}ger}, F_{N\text{-}DO}, F_{N\text{-}IO}]$ in either order, yielding true optionality in the relative order of the object enclitics. This is, in fact, what is obtained.[21]

(51) a. *dhinondas tu to*
giving him.GEN it.ACC
b. *dhinondas to tu*

(52) a. *ehondas tu to dhosi*
having him.GEN it.ACC given
b. % *ehondas to tu dhosi*

In imperatives, Rivero (1994) proposes that the verb raises to C° in the light of evidence for raising of the imperative verb to a position high in the clause. Following the treatment of Romance imperatives in section 2.3 above, we posit a feature [IMP] ranked below inflectional features, merged above all inflectional heads. By exact analogy with the argument for gerunds given above, with [IMP] in the place of $F_{V\text{-}ger}$, we expect ditransitive imperatives to exhibit enclisis of the object clitics in either order, and this is what is observed.

(53) a. *Stiltu* *to!*
send-him.GEN it.ACC
b. *Stilto tu!*

Thus, optionality in multiple clitic order directly results from the lack of relative ordering of feature matrices of features matching those on the object clitics, dictated by the Minimal Feature Ordering principle.

We don't expect this optionality in enclitic ordering of object clitics in gerunds and imperatives in languages in which there is any phonological conditioning of multiple pronominal clitics. For example, in Italian, indirect object clitics *gli*, *mi*, *ti*, *si*, *ci*, *vi* change to *glie*, *me*, *te*, *se*, *ce*, *ve*, respectively, when they occur with direct object clitics; this can be observed for *gli* and *glie* in (54).

(54) a. *dicendoglielo*
saying-him.DAT-it.ACC
'saying it to him'
b. * *dicendologli*

Along with the phonological conditioning of the multiple object clitics in (54), we observe the lack of optionality in their order with respect to one another. Thus, Italian is not a test case for the predictions which were explored for Greek above. See Laenzlinger (1993) and Manzini and Savoia (2004) for a discussion of the relative orders of multiple clitics in languages like Italian.

3. Problems with clitic climbing in a feature-based syntax

In Italian and Spanish, a clitic expressing the object of an infinitival verb can optionally appear as a clitic on a higher lexical verb (what would normally be considered the verb of a higher clause), as illustrated in the Italian data in (55), from Burzio (1986: 322).

(55) a. *Mario vuole leggerlo.*
Mario wants to-read it
b. *Mario lo vuole leggere.*
Mario it wants to-read

The higher verb in a clitic climbing structure can come from one of various classes of verbs (modal, raising, control, unaccusative) which can take an infinitival complement, but only certain verbs of each class permit clitic climbing; the ones which do are called restructuring verbs. Clitic climbing is not possible out of infinitival complements to nonrestructuring verbs, as in (56) below, from Burzio (1986: 322–323).

(56) a. *Mario odia leggerlo.*
Mario hates to-read-it
b. * *Mario lo odia leggere.*
Mario it hates to-read

Examples such as (55a) show that clitic climbing is not obligatory out of infinitival complements of restructuring verbs. But clitic climbing is one of a small set of operations which can only occur in the context of infinitival complementation with restructuring verbs, and which generally apply all together, or none at all, in contexts in which more than one of them can apply. This indicates that restructuring verbs can take a special kind of infinitival complement which conditions these operations, along with ordinary infinitival complements, which don't condition them. A clause with a restructuring verb together with this special kind of infinitival complement is called a restructuring context. The nature of restructuring will be discussed in section 4.1 below, and various other restrictions on clitic climbing will be taken up in section 4.3. For discussion in the literature, see Rizzi (1982), Luján (1980), Napoli (1981), Burzio (1986), LaPolla (1988), Kayne (1989a), Terzi (1993, 1994), Rooryck (1994), Roberts (1997), Wurmbrand (2001), and references cited therein.

In the present section, some problems in the mechanics of the formulation of clitic climbing on accounts in the literature will be identified without committing to any particular theory of restructuring contexts. The accounts discussed here are chosen for the explicitness of their mechanisms, for such explicitness makes it possible to raise the issues under consideration here. In the next section, some theories of restructuring contexts will be surveyed, and it will be shown that a feature-based account of clitic climbing in terms of the mechanisms of clitic placement developed earlier in this chapter is implicated by the simplest and most common view of restructuring contexts.

Rooryck (1994) analyzes clitic climbing as excorporation of the clitic out of a head complex, conditional upon government by the [V-T-Agr_S]

complex of the higher clause, but obligatory under these circumstances. In particular, Rooryck assumes that a clitic is invariably attracted to a governing T^o (or Inf^o) within the local infinitive. The highest verb in the infinitive, V_{inf}, moves to T, and the clitic moves to T, producing the $[_T$ cl-V_{inf}-T$]$ complex shown in (57), with the clitic analyzed as D^o.

(57)

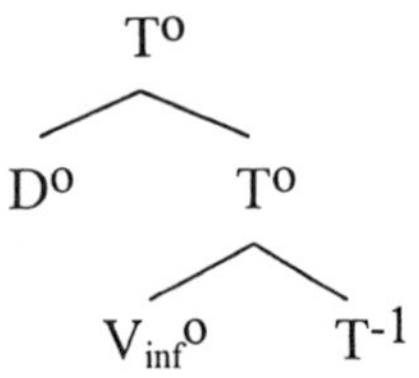

At this point, there are two possible lines of derivation. On one line of derivation, the lower T^o segment excorporates out of this complex and moves to Agr_S, stranding the clitic in the infinitival T^o; this yields a structure of enclisis within the local infinitival, and the clitic, which in this position is not vulnerable to government by a higher T^o, will not climb. On the second line of derivation, the higher T^o segment moves as a whole to Agr_S, which, in a non-*wh*-infinitive, Rooryck takes to be the highest functional head in the infinitival complement clause. Within this head complex, the clitic is governed by the [V-T-Agr_S] complex of the higher clause, and hence attracted to it.[22] On this analysis, the optionality of clitic climbing is tied to the option of moving the lower or the higher T^o segment in (57) to Agr_S. In the case of a *wh*-infinitive, which is a CP complement, the resulting derivation is essentially the same with respect to clitic movement, except that the embedded $[_{Agr_S}$ cl-V_{inf}-T-$Agr_S]$ moves to C, where the clitic is governed by the higher T and excorporates out of $[_C$ cl-V_{inf}-T-Agr_S-C$]$ to the higher [V-T-Agr_S].

The main problem in formulating Rooryck's account within a feature-based syntactic framework is in identifying the attraction of clitics to T^o in terms of feature-matching requirements. What sort of features would attract an object clitic to T^o in general? If the features are ones particular to the object clitic, such as case or N-features, then it is unclear why they should be projected twice, once in the local clause (on T, according to Rooryck) and once in the higher clause, on the higher T, and it is not clear why these features should be projected onto the higher T at all. Thus, even if we analyze away the role that Rooryck accords to government in conditioning this attraction, his account is problematic in a framework in which movement is driven by feature checking.

Similar issues arise in consideration of the analysis of clitic climbing given in Roberts (1994a). Clitic movement on Roberts' account is driven by a general requirement on the distribution of clitics, which Roberts expresses as in (58) below, assuming a unitary Agr head taking TP as its complement, in the phrase structure of Belletti (1990); by "successive-cyclic movement", Roberts means movement into, and excorporation out of, appropriate functional heads.

(58) Clitics adjoin to Agr, possibly via successive-cyclic movement.

Roberts proposes that, in clitic climbing, the clitic skips the local Agr and moves into the C node of the infinitival complement, then excorporates from C and moves to the higher Agr. The clitic does not move through the local Agr at all, and Roberts rules out excorporation of the clitic from Agr. To give this an implementation within a feature-based syntax, the features attracting the clitic must be present on the higher Agr, but not on the local Agr; otherwise, the clitic would be attracted to the local Agr. But the local Agr has object N-features that can be checked off by the clitic and which therefore attract the (features of) the clitic; as noted by Iatridou (1994), it is not clear how clitic climbing can skip the local Agr on Roberts' account. Furthermore, there are problems in conditioning clitic movement into the higher clause since there is no reason for object N-features that can be checked by the clitic, which are projected in the numeration onto the local Agr, to be redundantly projected onto an Agr head in a higher clause.

An approach along these lines deserves closer scrutiny. Reverting to the view of object clitic movement assumed here, as attraction to $F_{N\text{-}o}$ features matching those on the clitic, an analogue of the analyses proposed by Rooryck and Roberts would be to suppose that object N-features matching those of the clitic are present in the clause of origin of the clitic, and in the higher clause. In an infinitival clause, there are no object agreement V-features, so the $F_{N\text{-}o}$ features to be checked by the object enter the numeration as floating features, and are then associated with the V-features for tense, $F_{V\text{-}T}$, and projected onto the functional head $^\wedge[F_{V\text{-}T}, F_{N\text{-}o}]$, as proposed in section 2.1 above. In the analysis of clitic climbing presently under consideration, one or more additional sets of copies of the feature matrix $F_{N\text{-}o}$ would be projected higher in the sentence. For the example of clitic climbing in (55b), where the higher clause is a tensed clause with object V-features, the duplicate copy of $F_{N\text{-}o}$ would be projected together with $F_{V\text{-}o}$ in the higher clause. The relevant lexical and functional categories in the numeration are given in (59).[23]

(59)	"Agr_S	T	Agr_O	*Mario*	*vuole*	[T	PRO	*lo*	*leggere*]"
			$F_{V\text{-}o}'$		$F_{V\text{-}o}'$	$F_{V\text{-}T}$		$F_{N\text{-}o}$	$F_{V\text{-}T}$
			$\mathbf{F_{N\text{-}o}}$			$\mathbf{F_{N\text{-}o}}$			

Furthermore, suppose that the object N-features of the clitic can check off matching features on multiple functional heads without themselves deleting. Then clitic climbing could take place as follows: the clitic is attracted to the local ^[$F_{V\text{-}T}$, $F_{N\text{-}o}$], checking off the lower copy of $F_{N\text{-}o}$, and is then attracted to ^[$F_{V\text{-}o}'$, $F_{N\text{-}o}$] in the higher clause, checking off the higher copy of $F_{N\text{-}o}$.[24]

Inspiration for this analysis of clitic climbing might be taken from Chomsky's (1995a, 1995b) treatment of subject agreement with an adjective and copula in Spanish examples such as (60) below, discussed in Chapter 2 above.

(60)	*María*	*está*	*alt-a.*
	Maria	be.PRES.3.SG	tall-FEM.SG

Recall that the numeration for the example in (60) is that given in (61) below, with categories listed in right-to-left merge-order, and that, in the course of the derivation, the N-features of the subject NP *María*, $F_{N\text{-}s}$, successively check the matching features in the matrices [F_A, $F_{N\text{-}s}$] and [$F_{V\text{-}s}$, $F_{N\text{-}s}$], projected as the heads labeled here as Agr_A and Agr_S, through NP-movement to the specifiers of these two heads.

(61)	"Agr_S	T	V	[Agr_A	[NP	A]]"
			está		*María*	*alta*
	$F_{V\text{-}s}$	$F_{V\text{-}T}$	$F_{V\text{-}T}$	F_A	$F_{N\text{-}s}$	F_A
	$F_{N\text{-}s}$	[NOM]	$F_{V\text{-}s}$	$F_{N\text{-}s}$	[NOM]	

But, as discussed in Chapter 2, the derivation with multiple feature-checking based on the numeration in (61) is sensible precisely because the two separate copies of $F_{N\text{-}s}$ features, projected to match those on the subject, are needed to mediate two separate instances of NP-head agreement. This motivated the Economy of Feature Projection, repeated below.

(62) *Economy of Feature Projection*
Given the lexical categories in a numeration, a minimal suite of matching features is entered into the numeration to be projected onto functional categories.

Recall that "minimal" in this formulation was interpreted to mean that, given a nominal with N-features F_N, one copy of F_N could be projected to mediate each instance of NP-head agreement, and that otherwise only one copy can be checked against the lexical copy. Returning to (59), the copies of $F_{N\text{-}o}$ projected with $F_{V\text{-}T}$ in the complement clause and with $F_{V\text{-}o}'$ in the main clause do not mediate instances of NP-head agreement; thus, only one matching copy of $F_{N\text{-}o}$ can be projected at all. The derivation from (59) therefore violates the Economy of Feature Projection.[25]

4. A feature-based approach to clitic climbing

4.1. Restructuring

What is needed to support clitic climbing (CC) on a feature-based formulation of syntactic theory is a way for N-features of the clitic on the lower verb in a restructuring context to appear on a higher Infl-head *instead of* on a local Infl-head. Mechanisms for such an alternate association of object N-features should be formulated in such a way that they will operate only in restructuring contexts. For this reason, some major views of restructuring and the bases on which they rest will be surveyed before the mechanisms of clitic climbing are examined.

The hypothesis that some infinitival complements of restructuring verbs are structurally distinguished as restructuring infinitives rests on the co-occurrence of several processes. In addition to clitic climbing, these include a change of auxiliary by which an auxiliary verb accompanying the restructuring verb depends on the nature of the infinitival predicate, and a process promoting the object of the infinitive to subject position of the higher clause under conditions when the subject position of the higher clause is not filled by the external argument of the restructuring verb. These will be introduced in turn.

There is a widespread principle of Auxiliary Selection, by which transitive and unergative verbs take the auxiliary *HAVE*, while unaccusatives take the auxiliary *BE* (where capital letters are used for the class of corresponding verbs, cross-linguistically). This is seen in Italian with the choice of *avere* 'have' with the unergative main verb in (63a) below, and with the choice of *essere* 'be' accompanying the unaccusative main verb in (63b).[26]

(63)	a.	*Giovanni*	***ha***	*telefonato.*
		Giovanni	**has**	telephoned
	b.	*Giovanni*	***è***	*arrivato.*
		Giovanni	**is**	arrived

Restructuring verbs which normally select *HAVE* optionally select *BE* when their infinitival complement has a main verb which selects *BE*. This Change of Auxiliary (CA) phenomenon is illustrated for the restructuring verb *volere* 'want' in (64) below.

(64)	a.	*Mario*	***avrebbe***	*proprio*	*voluto*	*andare*	*a casa.*
		Mario	**would.have**	really	wanted	to-go	home
	b.	*Mario*	***sarebbe***	*proprio*	*voluto*	*andare*	*a casa.*
		Mario	**would.be**	really	wanted	to-go	home
		'Mario would have really wanted to go home.'					

The examples in (65) illustrate the fact that the verbs which permit CA are the same as those which permit clitic climbing: CA only occurs in clauses with restructuring verbs.

(65)	a.		*Mario*	***avrebbe***	*proprio*	*odiato*	*andare*	*a casa.*
			Mario	**would.have**	really	hated	to-go	home
	b.	*	*Mario*	***sarebbe***	*proprio*	*odiato*	*andare*	*a casa.*
			Mario	**would.be**	really	hated	to-go	home

Finally, restructuring verbs permit long-distance promotion of the object (LOP) of the infinitive to matrix subject position. This can happen under passivization in the higher clause (see Wurmbrand 2001 for many examples of this in German), and in Italian impersonal *si*-clauses, and it applies specifically to objects which would ordinarily be recipients of structural case in object position of the infinitival verb. Alongside the fully monoclausal example of the latter in (66a), there is the LOP example in (67a); both alternate with examples without object promotion in (66b) and (67b).

(66) a. *Alcuni articoli si leggeranno volentieri.*
a-few articles SI will.read-PL willingly
b. *Si leggerà volentieri alcuni articoli.*
SI will.read-SG willingly a-few articles

(67) a. *Questi libri si volevano proprio leggere.*
these books SI wanted-PL really to-read
'We really wanted to read these books.'
b. *Si voleva proprio leggere questi libri.*
SI wanted-SG really to-read these books

This, like CC and CA, is restricted to contexts with infinitival complements of restructuring verbs, as shown in (68).

(68) a. *Si odiava proprio leggere questi libri.*
SI hated-SG really to-read these books
b. * *Questi libri si odiavano proprio leggere.*
these books SI hated-PL really to-read

Regarded individually, each of these processes seems to be optional, applying or not in any context in which it could apply. However, in contexts in which more than one of them could apply, there are some mutual co-occurrence requirements on their application. Whenever CC has applied, and the lower verb is unaccusative, CA must occur as well, as shown by (69b,c), although both can fail to apply together, as in (69a).

(69) a. *Mario avrebbe proprio voluto andarci.*
Mario would.have really wanted go-INF-there
b. *Mario ci sarebbe proprio voluto andare.*
Mario there would.be really wanted go-INF
c. * *Mario ci avrebbe proprio voluto andare.*
Mario there would.have really wanted go-INF

And whenever LOP has occurred, a clitic object of the infinitival verb must undergo CC; see (70).

(70) a. *Questi libri gli si vorrebbero proprio dare.*
these books him.DAT SI would.want really give-INF

b. * *Questi libri si vorrebbero proprio dargli.*

LOP cannot co-occur with CA since an unaccusative infinitival verb does not have an object which would ordinarily be assigned structural case. Two combinations are missing from this paradigm of co-occurrence: LOP can fail to apply in the presence of CC, and CC can fail to apply in the presence of CA; see (71).

(71) a. *Gli si vorrebbero proprio dare questi libri.*
him.DAT SI would.want really give-INF these books

b. *Mario sarebbe proprio voluto andarci.*
Mario would.be really wanted go-INF-there

(71a) is accounted for by detailed theories of restructuring (see below). (71b) does not have such an account. But unaccusative verbs do not have object clitic arguments; therefore, the failure of CC in the presence of CA can only be attested for locative clitics such as *ci* in (71b).[27]

If CC, CA, and LOP applied independently of one another in the contexts of restructuring verbs, then there would be no reason to say that there is anything special about the infinitival complements in cases where they apply, but only about the restructuring verbs themselves, which condition these processes: given a restructuring verb with an infinitival complement, the processes in question would simply apply or not, as the case may be. Since these processes in fact exhibit positive co-occurrence requirements, this suggests that, alongside ordinary infinitival complements, restructuring verbs can take a special type of infinitival complement, a restructuring infinitive, which is required for these processes to apply, and which requires them to apply, so that the application of any one of them can be considered diagnostic of the presence of a restructuring infinitive, and therefore determinative of the application of the other processes (if they are applicable).

Various proposals have been advanced regarding the nature of restructuring contexts. At one extreme, restructuring infinitives are regarded as purely lexical (VP) structures, whether directly generated or derived; see Rizzi (1982), Burzio (1986), Wurmbrand (2001), and many others. On other accounts, restructuring infinitives have full clausal structure, but are more tightly tied to the higher verb and its functional projections through head movement of the lower verb (by covert movement) or of the lower clause T node (overtly) to a head position outside the infinitival complement (in the higher clause, if that is how the structure is conceived). Wurmbrand (2001) gives an extended argument for restructuring infinitives as lexical VP structures, citing extensive data from German, but countering arguments for more elaborate structures of restructuring infinitives in Romance languages as well. Applied to the Italian data cited above, the lexical VP proposal has the following ramifications for CC, CA, and LOP. To begin with, an object clitic of the infinitive must undergo CC in a restructuring context, assuming any account of clitic placement involving movement to functional heads, since there are no functional heads in the restructured infinitive. The obligatoriness of CA in a restructuring context is more subtle, resting on the analysis of the structure as essentially monoclausal, in which the infinitive verb counts as the main verb for purposes of auxiliary selection. Whenever the infinitive is unaccusative, it follows that auxiliary *BE* will occur. (In this case, the higher verb in a restructuring context is analogized to a modal or light verb, which is more plausible in the case of modal triggers of restructuring than in the case of lexical verbs such as *volere* 'want' featured in several of the examples above.) Finally, Wurmbrand adds significantly to the account of LOP in restructuring contexts. She argues that the restructured infinitive, lacking all functional projections, cannot provide for checking of accusative case on an object of the infinitive. But a full nominal object of the infinitive verb can check accusative case features under covert movement to functional projections of the higher verb, as in Minimalist accounts of Exceptional Case Marking suggested in Chomsky and Lasnik (1995) and developed in Johnson (1991), Koizumi (1993), Lasnik (1999: 137–140). Thus, a nominal object, unlike a clitic pronoun, can remain in its base position in the overt syntax.

In present terms, the lexical structure of the restructuring infinitive, without tense, aspect, or agreement heads, can be characterized as an infinitival clause without V-features on lexical items in the lexical array of the infinitival complement. (This is actually slightly more permissive than Wurmbrand's view that restructuring infinitives lack all functional projections, since the present account allows that a complementizer without morpho-syntactic V-features might occur in a restructuring infinitive; this aspect of the present account will be needed in section 4.3 below.) The mechanics of clitic climbing will be considered under this account of restructuring infinitives in the next section. The consequences of adopting more elaborate accounts of restructuring complements will be considered later, in section 4.4.

4.2. Mechanics of clitic climbing with feature-derived functional categories

Now return to the Italian examples in (55a,b), repeated below.

(55) a. *Mario vuole leggerlo.*
Mario wants to-read-it
b. *Mario lo vuole leggere.*
Mario it wants to-read

By the discussion in section 4.1 above, the complement without clitic climbing in (55a) is an ordinary infinitival clause. It therefore has infinitival tense V-features, $F_{V\text{-}T}$, but no V-features for object agreement. The object N-features $F_{N\text{-}o}$ matching those of the clitic associate with $F_{V\text{-}T}$ and are projected as a head $^\wedge[F_{V\text{-}T}, F_{N\text{-}o}]$, with the order $F_{V\text{-}T} < F_{N\text{-}o}$. As a result, the clitic is attracted and left-adjoins to this head first, and the verb is subsequently attracted to this head, and left-adjoins, producing the enclitic form *leggerlo* in (55a).

Following the discussion in section 4.1 above, (55b) is produced in the context of a restructuring infinitive complement of the verb *vuole* 'want'. The restructuring infinitive has no V-features whatsoever; hence it lacks $F_{V\text{-}T}$ as well as object agreement V-features. But, turning to the higher clause, verb raising proceeds internally within clauses with clausal complements exactly as it does in clauses with nominal complements. Thus, the higher verb in (55b) has a verbal matrix $F_{V\text{-}o}'$, and a matching copy of this matrix is introduced and projected into phrase structure as a head which will attract the higher verb. By the Economy of Projection of Infl-Categories, the feature matrix $F_{N\text{-}o}$ introduced to check features of the clitic must be associated with V-features in order to be projected onto a functional head. In the absence of any V-features in the restructuring infinitive, the features $F_{V\text{-}o}'$ introduced to check features on the higher verb are the nearest appropriate V-features with which the features attracting the clitic can associate. Assuming that they do so, the resulting numeration is depicted in (72). (Features attracting the clitic are in boldface; features irrelevant to the present discussion are suppressed.)

(72)	"Agr_S	T	Agr_O	*Mario*	*vuole*	[	*lo*	*leggere*]"
			$F_{V\text{-}o}'$		$F_{V\text{-}o}'$		$F_{N\text{-}o}$	
			$\mathbf{F_{N\text{-}o}}$					

In the syntactic derivation from (72), the clitic is attracted to ^[$F_{V\text{-}o}'$, $F_{N\text{-}o}$] in the higher clause, and this functional head is the only (hence the nearest) head with features to attract the clitic. Hence, the clitic moves to this head in accord with Minimalist constraints on movement, producing clitic climbing in (55b). Following Chomsky (1995a, 1995b) as before, the clitic is a lexical category which has not projected, and therefore can count as either a head or a maximal projection; its initial steps of movement are as a maximal projection, and it then adjoins to its target as a head. Well known facts about constraints on clitic climbing discussed in section 4.3 below implicate standard constraints on XP-movement.

The crucial question regarding the numeration in (72), and the derivation based on it, concerns the ordering of the floating $F_{N\text{-}o}$ with respect to the features $F_{V\text{-}o}'$. If the order of the $F_{N\text{-}o}$ features introduced to check features of the clitic were initially specified with respect to all other features in the numeration, then $F_{N\text{-}o}$ would be ordered higher than $F_{V\text{-}o}'$ in (72). As a result, in the derivation from (72), the clitic would move to ^[$F_{V\text{-}o}'$, $F_{N\text{-}o}$] first, after which *vuole* would be attracted to this head and would left-adjoin, producing enclisis with clitic climbing in (55b), contrary to fact. However, the feature orderings assumed in this derivation violate the Minimal Feature Ordering principle in (44) above. Given the transitivity of the ordering relation, it would be unnecessary to stipulate the relative order of F_i and F_j for all pairs of features {F_i, F_j} within the numeration. The ordering of features with respect to one another within the Infl-system of a clause, or within a particular nominal, needs to be specified in order to guide the projection of functional categories for that clause or nominal, and thus in order to guide the derivation of that clause or nominal. But the ordering of all pairs of features does not need to be stipulated across clausal or nominal boundaries. The cluster of operations needed to construct a clausal or nominal system will be ordered as a whole by selectional relationships with respect to the clusters of operations needed to construct other clausal or nominal systems. In the construction of (55a,b), for example, the cluster of operations needed to construct the infinitival complement clause needs to be internally ordered by the order of features for that clause within the numeration; likewise, the cluster of operations needed to construct the higher, finite, clause needs to be internally ordered by the order of features for that clause. But the ordering of the two clusters of operations as a whole, by which the entire complement clause is constructed first, and then the matrix clause is constructed, does not require initial specification of the ordering on all pairs of features within the numeration. It requires only that features be ordered at the clausal interface by selectional relationships; the ordering of remaining pairs of features across the clausal boundary follows by the transitivity of the ordering relation. The verb *vuole* in (55a,b) selects the infinitival clause as its complement; it is therefore enough to order $F_{V\text{-}o}'$ lower than the lowest feature of the complement clause. Therefore, by the Minimal Feature Ordering principle, the $F_{V\text{-}o}'$ features in the main clause will not be initially ordered in the numeration with respect to the $F_{N\text{-}o}$ features matching features on the clitic.

In line with these considerations, the order of $F_{N\text{-}o}$ features with respect to the V-features $F_{V\text{-}o}'$ in the higher clause is initially unspecified in the numeration; the order between these two feature matrices will be specified only when they are put together in a single feature matrix. Assuming that the specification of order treats the $F_{N\text{-}o}$ the same as it would local object features, the order $F_{N\text{-}o} < F_{V\text{-}o}'$ will result in (72). Thus, in the derivation from (72), *vuole* moves to ^[$F_{V\text{-}o}'$, $F_{N\text{-}o}$] first, and the clitic, undergoing clitic climbing, subsequently left-adjoins to [V-^[$F_{V\text{-}o}'$, $F_{N\text{-}o}$]], producing proclisis in (55b). It is pertinent to this account that when the $F_{N\text{-}o}$ feature is projected with $F_{V\text{-}o}'$ as a functional head in the higher clause and is ordered with respect to the local features of the higher clause, it is then ordered lower than features in the complement clause. This is possible if the order of the feature matrix $F_{N\text{-}o}$ is not defined until it is associated with V-features within the numeration.[28]

When the higher verb is a participle, the local object V-feature matrix $F_{V\text{-}o}'$ is projected above the associated auxiliary. If the $F_{N\text{-}o}$ features to be checked off by the clitic are projected with $F_{V\text{-}o}'$ in this case, the clitic will move to ^[$F_{V\text{-}o}'$, $F_{N\text{-}o}$] only after movement of the auxiliary to this head has checked off $F_{V\text{-}o}'$; this yields cl-Aux order, as in (73) below (from Rizzi 1982: 4).

(73)	*Gianni*	*gli*	*ha*	*potuto*	*parlare*	*personalmente.*
	Gianni	him.DAT	has	been-able	to-speak	personally

With clitic climbing into a higher infinitival, enclisis is produced, as illustrated in (74b) below (adapted from Napoli 1981: 874).

(74)	a.	*Bisognava*	*andare*	*a cercarli.*
		It-was-necessary	to-go	to-look-for-them
	b.	*Bisognava*	*andarli*	*a cercare.*
		It-was-necessary	to-go-them	to-look-for

Within an infinitival clause in Italian, as discussed in section 2.1 above, object N-features are not accompanied by local $F_{V\text{-}o}$ features; ordinarily, they are associated and projected with the infinitival tense features, $F_{V\text{-}T}$. In (74a), the complement is not a restructuring infinitival, so the $F_{N\text{-}o}$ features entered into the numeration to check features of the clitic are associated with $F_{V\text{-}T}$ in the lower infinitival clause. But the lower infinitive in (74b) is a restructuring infinitive, which lacks any V-features. The nearest V-feature matrix with which $F_{N\text{-}o}$ can associate is $F_{V\text{-}T}'$ of the higher infinitive (the intermediate clause in the tri-clausal structure of (74b)), and the two feature matrices can be projected as a functional head $\hat{}[F_{V\text{-}T}', F_{N\text{-}o}]$ in the higher clause. The $F_{N\text{-}o}$ will be assigned the order appropriate to object N-features within this clause, which is an order higher than that of the local V-features $F_{V\text{-}T}'$. The resulting numeration is shown in (75) below, with $F_{V\text{-}T}' < F_{N\text{-}o}$.

(75)	"... Agr_S	T	PRO	*andare*	[*a*	*li*	*cercare*]"
		$F_{V\text{-}T}'$		$F_{V\text{-}T}'$		$F_{N\text{-}o}$	
		$\mathbf{F_{N\text{-}o}}$					

In the derivation from this numeration, once the head $\hat{}[F_{V\text{-}T}', F_{N\text{-}o}]$ is merged into phrase structure in the intermediate clause, the clitic *li* will move and left-adjoin to it, checking $F_{N\text{-}o}$, and then the verb *andare* will move and left-adjoin to this [cl-$\hat{}[F_{V\text{-}T}', F_{N\text{-}o}]$], producing enclisis, *andarli*.

Modern French does not have clitic climbing except in contexts of infinitival complements to causative verbs. The complements of causative verbs are arguably bare lexical infinitives of the sort proposed in the literature for restructuring complements in Italian and German, adopted here. Other verbs in French evidently do not take such bare lexical infinitive complements. However, on the present account, it would not be necessary to assume that infinitival complements in French are always full clausal structures, with infinitival tense. It is sufficient to suppose that the aspectual V-features proposed in section 2.2 above, which drive short verb movement, are always present in French infinitives (except for complements of causative verbs), and that the $F_{N\text{-}o}$ entered into the numeration to check features of the clitic will obligatorily associate with these V-features. Therefore, the feature matrix $F_{N\text{-}o}$ attracting the clitic will never associate with V-features of the higher verb, so clitic climbing will never occur.

The account of clitic climbing presented here bears some resemblance to the feature-passing account of clitic climbing developed in LaPolla (1988), which discussed primarily Spanish data in a rather different theoretical setting. In LaPolla's account, as in the present one, clitic climbing depends on whether or not a bundle of features or a feature matrix is passed to a higher clause or kept within the local clause to which the clitic thematically belongs; however, for LaPolla, the clitic is not attracted to these features, but is itself the spell-out of these features. There are other crucial differences of detail between the two accounts, in that LaPolla formulates the feature-passing as a direct and free transfer of features from the infinitival verb to the higher verb, rather than as an obligatory association of these features with features of the higher verb, necessitated by the lack of local V-features, in the context of a more general theory of the distribution of features onto functional categories such as that presented here. LaPolla rejects a restructuring view of the context for clitic climbing, in part on the basis of the existence of cases in which complementizers and other elements intervene between the lower and higher verbs in a clitic climbing construction, as discussed in section 4.3 below. However, these can be accommodated on the account offered here so long as the intervening material does not contain any V-features and (as discussed further in section 4.3 below) does not interfere with the XP-movement phase of clitic movement.

4.3. Some properties of clitic climbing

Standard constraints on clitic climbing, illustrated in (76)–(78), that it is blocked by negation, by the *se* 'if' complementizer, and blocked out of most *wh*-infinitivals, are on the present approach not due to constraints on the association of N-features matching those of the clitic with V-features within a higher clause, but are, rather, constraints on the XP-movement phase of clitic movement.[29]

(76) a. *Non lo voglio fare.*
(I) NEG it want to-do
b. *Voglio non farlo.*
(I) want NEG to-do-it
c. * *Lo voglio non fare.*
it I-want NEG to-do

(77) a. *Non so se farli.*
(I) NEG know if to-do-them
b. * *Non li so se fare.*
(I) NEG them know if to-do

(78) a. * *Non lo saprei a chi dire.*
NEG it would.know to whom to-say
b. * *Non ti saprei come dire che la macchina era rotta.*
NEG to-you would.know how to-tell that the car was broken

There are some cases in which clitic climbing is permitted out of *wh*-infinitives.

(79) *Non ti saprei che dire.*
(I) NEG you.DAT would.know what to-say

Rooryck (1994) argues that the *wh*-word *che* is a clitic located in C^{o}, allowing for XP-movement of the object clitic through spec-CP into the higher clause in cases like (79).[30] Rooryck argues that other well known cases of clitic climbing out of *wh*-infinitivals, involving left-dislocation of an NP with which the clitic is construed, are structures of clitic left-dislocation, as studied by Cinque (1990), and have different properties from structures of clitic movement.

In the languages considered here, multiple object clitics either climb together, or are placed together in their clause of origin, as illustrated by (80), from Rizzi 1982: 44).

(80) a. *Piero voleva dar-me-lo.*
Piero wanted to-give-me-it
b. *Piero me lo voleva dare.*

c. * *Piero lo voleva darmi.*
d. * *Piero mi voleva darlo.*

This follows directly since the infinitival complement is either a restructuring infinitive, or not. If it is, then all object clitics must climb, and if it isn't, then all of them will associate with V-features within the infinitive, so none of them will climb.[31]

Finally, clitic climbing is blocked out of finite (subjunctive) complements of restructuring verbs, as illustrated by the following example from Kayne (1989a: 243).

(81)	* *Gianni*	*li*	*vuole*	*che*	*(Maria)*	*veda.*
	Gianni	them	wants	that	Maria/she	see-SUBJ

This follows since N-features are linked to a head with V-features in a finite clause and are therefore not floating. The intervention of the complementizer in (81) should evidently not be implicated in the failure of clitic climbing, since, as pointed out and discussed in LaPolla (1988) (see also Terzi 1993, 1994), clitic climbing can take place out of infinitival complements introduced by the indicative 'that'-complementizer in Spanish, as in (82) below (from Terzi 1993).

(82)	*Juan*	*los*	*tiene*	*que*	*ver.*
	Juan	them	has	that	to-see
	'Juan has to see them.'				

The numeration for (82) will be formed with the features matching those of the clitic associated with V-features in the higher clause, provided the complementizer has no V-features itself. The example in (82) can then be derived from this numeration if clitic movement in the XP stage has at least some of the characteristics of A′-movement.[32]

In summary, the basic constraints on clitic climbing are accounted for by the following aspects of the present proposals:

- There is no clitic climbing out of finite clauses since the finite complement has $F_{V\text{-}o}$, which ties down the features $F_{N\text{-}o}$ matching those on the clitic.[33]
- All but the last step of clitic movement is XP-movement. The XP movement of the clitic is blocked by negation.

– *Se*-complements and *wh*(XP)-complements are islands for all XP movement, hence for clitic movement out of a clause.

4.4. Other accounts of clitic climbing

The account of clitic climbing given in section 4.2 above, and its consequences for the various properties of clitic climbing mentioned in section 4.3, rested on the hypothesis that restructuring infinitives lack V-features introduced into the numeration to match V-features on the lexical infinitive; this is an adaptation of the bare lexical structure for the restructuring infinitive which is argued for by Wurmbrand (2001). We found that on this structure for the restructuring infinitive, no special principles were required to account for clitic climbing with the exact suite of properties it exhibits. The $F_{N\text{-}o}$ feature matrix introduced into the numeration must associate with V-features in order to be projected onto a functional head, there are no V-features in the restructuring infinitive, and so the $F_{N\text{-}o}$ matrix associates with V-features introduced to match features on the higher verb, and attracts the clitic, producing proclisis or enclisis, depending on the ordering of $F_{N\text{-}o}$ with respect to the V-features with which it associates.

If a fuller clausal structure is adopted for restructuring infinitives, a feature-based account of clitic climbing is not so straightforward and cost-free. Suppose, for the moment, that restructuring infinitives have V-features, and are therefore distinguished from other infinitival complements not by their complete lack of V-features, but by some other property, such as a deficient tense node, or head movement of the infinitival tense node of the infinitive complement to a functional head associated with the higher verb. (Accounts positing such head movement as the distinguishing property of restructuring will be cited below.) Thus, on this view, restructuring infinitives have some V-feature matrix $F_{V\text{-}X}$ entered into the numeration to match features on the infinitive verb. For concreteness, suppose that $F_{V\text{-}X}$ consists of (possibly deficient) tense features, $F_{V\text{-}T}$.

Under these assumptions, the $F_{N\text{-}o}$ feature matrix introduced to match features of the clitic would be initially floating, as shown in (83), and would normally associate with the local tense matrix $F_{V\text{-}T}$, as in (84), and the derivation from (84) would produce enclisis on the infinitive verb.

(83)

"Agr_S	T	Agr_O	*Mario*	*vuole*	[	T	PRO	*lo*	*leggere*	]"
		$F_{V\text{-}o}'$		$F_{V\text{-}o}'$		$F_{V\text{-}T}$		$F_{N\text{-}o}$	$F_{V\text{-}T}$	
								($\mathbf{F_{N\text{-}o}}$)		

(84)

"Agr_S	T	Agr_O	*Mario*	*vuole*	[	T	PRO	*lo*	*leggere*	]"
		$F_{V\text{-}o}'$		$F_{V\text{-}o}'$		$F_{V\text{-}T}$		$F_{N\text{-}o}$	$F_{V\text{-}T}$	
						$\mathbf{F_{N\text{-}o}}$				

In order to derive a structure with clitic climbing, the $F_{N\text{-}o}$ matrix in (83) would have to have the additional option of associating with the V-features $F_{V\text{-}o}'$ of the higher verb instead of with the local V-features, producing the numeration in (85).

(85)

"Agr_S	T	Agr_O	*Mario*	*vuole*	[	T	PRO	*lo*	*leggere*	]"
		$F_{V\text{-}o}'$		$F_{V\text{-}o}'$		$F_{V\text{-}T}$		$F_{N\text{-}o}$	$F_{V\text{-}T}$	
		$\mathbf{F_{N\text{-}o}}$								

But there is no provision in the theory, articulated to this point, for the $F_{N\text{-}o}$ matrix in (83) to optionally associate with non-local V-features. The only instances of optional association which we have seen were with local V-features, immediately adjacent in the partial linear ordering of features in the numeration, which figured in the account of the optionality of proclisis and enclisis in Italian indicative suppletive imperatives (some dialects), exhibited in (42) in section 2.3. The option of associating the $F_{N\text{-}o}$ matrix with V-features of the higher verb in (85) would be a special dispensation granted to the $F_{N\text{-}o}$ matrix specifically to permit the derivation of clitic climbing. This special dispensation would have to be assumed for a feature-based account of clitic climbing on any theory of restructuring infinitives which did not assume a complete lack of V-features in the restructured infinitive, in other words, any theory of restructuring infinitives other than the one adopted in sections 4.1 and 4.2 above. Thus, the theory of restructuring infinitives as lacking all V-features seems to be the best foundation for a feature-based account of clitic climbing.

Among head movement accounts of clitic climbing, one type posits head movement of the clitic through C^o into the higher clause, independently of the movement of any other heads out of the clause of origin of the clitic. Accounts of this sort include those of Kayne (1989a) and Roberts (1994a). One concern with these accounts is that they would not block clitic climbing out of *wh*-infinitivals with a full XP *wh*-phrase in spec-CP, such as (78a) above. A deeper property of these accounts is that they need to address the question why some heads block clitic climbing, and not others. Attempts to answer this question have led to elaborate typologies of types of head movement, such as that of Roberts (1994a). On another type of head movement account (see Roberts 1997), clitic climbing is effected through restructuring realized as head movement of the local Infl into the higher Infl. In this case, again, it is not clear why head movement should be blocked out of *wh*-infinitivals such as those in (78a) short of a more elaborate typology of heads.

At great variance with all other accounts discussed here, a lexical account of clitic climbing forms the [V-cl] or [cl-V] complex as part of the lexical morphology, prior to "lexical insertion," that is (in the terms adopted here), prior to selection of lexical items for inclusion in the lexical array, and hence, in the numeration. Such an account is strained by the fact that clitic climbing is potentially unbounded; see (73) above. Furthermore, on a lexical account, there is no particular reason why the clitic should form [cl-Aux] and [Aux-cl] complexes in participial constructions, since Aux bears no thematic or other discernible lexical relation to the clitic.

4.5. Clitic climbing out of finite clauses in Salentino

Terzi (1993, 1994) addresses cases of clitic climbing out of finite (subjunctive) clauses in Salentino, which are of particular interest to any account of clitic climbing. Subjunctive complements in Salentino can be introduced by the mood particle *ku*, in which case the complement admits of a full range of inflections. (All examples in this section are from Terzi (1993)).

(86)	*Ulia*	*ku*	*benne.*
	want-1.SG-PAST	PRT	come-3.SG-PRES

The mood particle can be missing, in which case the lower subject must be construed in reference (and features) with the higher subject, which Terzi takes to be due to subject control, as indicated in (87) below.[34]

(87)	*pro*$_i$	*voggyu*	*pro*$_{i/*j}$	*lu*	*kkattu.*
		want-1.SG		it	buy-1.SG

When the mood particle is missing, clitic climbing can (optionally) occur.

(88)	*Lu*	*voggyu*	*kkattu.*
	it	want-1.SG	buy-1.SG

Terzi proposes that movement of the clitic imposes coindexation of intervening specifiers, which is only possible under control of the lower subject by the higher subject. On the present approach, when *ku* is present, we would have a numeration of the sort given in (89) below, from which there can be no clitic climbing. (Tense and complementizer features omitted here.)

(89)	“Agr_S	T	Agr_O	*pro_i*	*voggyu* [*ku*	Agr_S	T	Agr_O	*$pro_{i/j}$*	*lu*	*kkattu*]”
	$F_{V\text{-}s}'$		$F_{V\text{-}o}'$	$F_{N\text{-}s}'$	$F_{V\text{-}o}'$	$F_{V\text{-}s}$		$F_{V\text{-}o}$	$F_{N\text{-}s}$	$F_{N\text{-}o}$	$F_{V\text{-}o}$
	$F_{N\text{-}s}'$				$F_{V\text{-}s}'$	$F_{N\text{-}s}$		$F_{N\text{-}o}$			$F_{V\text{-}s}$

When *ku* is absent, the higher subject controls the lower subject, as noted by Terzi. This will follow if, when *ku* is absent, the values of subject and object N-features and V-features in the lower clause are anaphoric to the values of the corresponding features in the higher clause. Note that this anaphoricity would exclude $F_{N\text{-}o}$, the feature matrix introduced into the numeration to match features on the clitic, since there are no $F_{N\text{-}o}$ features in the higher clause for the $F_{N\text{-}o}$ features matching those of the clitic to be anaphoric to. Furthermore, the feature matrix $F_{N\text{-}o}$ is not entered into the numeration in conjunction with object V-features $F_{V\text{-}o}$, since the object V-features of the lower clause get their value anaphorically from the higher clause. Thus, the matrix of features $F_{N\text{-}o}$, introduced into the numeration to match features on the clitic, are initially floating. The resulting numeration is shown in (90), where the primes indicate identity of the lower subject V-features and N-features and object V-features under anaphoric relation to the higher clause.

(90)	“Agr_S	T	Agr_O	*pro_i*	*voggyu*	[Agr_S	T	Agr_O	*$pro_{i/*j}$*	*lu*	*kkattu*]”
	$F_{V\text{-}s}'$		$F_{V\text{-}o}'$	$F_{N\text{-}s}'$	$F_{V\text{-}o}'$	$F_{V\text{-}s}'$		$F_{V\text{-}o}'$	$F_{N\text{-}s}'$	$F_{N\text{-}o}$	$F_{V\text{-}o}'$
	$F_{N\text{-}s}'$				$F_{V\text{-}s}'$	$F_{N\text{-}s}'$					$F_{V\text{-}s}'$
										$\mathbf{F_{N\text{-}o}}$	

As always when $F_{N\text{-}o}$ features of the clitic are left floating, they can be associated with the nearest suitable V-features. In (90), the nearest V-features are $F_{V\text{-}o}'$, but there are two copies of these (in addition to the copies on the verbs), one in the local clause, and one in the higher clause. The

$F_{N\text{-}o}$ matrix can be associated with $F_{V\text{-}o}'$ in either of its two occurrences, in the lower clause or in the higher clause. Choice of the lower clause $F_{V\text{-}o}'$ matrix, resulting in the projection of ^[$F_{V\text{-}o}'$, $F_{N\text{-}o}$] in the lower clause, yields the form without clitic climbing in (87), with proclisis produced through left-adjunction, given that $F_{N\text{-}o} < F_{V\text{-}o}'$. Choice of the higher clause $F_{V\text{-}o}'$ matrix, resulting in the projection of ^[$F_{V\text{-}o}'$, $F_{N\text{-}o}$] in the higher clause, yields the numeration in (91).

(91)	"Agr_S	T	Agr_O	*pro_i*	*voggyu*	[Agr_S	T	Agr_O	*$pro_{i/*j}$*	*lu*	*kkattu*]"
	$F_{V\text{-}s}'$		$F_{V\text{-}o}'$	$F_{N\text{-}s}'$	$F_{V\text{-}o}'$	$F_{V\text{-}s}'$		$F_{V\text{-}o}'$	$F_{N\text{-}s}'$	$F_{N\text{-}o}$	$F_{V\text{-}o}'$
	$F_{N\text{-}s}'$		$\mathbf{F_{N\text{-}o}}$		$F_{V\text{-}s}'$	$F_{N\text{-}s}'$					$F_{V\text{-}s}'$

The features $F_{N\text{-}o}$ are then ordered as appropriate for object N-features in the higher clause in (91), as $F_{N\text{-}o} < F_{V\text{-}o}'$, so that *voggyu* moves to ^[$F_{V\text{-}o}'$, $F_{N\text{-}o}$] first, checking $F_{V\text{-}o}'$, and then the clitic *lu* moves to this head, left-adjoining, producing the proclisis in (88).

5. Conclusion

In the course of developing consistent feature-based accounts of clitic placement in a variety of contexts, including clitic climbing, the present chapter provides support (albeit, under a new implementation) for proposals of Madeira (1993), Manzini (1994), and Belletti (1999) that object clitics are Infl-oriented in varieties of Modern Italian, Spanish, and French, and that the alternations between proclisis and enclisis in different types of clauses depend on different sequences of verb and clitic movement to an appropriate Infl-head.

The effort to formulate feature-based accounts of clitic placement in a wide variety of different contexts with minimal appeal to construction-specific principles provided motivation or further support for certain general principles regulating the selection and distribution of features projected onto functional categories to check features on lexical items in a numeration. The Economy of Projection of Infl-Categories was found to underwrite an account of clitic placement with respect to the verb (proclisis versus enclisis) in terms of the difference in the availability of object V-features in finite and infinitival clauses, with direct consequences for the sequencing of verb and clitic movements in the two clause types which yield the observed facts. The Economy of Feature Projection was found to rule out theoretically unparsimonious accounts of clitic climbing which would project copies of features matching those of an object clitic in duplicate, on functional categories associated with the infinitive verb and, in the same derivation, on ones associated with the higher verb. Finally, a principle of Minimal Feature Ordering was found to underwrite an account of the fact that multiple object clitics have a fixed order with respect to one another in Greek finite clauses, but exhibit optionality in order with respect to one another in Greek gerunds and imperatives. The most general form of this principle was the following, repeated from (44b).

(92) *Minimal Feature Ordering*
The partial linear order defining the checking order of features in a numeration is minimal to determine a convergent derivation of a syntactic structure from the numeration.

The corollary of this required for the account of multiple object clitic placement in Greek was the following.

(93) *Minimal Feature Ordering: Corollary for N-features*
The partial linear order defining the checking order of features in a numeration does not specify the checking order of N-features with respect to one another, but only with respect to V-features.

The Minimal Feature Ordering principle was also appealed to in order to account for the fact that when a matrix of N-features matching those on an object clitic associates with a V-feature matrix of a higher verb, the relative checking order of the two feature matrices is not specified beforehand, but is determined upon association together as appropriate for features within a single clause. This, in turn, was taken to be a consequence of the Minimal Feature Ordering principle on the grounds that it would not be necessary to specify the checking order of all pairs of features in a numeration which will be projected across clausal boundaries; it suffices to specify feature orders on features which will be projected at the boundary of a clause and on features which will be projected within each clause. (The same would be true with complex nominals in place of clauses.) This is a second corollary of the Minimal Feature Ordering principle stated in its most general form in (92). This second corollary can be formulated more concisely in terms of the notion of a derivational phase, from Chomsky (2000, 2001). A derivational phase is, roughly, a set of derivational steps which effect the construction of a clause (or complex nominal); the equivalence is only rough since Chomsky defines a phase for the derivation of a clause in terms of the projection of *v*, T, and C. But making allowance for this disparity, the desired corollary can be understood to assert that features need to be ordered with respect to one another within a numeration only when they will be accessed during the same derivational phase, or at the edge of a phase, in the derivational transition from one phase to the next. This formulation is recorded in (94).

(94) *Minimal Feature Ordering: Corollary for phases*
Feature matrices F_i and F_j within a numeration are ordered with respect to one another only if there is a phase α such that F_i and F_j are both projected in α, or there are phases α and β such that β immediately follows α, and one of F_i and F_j is the last feature matrix projected in α, and the other is the first feature matrix projected in β.

To express this more casually, F_i and F_j within a numeration are ordered with respect to one another only if they are projected within the same derivational phase, or if they straddle a phase edge. There is no reason to think that there are no other corollaries of the general principle of Minimal Feature Ordering. Any such corollary should reflect a plausible respect in which the partial linear checking order can be partial; the empirical payoff of any such further corollary is a matter of discovery, to the extent that it might be found to play a role in feature-based syntactic analysis.

Notes

1. For discussion of imperatives in these languages, see section 2.3 below.
2. Example (1a) is from Manzini (1994: 300), (1b) is from Kayne (1991a: 648), and the example in (2) is from Lepschy and Lepschy (1988: 194).
3. Example (3a) is from Kayne (1991a: 648) and (3b) is from Manzini (1994: 300). Examples (5) and (6) are from Lepschy and Lepschy (1988: 120, 118), respectively.
4. Roberts (1994a) also assumes that object clitics adjoin to Agr in the phrase structure of Belletti (1990).
5. These representations assume that the clitic is generated as a DP, but that its final step of movement is as a head. This suggestion is made in Chomsky

(1995a) and adopted by a number of researchers. It will be adopted in the account developed here as well.

6. These structures are spelled out in detail by Belletti (1999). Arguments for the presence of a participial Agr, distinct from Agr_o, and other aspects of the participial structure given in (11), were also given by Uriagereka (1995b), Friedemann and Siloni (1993), and Laenzlinger (1993).
7. Uriagereka, but not Belletti, assumes that the clitic D takes an empty NP as complement. No position on this issue will be taken here.
8. This is a formulation of Kayne's (1991a) assumption that the finite verb moves through all higher Infl-heads.
9. The order in (15), and its counterpart for subject features on ^[$F_{V\text{-}s}$, $F_{N\text{-}s}$], is only operative if the N-features and the V-features are of the same strength, that is, both strong or both weak. In English finite clauses, for example, the N-features $F_{N\text{-}s}$ (whether subject φ-features, or an EPP feature) are strong, while the V-features $F_{V\text{-}s}$ are weak, so $F_{N\text{-}s}$ are checked before $F_{V\text{-}s}$; therefore, the ranking of V-features above N-features is not operative in such a case when they are not of the same strength.
10. Chapter 5 argues at length that [EPP] can be projected on its own as a functional head in certain reduced clauses in English, such as "bare infinitive" complements of perception verbs.
11. In some varieties of Romance, an object clitic can appear as enclitic on a participle, as in the following example from Franco-Provençal Valdôtain, cited in Roberts (1994b: 377), where SCL is a subject clitic:

    (i) *Pa gneun l'a vuu-me.*
    Nobody SCL-has seen-me

    As Roberts shows, the enclisis gives way to the more common pattern of proclisis to the auxiliary when no subject clitic is present. One account of the enclisis in (i) would be that the object clitic is not attracted to $F_{N\text{-}o}$, but rather to a feature on a lower functional head, closer to the projection of the participle. This might be an Agr head local to the participle (as proposed by Kayne 1989b for cases of participle agreement with a clitic in French), but distinct from Agr_o (as suggested for French participle agreement by Uriagereka 1995b), to which the participle moves. However, as Roberts stresses, the enclisis in forms like (i) is not accompanied by participle agreement in Valdôtain. A lower Agr head would therefore have no V-features for the participle, and so, by the Economy of Projection of Infl-Categories, it should not be projected. However, the object enclitic in (i) does seem to be positioned on a lower head than the tense and agreement heads. A clue to the status of the object clitic is the fact that the enclisis pattern in (i) is obtained only in the presence of a subject clitic doubling the subject. This suggests that the subject and object clitics in (i) are merely spell-outs of subject and object N-features on appropriate heads. If the object clitic in (i) is a spell-out of *v*, where its case is checked, then the movement of the participle to *v* will produce enclisis. In support of the supposition that the object enclitic in (i) is on a lower functional head than an object proclitic, there are cases of split clitics in participial clauses in Franco-Provençal Valdôtain, such as in (ii) below, cited by Kayne (1991a: 661) from Chenal (1986: 398, 399).

(ii) a. *T'an-* *të* *prèdzà-nen?*
you-DAT-have they spoken of-it
b. *T'an-* *të* *deut- lo?*
you-DAT-have they said it

The dative clitic behaves as expected here, left-adjoining to [Aux- Agr_o], that is, [Aux-^[$F_{V\text{-}o}$, $F_{N\text{-}o}$]], yielding proclisis. The other clitics are enclitics on the participle, suggesting that they are spelled-out on *v*, where they emerge as enclitics upon participle movement to *v*.

12. Example (23a) is from Sportiche (1996: 221), and (23b) from Kayne (1991a: 658). The examples in (24) are from Kayne (1991a: 648).
13. As noted by Pollock, the behavior described here for auxiliaries is shared by main verb *HAVE* and *BE*; as Pollock expresses the distinction, verbs with thematic roles (which he calls lexical verbs) have the behavior attributed here to main verbs, while verbs without thematic roles behave according to the description of auxiliaries.
14. This account is not directly compatible with Cinque's (1999) proposal that adverbs of a given class appear in the specifier of a particular functional head unless subject to topicalization or other movement operations. However, the bulk of Cinque's argument is distributional, and the restrictions on adverb position which he cites in support of it could be interpreted as demonstrating not that the adverb resides exactly in the specifier of a particular functional category, but that the functional head defines the locus of that class of adverb in phrase structure, relative to other classes of adverbs and other scope-bearing elements. This generalizes the possible attachment sites of the adverb slightly, making the proposal more in line with Travis' (1988) proposal that adverbs of a given class have a particular locus of attachment in a clause, rather than a particular phrase structure position.
15. If the floating $F_{N\text{-}o}$ feature matrix were to be projected with the lower ranked tense features, instead of with the higher ranked aspectual features, then it would be possible for a clitic, appearing in ^[$F_{V\text{-}T}$, $F_{N\text{-}o}$], to be separated from the infinitive verb, in Asp, by an adverbial adjoined to AspP. In Modern French, such a structure would presumably crash at the PF interface due to morpho-phonological requirements of the clitic. However, Kayne (1991a) notes that the order produced in this way, shown in (i) below, is attested in Old French, although it is antiquated in Modern French.

(i) ... *en* *bien* *parler* ...
of-it well to-speak

This suggests that Old French was more permissive in the association of the floating features, as well as in morpho-phonological conditions allowing the clitic to be separated from the verb.

16. See Uriagereka (1995b) for arguments for this position, including the availability of participle agreement in various varieties of Romance in forms such as unaccusatives and passives, in which Agr_O would not be expected to play a role. Within the theoretical context developed here, the participial Agr is a viable hypothesis for French, in contrast to Franco-Valdotâin, discussed in note 11 above, since the French participle exhibits agreement (with object clitics and other leftward-moved objects), which would result from checking V-feature(s), $F_{V\text{-}prt}$, against the participial Agr. Due to these V-features, the projection of the French participial Agr would accord with the Economy of Projection of Infl-Categories.
17. Sportiche (1996) addresses problems posed by the optionality of participle agreement for an analysis of the sort adopted here. For Sportiche, participle agreement is established in the spec-head relation at Agr_O, as part of an extensively worked out system of assumptions which differ significantly from those adopted here, with consequences for ordinary verb movement and clitic placement. On Sportiche's account, given the role assigned to Agr_O in participle agreement, Pollock-type distinctions in ordinary verb movement are made higher in the clause, leading to the postulation of additional Infl-level functional heads beyond the Agr_S-T-Agr_O-Asp/Agr_{prt} sequence adopted here (that is, reconstructed here in terms of projection of feature matrices).
18. Examples (35)–(36), (37a), (38)–(40) are from Zanuttini (1997: 143–144, 130, 132, 180); (37b) is from Martins (1994: 194).
19. In Italian and Spanish infinitival imperatives, discussed in Kayne (1991b) and Rooryck (1992), the imperative verb checks infinitival tense features $F_{V\text{-}T}$ as well as a low ranked [IMP] feature. This treatment will regard French infinitives used as instructions as morphologically and syntactically infinitive forms, not as morphologically and syntactically imperative. They exhibit proclisis (Jones 1996: 255), as is normal for French infinitives.
20. Zanuttini supposes that a supra-Infl feature must be checked in negative suppletive imperatives, as well as in positive true and suppletive imperatives. However, she assumes that Neg itself, rather than the verb, checks this feature in a negative imperative; as a result, the verb remains within the Infl system in negative imperatives. Our assumption that [NEG] is incompatible with [IMP] is a more straightforward way to explain why true imperatives cannot occur with preverbal negation, along the same lines according to which Laka (1990) assumes that [NEG] and [IMP] are mutually exclusive since they compete for the same site of expression in clausal phrase structure, Laka's Σ node. This

difference with Zanuttini's proposal does not have any evident empirical consequences, and we will follow Zanuttini's proposals regarding negative imperatives in all other respects, as discussed below.

21. The ACC-GEN order of enclitics on the auxiliary in the participial gerund in (52b) is good for some speakers, but not for others. For some speakers of each sort, the judgment is not very robust.
22. Rooryck assumes as well that [T-Agr_S] raises out of the embedded [$_{Agrs}$ cl-V_{inf}-T-Agr_S] to the higher verbal complex in order that the clitic, on a slight reformulation of Relativized Minimality, can antecedent-govern its trace within the embedded Agr_S complex; this effects tense coindexation of the embedded infinitive and the higher clause.
23. These categories are merged into the tree from right-to-left. For clarity, features not relevant to the present discussion are suppressed, and the features introduced by lexical items in the higher clause and their matching features are marked with primes. As usual, the top line is not part of the numeration, but is put in purely for expository convenience.
24. A version of this analysis, formulated within a precursor to the present framework, was suggested to me by Kazumi Matsuoka and Roger Martin.
25. Cases of past participle agreement between a clitic and a participle in the local clause under clitic climbing, alongside cases with agreement between a clitic and a participle in a higher clause, might make it look like there can be multiple functional categories in a numeration with N-features of the clitic in cases of clitic climbing. However, as discussed in section 4.2 below, these are not cases of duplication of N-features attracting the clitic; participle agreement is established with a local participial Agr node under XP-movement of the clitic through spec-AgrP in the course of its movement under attraction by N-features on a functional category within the local or a higher clause. Also, cases of clitic climbing in certain dialects of Italian in which a copy of the clitic appears in the local clause as well as in the higher clause might look like they are produced by a numeration containing duplicate copies of N-features attracting the clitic, but are best analyzed otherwise, as discussed in note 28 below.
26. Data in (63)–(71) are from Burzio (1986: 46, 53, 322–323, 327).
27. In a context such as (i) below, from Rizzi (1982: 4), where the lower verb takes *HAVE*, not *BE*, CA is not possible, so CC has no implications for CA in such a context.

    (i) *Gianni gli ha potuto parlare personalmente.*
    Gianni him.DAT has been-able to-speak personally.

28. Certain Northern Italian varieties exhibit examples of the form given in (i) below, in which, upon clitic climbing, an enclitic copy of the clitic is left in the lower clause. (These facts were called to my attention by an anonymous reviewer.)

(i) *Lo voglio vederlo.*
it I-want to-see-it

It might be argued that the enclitic order in the complement in (i) implicates functional structure in the infinitive complement, contrary to the view of restructuring infinitives as purely lexical, adopted here. But appealing to Chomsky's (1993, 1995a, 1995b) copy theory of traces, the lower copy of the clitic could be simply a spelled-out trace of the climbed clitic in the object position to the infinitival verb, where the clitic is generated. Upon phonological merger with the adjacent verb, the spelled-out copy would be pronounced as an enclitic on the verb.

29. Examples (76a–c) are from Roberts (1994a: 223); (77a,b) and (79) are from Kayne (1989a: 245–246); and (78a,b) are from Rooryck's (1994) example (4).
30. Rooryck's account of (79) would apparently apply as well to Spanish examples of this sort, presented and discussed by LaPolla (1988). As Rooryck notes, the position of Italian *che* 'what' in the clausal syntax on his account is similar to that proposed by Bouchard and Hirschbüler (1986) for its French cognate *que*.
31. A reviewer urges consideration here of the Franco-Provençal split-clitic data cited in Kayne (1991a), discussed in note 11 (example (ii)) above. These data involve split clitics in a participial clause, not under clitic climbing of the sort addressed here, out of complements of lexical restructuring verbs. The difference, as conceived here, is that in the participial case, one clitic is attracted to $F_{V\text{-}o}$, and, at least in Franco-Provençal, the other clitic is spelled-out on *v*. Split clitics are not obtained with clitic climbing out of complements of lexical restructuring verbs of the sort considered here in languages with infinitive-clitic order. Split clitics are attested with clitic climbing out of complements of lexical restructuring verbs in certain dialects with clitic-infinitive order, that is, with proclisis of object clitics in infinitival clauses; these are mentioned, and relevant sources are cited, in Kayne (1989a). These dialects are obviously very different from those discussed here and would require a close, detailed examination beyond the scope of the present work.
32. Burzio (1986: 369) reports the (marginal) agreement of a clitic with a higher participle upon clitic climbing given in (i) below, and a reviewer of an early version of this chapter notes the agreement of a clitic with the lower participle in (ii).

(i) *Maria li è ?andata/??andati a prendere.*
Maria them *essere* gone-FEM/gone-PL to fetch

(ii) *Li vorrei aver visti.*
them.MASC.PL I-would-like to-have seen-MASC.PL

Following Kayne (1989b), we take agreement between a clitic and a participle to be obtained as a consequence of clitic movement past the participle, except that we cast the proposal in feature checking terms and require it, more specifically, to be the result of clitic movement (in its XP-movement phase) through spec-AgrP of an Agr that attracts the participle. The agreement with the subject in (i) would be the normal consequence of the raising of the subject of an unaccusative verb. The participle agreement with the clitic in (i) and (ii) might be established by clitic movement through the spec of an Agr or other head more local to the participle than the projection site of $F_{V\text{-}o}$ (such as the Agr postulated in French participle agreement in section 2.2 above, following Kayne 1989b, and relying on the proposal of Uriagereka 1995b that this Agr is distinct from Agr_O). However, the presence of such a participial Agr in (ii) would mean that the restructuring infinitive in (ii) is not entirely lexical. The claim that restructuring infinitives are entirely lexical would therefore have to be amended to the claim that they lack infinitival tense features and any other basic clausal features with which object N-features might associate, while allowing participial features. The participial Agr, on this view, would constitute inflection for the participial structure, not for the infinitival clause. The lack of clausal inflectional structure, as opposed to participial inflectional structure, would then be considered definitive of restructuring infinitives. Thus, the agreement of the higher participle with the clitic under clitic climbing in (i) and (ii) does not necessarily have anything to do with the mechanism driving clitic climbing, namely, the association of $F_{N\text{-}o}$ features (matching those of the clitic) with V-features of the higher clause, but might be a consequence of clitic movement past intervening Agr heads on its way to $F_{N\text{-}o}$ projected with V-features in the higher clause. Thus, the mechanisms of clitic climbing proposed here do not necessarily preclude clitic agreement with a participle, in either the higher clause or the infinitival complement.

33. Except in the special circumstances of Salentino; see section 4.5 below.
34. Terzi gives (87) (her (35)) with the opposite order of the lower *pro* and the clitic. The order has been changed here to reflect the proposals about clitic placement developed here.

Chapter 5
Tenseless clauses and coordination

1. Accusative subject conjuncts

1.1. Properties of the accusative subject conjunct construction

In colloquial (North American) English, a small clause-like structure, with an accusative subject, and a verb without tense or subject agreement inflection, can occur in coordinate structures such as those in (1)–(2) below, with the interpretations indicated.

(1) *He should check out the book tomorrow and her return it on Saturday.*
'It should be the case that: he checks out the book tomorrow, and she returns it on Saturday.'

(2) a. *He won't check out the book tomorrow and her return it three months later.*
'It won't be the case that: he checks out the book tomorrow and she returns it three months later.'
b. *He didn't check out the book a week ago and me return it yesterday.*
'It wasn't the case that: he checked out the book a week ago and I returned it yesterday.'
c. *We can't redirect seven different shipments and them be totally unaware of it.*
'It can't be the case that: we redirect seven different shipments and they remain totally unaware of it.'

Nonpronominal NPs and DPs can occur in the position of the accusative subject, although they won't show accusative case.

(3) a. *He should check out the book tomorrow, and Susan return it on Saturday.*

b. *He won't check out the book tomorrow and the other guy return it three months later.*
c. *We can't redirect seven different shipments and the guard be totally unaware of it.*

It remains to determine what constituents are actually coordinated in these examples. For descriptive purposes, we can refer to the full clause which appears first in linear order as the first clause, and the small clause-like second clause, which is the second conjunct of the coordinate structure, as the ASC, for "Accusative Subject Conjunct." The distinctive construction in (1)–(3) will be called the ASC construction.

The ASC structure is particularly natural with negation or a modal auxiliary in the first clause, as in the examples above. It also occurs when the first clause is perfect or progressive. In (4), where the first clause has perfective aspect, the second clause, while showing no tense, has a perfect participle form of the verb.

(4) a. *He has checked out the book and her returned it, just as he said would happen.*
b. *He has checked out the book on Friday and her returned it on Saturday many times in the past.*
c. *He has often checked out the book on Friday and her returned it on Saturday.*
d. *We have often redirected a shipment and them been totally unaware of it.*

In (5a), where the first clause is progressive, the second has a progressive participle; and in (5b), where the first clause is perfect progressive, the second clause has morphology for the perfect and the progressive, but, as in (4), lacks perfective *have*.[1]

(5) a. *He is checking out the book on Tuesday and her returning it on Saturday.*
b. *He has been stealing silverware and her been covering up for him for years.*

But the ASC is impossible when the first clause lacks an overt auxiliary altogether. This is shown by the examples in (6)–(7) below, which are ungrammatical when the second clause is untensed as in ASC examples above, and equally ungrammatical when the second clause has tense matching that of the first clause.

(6) a. * *He checked out the book on Tuesday and her return(ed) it on Saturday.*
b. * *We redirected seven different shipments and them be/were totally unaware of it.*

(7) a. * *Every week, he checks out the book on Thursday and her return(s) it on Saturday.*
b. * *We redirect three shipments per day and them be/are totally unaware of it.*

However, auxiliary *will*, used to express periphrastic future (but historically derived from a modal) does license an ASC, as shown in (8).

(8) *He will check out the book tomorrow and her return it on Saturday.*
'It will be the case that: He checks out the book tomorrow and she returns it on Saturday.'

Thus, the second conjunct of the ASC is licensed not just within the scope of negation or a modal auxiliary: it can occur whenever the first clause has an overt auxiliary of any sort.

When semantically scopal elements such as negation or a modal auxiliary appear in the first clause, the effect of the ASC is to give this element scope over the second conjunct as well as the first. In a structure of full IP coordination, such as (9)–(10), this does not happen.

(9) a. *He must check out the book tomorrow and she might return it on Saturday.*
b. *We should redirect seven different shipments and they must be totally unaware of it.* [*it* = the event of us redirecting seven shipments]

(10) a. *He won't check out the book tomorrow and she will return it on Saturday.*
b. # *We can't redirect seven different shipments and they must be totally unaware of it.* [*it* = the event of us redirecting seven shipments]

(9a,b) might be understood in such a way that the possibility expressed by the second clause is conditional upon the realization of the event described in the first clause. But the second clause is not interpreted with the modal force of the modal verb of the first clause: (9a) does not mean that the event of her returning the book on Saturday is something which the speaker is asserting must happen; and in (9b), the situation of them being totally unaware of the redirection of shipments is not something which the speaker is asserting should happen. In (10a,b), the second clause is outside the scope of negation, not within it. As a result, (10a) is only sensible if it is known that she has checked out the book independently of him, or that she will do so before Saturday. And because the second clause of (10b) is outside the scope of negation, the pronoun *it* in (10b) does not have a suitable event antecedent through which it can have the referent indicated by anaphoric linking. Contrast (10a,b) with parallel examples involving VP coordination within the scope of negation:

(11) a. *He won't check out the book tomorrow and give it to Bill to photocopy.*
'It won't be the case that: he checks out the book tomorrow and gives it to Bill to photocopy.'
b. *We can't redirect seven different shipments and expect them to remain unaware of it.*
'It can't be the case that: We redirect seven different shipments and they remain unaware that we have done so.'

So the ASC structures in (1)–(2) serve as a concise means to give the modal or negation scope over the entire coordinate structure, including the accusative subject of the ASC. As a result, the ASC cannot have an independent modal: contrast (9a,b) with the examples in (12) below.

(12) a. * *He must check out the book tomorrow and her might return it on Saturday.*
b. * *We can't redirect seven different shipments and them could be totally unaware of it.*

Could the structures in (1)–(2) be produced by ellipsis (or gapping), as indicated in the structure (13) for (1)?

(13) *He should check out the book tomorrow and ~~he should~~ [have] her return it on Saturday.*

This involves a simple coordination of two IPs, each starting with the subject *he* and the modal *should*; the repeated material in the second clause would be elided in the derivation of (1). In addition, the causative *have* in (13) would have to delete in the derivation of (1), but be interpreted implicitly. But on this derivation, (1) would have the meaning given in (14) below.

(14) 'It should be the case that: he checks out the book tomorrow and he has her return it on Saturday.'

And this is incorrect. The meaning specified in (14) invokes causal power on the part of the referent of *he* in bringing about the state of affairs in which she returns the book on Saturday. But (1) can be used to assert simply that it should be the case that there is an event of him checking out the book tomorrow, followed by an event in which she returns it on Saturday, without necessarily imputing any causal power to the male person under discussion in bringing about this second event. For example, (1) could be a statement of a belief in pre-established harmony, with *should* interpreted as alethic modality. Likewise, on an account based on ellipsis, (15) would have to mean the same as (16).

(15) *He won't check out the book tomorrow and her return it on Saturday.*
'It won't be the case that: he checks out the book tomorrow and she returns it on Saturday.'

(16) *He won't check out the book tomorrow and ~~he won't~~ [have] her return it on Saturday.*
'It won't be the case that: he checks out the book tomorrow and he has her return it on Saturday.'

But (16) has the meaning indicated below the example sentence, which need not be the meaning of (15). So an account based on ellipsis of the sort exhibited in (13) and (16) is incorrect.

Examples corresponding to some of those in (1)–(2), but with a nominative subject in place of the accusative, are marginally acceptable. This is the case with (17) below.

(17) *He should check out the book tomorrow, and she return it on Saturday.*
'He should check out the book tomorrow, and she should return it on Saturday.'

Similar examples corresponding to (2a,b,c) run into coherence issues if we understand the event described in the second conjunct to be dependent on the occurrence of the event whose occurrence the first clause effectively denies. But similar examples without this drawback can be constructed, such as (18).

(18) *He won't tunnel under the moat and she climb the tower.*
'He won't tunnel under the moat and she won't climb the tower.'

To the extent that (17)–(18) are good, they favor a slight pause after the subject of the second clause, unlike the corresponding examples with accusative subjects. There is also a difference in meaning: to the extent that it is good, (17) means that he should check out the book tomorrow, and that she should return it on Saturday, with the force of the modal, *should*, applying independently to each of the two subjects; this is distinct from the interpretation of (1), which can be used to assert that the entire situation of him checking out the book and her returning it on Saturday is one which should obtain. The examples in (17)–(18) can, in fact, be derived as products of ellipsis.

(19) a. *He should check out the book tomorrow, and she ~~should~~ return it on Saturday.*
b. *He won't tunnel under the moat and she ~~won't~~ climb the tower.*

These exemplify a quite different phenomenon, more literary in flavor than examples of the type in (1)–(2), and more readily accounted for theoretically, so they will not be discussed further here.

Another variant of the pattern discussed to this point is provided by examples in which the first clause is infinitival.

(20) *To check out the book tomorrow and her return it on Saturday would be a bad idea.*
'To arrange a situation in which one checks out the book tomorrow and she returns it on Saturday would be a bad idea.'

(21) a. *To check out the book tomorrow and her ask for that very book on Saturday would be a great coincidence.*
'It would be a great coincidence for one to check out the book tomorrow and her to ask for the same book on Saturday.'
b. *We were amazed to check out the book on Tuesday and her ask for that very book on Saturday.*
'We were amazed that it transpired that we checked out the book on Tuesday and she asked for that very book on Saturday.'

(22) *I want him to check out the book tomorrow and her return it on Saturday.*
'I want it to be the case that: he checks out the book tomorrow and she returns it on Saturday.'

We can assimilate these to examples with a modal auxiliary in the full clause by identifying infinitival tense as a modal operator. The interpretation of infinitival tense as expressing a futurate unrealized eventuality puts it in a natural class with the standard modals and futurate *will*, making this identification plausible. Thus, the class of elements licensing ASCs includes infinitival tense. So the class of licensing elements is not just the set of overt auxiliaries, but, more broadly, the set of overt elements occurring in T^{o}.

A mechanical account of (20)–(22) would involve elision of the infinitival *for* complementizer and the infinitival *to* marker in the second clause; on this view, the second conjunct in (20)–(22) would be an infinitival CP. In particular, (20) would be derived from (23).

(23) *To check out the book tomorrow and ~~for~~ her ~~to~~ return it on Saturday would be a bad idea.*
'It would be a bad idea for one to check out the book tomorrow and for her to return it on Saturday.'

But this proposal fails to account for scope facts in examples such as (24) under the interpretation indicated, on which she is responsible for collating and reporting the information collected by others. On this interpretation, the ASC clause in (24) is within the scope of the negative subject, *nobody*.

(24) *For nobody to get the information and her report it would be unfortunate.*
'It would be unfortunate if it is not the case that: someone gets the information and she reports it.'

If the analysis in (23) is correct, (24) should be derived from the structure in (25), and should have the same meaning.

(25) *For nobody to get the information and for her to report it would be unfortunate.*
'It would be unfortunate if nobody got the information and if she were to report it.'

But (24) doesn't mean the same as (25), and the structure in (25) would not put the second clause within the scope of the negative subject of the first clause. As a result, (25) is incoherent on the understanding that she is supposed to collate and report information collected by the others, since *it* would have no referent if nobody gets the information, whereas (24) is fully coherent on that understanding. Thus the proposal in (23) should be rejected.

Rejecting a simple derivation-by-ellipsis account of (20)–(22), the ASC construction in these sentences looks very much like those observed in (1)–(3).

Turning now to an investigation of the coordination site in examples of the sort in (1)–(2), Aux-fronting in I-to-C movement shows that the coordination site of the ASC is below the position of I′ in the first clause.

(26) a. *Could he check out the book tomorrow and her return it on Saturday?*
'Could it be the case that: he checks out the book tomorrow and she returns it on Saturday?'

b. *Didn't he check out the book a week ago and me return it yesterday?*
'Wasn't it the case that: he checked out the book a week ago, and I returned it yesterday?'

c. *Can't we redirect seven different shipments and them remain unaware of it?*
'Couldn't it be the case that: we redirect seven different shipments and they remain unaware of it?'

Further evidence of the low coordination site of the ASC comes from examples in which the subject of the first clause has scope over the ASC. An example of this was seen in (24) above, but the scope of the subject of the first clause is revealed even more clearly by licensing of a negative polarity item (NPI) in the ASC.

(27) a. *Nobody had better check out a book today and anybody return it on Saturday.*
'It had better not be the case that: someone checks out a book today and somebody returns it on Saturday.'

b. *Nobody had better steal a book and her lift a finger to help them.*
'It had better not be the case that: someone steals a book and she does anything to help them.'

In (27a,b), *anybody* and *lift a finger* have negative polarity interpretations, indicating that they are within the scope of negation. These results are not obtained when a clause coordinates with another at the level of IP (or higher), as shown in (28).

(28) a. # *Nobody had better check out a book today and anybody had better return it on Saturday.*

b. # *Nobody had better steal a book and she had better lift a finger to help them.*

In (28a), *anybody* does not have an NPI interpretation; furthermore, since processing of the first clause is completed at the end of the first IP conjunct, the second IP conjunct is not within the scope of the modality of the first clause, and so the second conjunct, referring to the return of a book, is not sensible. In (28b), the expression *lift a finger* does not have its NPI interpretation; furthermore, since the second clause in (28b) is not within the scope of the subject and modality of the first, the pronoun *them* cannot be interpreted as bound by the subject of *steal*.

However, it is also possible to show that the coordination site is higher than the main VP, and indeed, higher than NegP. Examples such as those in (1)–(2) are obtained with overt aspectual material (perfective or the progressive) in the ASC, as in (29)–(30) below.

(29) a. *He should have checked out the book on Tuesday and her have returned it on Saturday. That would have left everyone happy.*
  b. *He won't have checked out the book on Thursday and her have returned it on Friday. That wouldn't have left them with time to get the information they needed from it.*
  c. *We can't have redirected seven different shipments and them not have noticed it.*

(30) a. *He should be checking out the first copy of the book and her returning the second copy at the same time.*
  b. *He won't be checking out the book on Tuesday and her returning it on Saturday. That plan has been scrapped in favor of a new one.*
  c. *They can't have been redirecting seven different shipments and the guards have been watching the whole time unawares.*
  d. *He may have been being followed and her have been following him.*

The second conjunct in these examples carries its own marking for aspect (perfective, progressive, or, as in (30c), perfect progressive). The aspect of the second conjunct might match that of the first clause for purposes of parallelism under coordination, but they can diverge when the result is sensibly interpretable, as in (31)–(33).

(31) a. *He should check out the book on Tuesday and her have already returned it on Wednesday. Only in this way can they get the information they need, while making the book available for use by others in time for the exam.*

b. *He won't check out the book on Tuesday and her have returned it already on Wednesday. They couldn't process the information in the book that quickly.*

(32) a. *He should check out the book on Tuesday and her be returning it when the library opens first thing Wednesday morning.*

b. *He won't check out the book on Tuesday and her be returning it when the library opens on Wednesday. We have discarded that plan.*

(33) *To submit the report tomorrow and her have already countered it would undermine our credibility.*

Thus, the ASC in examples such as (1)–(2) can have aspectual material which matches that in the first clause, or independent aspectual material. Furthermore, the ASC can have an independent clausal negation, as shown in (34) below.

(34) a. *He should check out the book tomorrow, and her not return it for six months. That will teach the library a lesson!*
'It should be the case that: he checks out the book tomorrow, and she doesn't return it until six months later.'

b. *He won't have checked out the book and given it to her, and her not ever have returned it. The two of them are better coordinated than that.*
'It couldn't have been the case that: he checked out the book and gave it to her, and she never returned it.'

c. *We can't have redirected seven different shipments and them not have noticed it.*
'It can't be the case that: we redirected seven different shipments, and they didn't notice it.'

d. *He may have been following her and her not have seen him.*
'It may have been the case that: he was following her and she didn't see him.'

e. *To submit the report tomorrow and her not have read it beforehand would be irresponsible.*
'It would be irresponsible to allow it to be the case that: one submits the report tomorrow when she has not read it beforehand.'

Looking just at (34a), one might suspect that the negation in the second conjunct is an instance of constituent negation on the V or VP, rather than clausal negation. But (34b–e) show that a full, clausal negation can occur in this position.

The examples in (31)–(34) show that the ASC has at least the phrase structure of an AspP (ProgP or PerfP) or NegP. Furthermore, these examples serve to disconfirm a simple and theoretically natural hypothesis for the syntactic structure of examples such as (1)–(2). Looking at (1)–(2) and the other early examples, it would be natural to suppose that the ASC is a bare VP with a subject in spec-VP receiving default accusative case. This would comport with widely accepted accounts of child language data for young children (typically of age 1;10 to 2;6) in Radford's (1990) VP stage, whose utterances typically consist of a VP with uninflected verb, sometimes accompanied by a subject, and sometimes not. When the subject is a pronoun, it typically exhibits accusative or genitive case (see Vainikka 1993/94 and Chapter 7 below). The specifier of the main VP is accordingly taken to be a position of default accusative case for this stage of child language. In light of this account of child language facts, it is reasonable to propose that the accusative subject in the ASC of (1)–(2) is likewise a recipient of a default accusative case. In fact, this proposal will be adopted in section 1.3 below. But there has to be more to the account since in (31)–(34) the subject of the ASC cannot surface in the specifier of the main VP, and in the examples in (34), the subject cannot surface in the spec of any VP since it appears before a clausal negation.

It is easy to see that the accusative case on the subject of the ASC is not assigned or checked by Exceptional Case Marking (ECM). In the examples with transitive verbs in the first clause, the accusative case of the first clause is checked by the object of that verb. Furthermore, ASC structures are obtained with an unaccusative verb in the first clause, as in (35).

(35) *He must arrive late and her pretend not to notice him.*
'It must be the case that: he arrives late, and she pretends not to notice him.'

Altogether, the facts regarding the ASC construction given so far present a paradox. Most of the facts exhibit scope of the first clause tense, negation, and subject over the ASC clause, showing that the ASC should be coordinated below Tense, negation and the subject of the first clause. Yet the facts in (29c) and (31)–(34) show that the ASC can have its own independent negation and its own independent aspect, and these, along with (29a,b) and (30), show that the subject of the ASC appears in a position external to the main VP of that clause, and external to aspectual auxiliaries and clausal negation. How can the ASC be coordinated with the first clause at a position below Neg, yet (1.) have its own clausal negation, and (2.) have its subject appear in the specifier of a functional projection above the lexical projections of its clause, and above its local Neg? Furthermore, how can the accusative case feature on this subject be checked, given that it is not in an ECM environment? Finally, why is an overt tense element required to appear on T^{o} in the first clause of the ASC construction?

The surface position of the subject of the ASC, outside the projections of its lexical categories and outside its aspectual and Neg projections, indicates that the ASC has a functional category (at least one) above Neg. The identity of this category (or these categories) is a question which we can add to those raised in the previous paragraph.

1.2. The structure of coordination in the ASC construction

One horn of the dilemma sketched above is that the ASC, which has a subject in the specifier of a functional category and which can have its own negation, should have some clausal structure. This favors coordination of supra-Neg functional categories at a mid or fairly high position in the first clause. The second horn of the dilemma is that the ASC cannot have an independent T node supporting a nominative case feature for its subject, and must be within the scope of negation in the first clause. This favors coordination of sub-Neg categories at a relatively low point in the first clause.

Johannessen (1998) develops a theory of coordinate structures which responds to this sort of dilemma, as well as to other puzzles about coordination. An instance of this sort of dilemma, which can serve to help motivate the mechanisms of her theory of coordinate structures, is presented by the interrogative in (36) below, one of many apparent violations of Ross's

(1967) Coordinate Structure Constraint (CSC) discussed by Lakoff (1986); contrast with a typical violation of the CSC in (37).

(36) *What kind of herbs can you eat and not get cancer?*

(37) (from: *Sam likes surfing and lives in a VW van.*)
a. * *What does Sam like and live(s) in a VW van?*
b. * *In what does Sam like surfing and live?*

On the one hand, (36) appears to involve a coordination of two VPs (if *not* is a form of local, or constituent, negation), or a coordination of two categories just below T in the hierarchical structure of the clause, specifically, coordination below the site which modal *can* occupied before it raised to C. But on this structure, shown in (38) with the coordinate structure indicated neutrally as 'CoP', the *wh*-phrase is extracted out of the first of the coordinated constituents, and not the second, a violation of the Coordinate Structure Constraint.

(38) [$_{CP}$ *what kind of herbs* [$_{C}$ *can*] [$_{IP}$ *you* t_T [$_{CoP}$ [*eat* t_{wh}] [$_{Co'}$ *and* [*not get cancer*]]]]]

On the other hand, (36) could involve coordination at a much higher level, a coordination of two CPs, so that the *wh*-chain is contained entirely within one conjunct, thus avoiding any violation of the CSC. The second conjunct can be construed as a full CP if it contains material deleted under identity, as shown in (39). The problem with (39) is that the *wh*-phrase does not have scope over both conjuncts, the second as well as the first, as it should.

(39) [$_{CoP}$ [$_{CP}$ *what kind of herbs* [$_{C}$ *can*] [$_{IP}$ *you* t_T *eat* t_{wh}]] [$_{Co'}$ [$_{Co}$ *and*] [$_{CP}$ [$_{C}$ ~~*can*~~] [$_{IP}$ ~~*you*~~ t_T *not get cancer*]]]]

A third structure, similar to (39) but with coordination at the level of C′, would be a structure of across-the-board extraction of the *wh*-expression *what kind of herbs*; this is incorrect since the *wh*-expression is not being extracted out of the second conjunct at all.

Johannessen (1998: 229–230) resolves this dilemma by generating coordinate structures with shared material, such as (39), and deriving a structure in which anything preceding the shared material within the CoP gets scope over the entire structure through an operation of tree restructuring. In particular, (36) is generated as a coordination of two CPs in a right-branching structure of coordination with the coordinate particle as head. (See Munn 1987, Munn 1993, and Grootveld 1992 for further support for such a structure of coordination.) The category of the projections of the coordinate particle, Co′ and CoP, are indexed for the category of the coordinated constituents.[2]

(40)

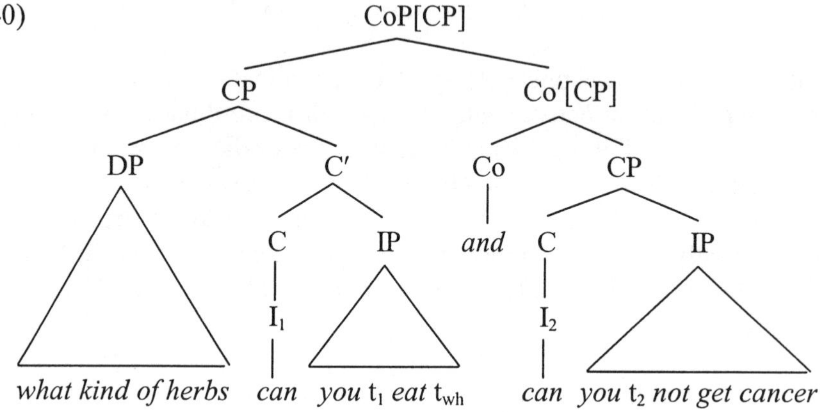

Restructuring applies so that the coordinate structure begins at C′, of which the shared material *can you* is the left-periphery in (40); with deletion-under-identity of this shared material in the second conjunct, the tree in (41) is obtained.

(41)

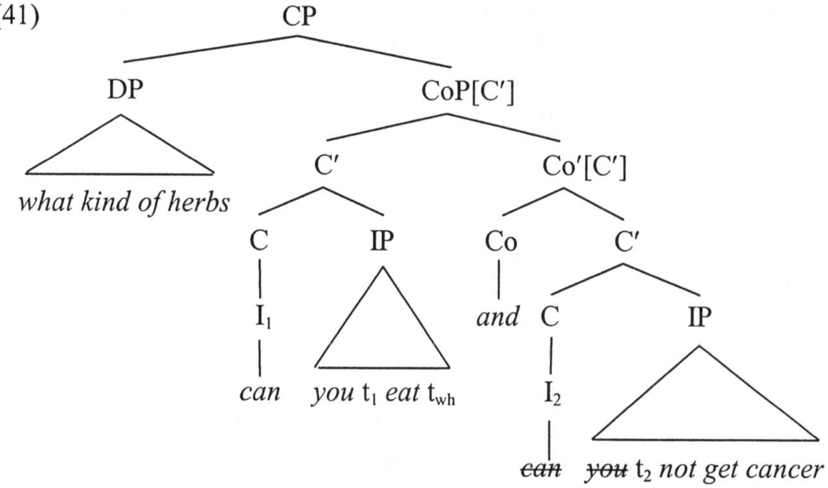

Critically, although (41) looks like a CSC violation, it was derived without movement of a constituent over the boundary of a conjunct in a coordination structure at any point in the derivation. Provided the tree restructuring process which converts (40) to (41) can be confined to use in cases which involve relations of causation, logical dependence, or temporal succession of the sort characterizing the Lakoff examples, this derivation circumvents the CSC for such examples while leaving it in force for examples such as (37) above. Furthermore, the tree restructuring operation proposed by Johannessen embodies a choice to keep the syntactic category of the coordinated constituents essentially unchanged between the input tree and the output tree by having the operation output a structure coordinating the largest possible constituents.[3]

An alternative formulation of the tree restructuring operation would output a structure in which the shared material would be given scope over the entire CoP, along with material preceding the shared material, by trimming the phrase structure of the two conjuncts to prune out the shared material and its associated phrase structure. Returning to (36), the structure in (39) would be formed through movement and merger as before. Taking (39) as input, the alternative formulation of the tree restructuring operation would give the shared material *can you*, and its associated phrase structure, scope over the coordinate structure CoP, while trimming the conjuncts to VP (or VP and NegP, if *not* is clausal negation). The resulting output is the tree shown in (42), which is just (38), but derived without the CSC violation.

(42) $[_{CP}$ *what kind of herbs* $[_{C}$ *can*$]$ $[_{IP}$ *you* t_T $[_{CoP}$ $[$*eat* $t_{wh}]$ $[_{Co'}$ *and* $[$*not get cancer*$]]]]]$

The additional burden of this approach over Johannessen's is to specify that the VP [eat t_{wh}] and the constituent [not get cancer] are suitable for coordination. But this follows from compatibility of semantic function, and should not need a special syntactic specification; in this respect, it is similar to standard instances of coordination of unlike categories, such as, *She is very smart and an excellent engineer*, or, *The recorder is ready and on the table*. The alternative formulation of the tree restructuring operation will be invoked here, but the consequences of reverting to Johannessen's formulation will be explored along the way.

The tree restructuring operation is constrained by the fact that the shared material must be at the left periphery of the right conjunct. But it must also be constrained by the specific semantic relationships involved in an example such as (36). (Following Kehler 2002, these semantic relationships might, in fact, amount to conditions of textual coherence.) Clearly the restructuring of coordination cannot apply in (37). We don't want to claim that whenever we generate a coordination $[[\alpha[\beta\delta]]$ and $[\beta\gamma]]$, for constituents α, β, δ, and γ, where α c-commands $[\beta\delta]$ and β c-commands δ in the first conjunct, and β c-commands γ in the second conjunct, we can (optionally) reformulate it as $\alpha[\beta[\delta$ and $\gamma]]$. However, we do want to claim that this restructuring can occur when $[\alpha[\beta\delta]]$ and $[\beta\gamma]$ describe coherent parts of a complex event or state. This coherent part structure on events or states is what distinguishes (36) from (37), and it characterizes the relationship between the events described by the first clause and the ASC clause in an ASC coordinate structure.

Returning to the problem at hand, (43) below can be generated as (44), where X is the functional category in whose specifier the subject of the ASC will surface.

(43) *He should check out the book and her return it.*
'It should be the case that: he checks out the book and she returns it.'

(44)

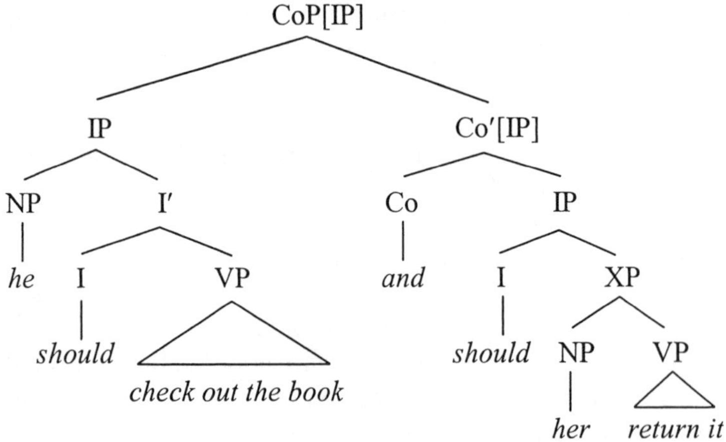

XP is suitable for coordination with functional projections between VP and T. Given that the two IPs in (44) describe coherent parts of a complex event, tree restructuring can apply under the alternative formulation given above, lifting the shared material and everything before it to a position having scope over the entire coordinate structure; this yields the tree in (45), where YP represents the functional layer between VP and T in the first clause.

(45)

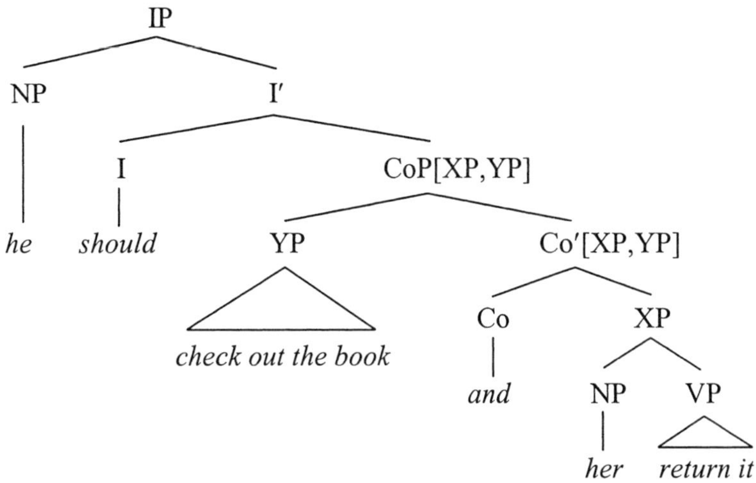

Likewise, (2a), repeated in (46) below, will be generated as (47), which, with tree restructuring and deletion, produces the structure in (48).

(46) *He won't check out the book tomorrow and her return it three months later.*

(47)

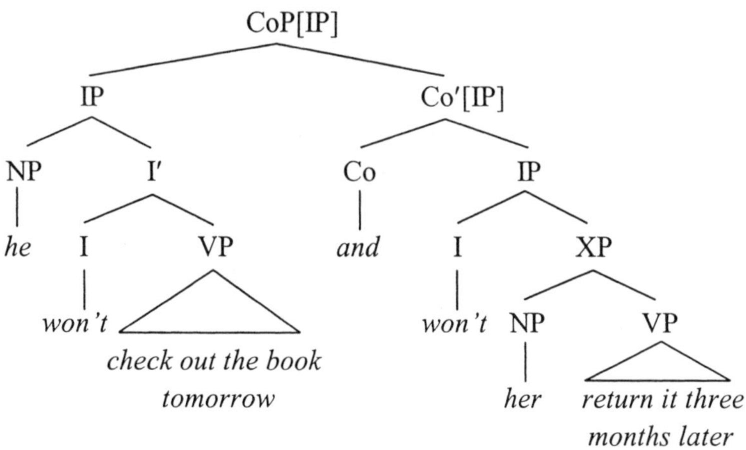

(48)

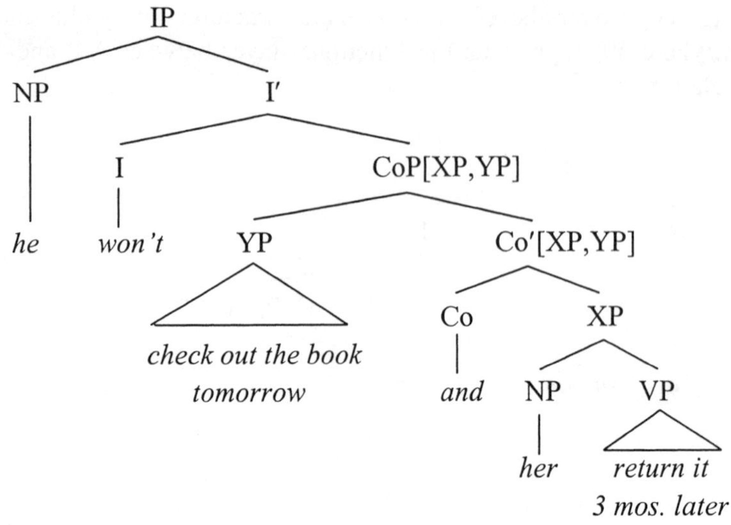

These structures account for why negation or a modal auxiliary have scope over the ASC clause in examples such as (1)–(3): these elements precede the shared material and are given a position c-commanding CoP by the tree restructuring operation. Similarly, the subject of the first clause is elevated to a position c-commanding the whole CoP, giving the subject scope over the ASC, accounting for (24) and (27). By merging an interrogative C to the output of the tree restructuring of the IPs, I-to-C movement can take place in examples such as (26) without violating the CSC. Finally, in these structures, the ASC is an XP containing aspectual auxiliaries and, potentially, Neg, accounting for the examples in (29)–(34).

Before turning in section 1.3 below to questions concerning the internal structure of XP in (44)–(45) and (47)–(48), note that facts of pronoun and r-expression binding provide further evidence that the ASC is within the scope of the subject of the first clause. This is shown by the Binding Theory Condition B and Condition C effects in (49) below.

(49) a. * *Max*$_i$ *should check out the book today and him*$_i$ *return it on Saturday.*

b. * *He*$_i$ *should check out the book today and Max*$_i$ *return it on Saturday.*

Contrast (49b) with results when the second clause is a full, finite clause, as in (50).

(50) a. *He$_i$ should check out the book today and Max$_i$ should return it on Saturday.*
b. *He$_i$ should check out the book today and Max$_i$ should study it all night.*

Interestingly, a reflexive subject of the ASC clause fares no better than a pronoun.

(51) * *Max$_i$ should check out the book today and himself$_i$ return it on Saturday.*

This follows if anaphor binding relies on a form of A-movement of features (or LF A-movement) to the antecedent, as discussed in Chomsky (1993, 1995b, 2000); for movement is not possible out of the ASC: the ASC remains wholly coordinated throughout the derivation discussed above, and movement of anything out of it therefore violates the Coordinate Structure Constraint.

If we use Johannessen's (1998) formulation of the tree restructuring operation, with (44) as input for the structure of (43), we obtain the output tree given in (52) below, rather than that in (45).

(52) [$_{\text{IP}}$ *he* [$_{\text{CoP[I']}}$ [$_{\text{I'}}$ *should check out the book*] [$_{\text{Co'}}$ *and* [$_{\text{I'}}$ ~~*should*~~ *her return it*]]]]

The effects of this depend on the nature of the elision process. If the modal auxiliary in the second conjunct in (52) is deleted entirely, without recoverability, then, since the common material is not exported on Johannessen's formulation of tree restructuring, the modal in the first conjunct will not have scope over the second conjunct, contrary to fact. If the modal in the second conjunct has only its phonetic matrix deleted, so that it is semantically interpreted as present, then (52) is interpreted as a conjunction of modal statements: it should be the case that he checks out the book, and it should be the case that she returns it. This is semantically coherent, but, although the distinction is somewhat subtle, this is not quite the correct interpretation of (43). The difference is roughly as follows. The interpretation of (43) can be represented as in (53) below, asserting the existence of a complex event consisting of two, related, parts, one in which he checks out the book, and another in which she returns it. (x_1 and x_2 are constants determined by pronominal reference, and b a constant determined by definite description.)

(53) should ($[\exists e, e', e'']$ $[(e = e' + e'') \wedge \text{check-out}\,(x_1, b, e') \wedge \text{return}\,(x_2, b, e'')]$)

In contrast, (52) with parallel modals, would be interpreted as:

(54) should ($[\exists e]$ $[\text{check-out}\,(x_1, b, e)$) $\wedge$ should ($[\exists e']$ $[\text{return}\,(x_2, b, e')]$)

The interpretation in (54) does not constrain the two events to be components of a larger coherent event, as (53) does. Thus, Johannessen's formulation of the tree restructuring operation would not yield results as satisfactory as those obtained under the alternative formulation presented above.

1.3. The internal structure of the ASC clause

Finally, what sort of clausal structure is the XP in (44)–(45) and (47)–(48)? The head X doesn't fit into the standard inventory of fixed functional categories, {C, Agr_S, T, Agr_O, Neg, Asp}. It is projected above aspectual categories and clausal negation, as shown in (29)–(30) and (34) above, some examples of which are reproduced in (55) below.

(55) a. *He may have been being followed, and her have been following him.*
b. *The book must have been checked out and her not have recorded it.*
c. *He may have been following her and her not have seen him.*

If the case on the ASC subject is a structural case, then, since it cannot be nominative (due to the association of nominative Case with finite Tense), it must be accusative. The most commonplace example of this in more familiar syntactic constructions is the small clause of the sort given in (56).

(56) *We consider* [*her intelligent*].

But the subject of a small clause checks a case feature in the higher clause, more specifically, against a feature bundled onto a functional category, namely Aspect, Agr_O, or *v*, projected in the higher clause, as in (57) below; the small clause does not have a matching case feature for its own subject.[4]

(57) *We* [$_{AspP/Agr_OP/vP}$ *her* [$_{Asp'/Agr_O'/v'}$ [$_{Asp/Agr_O/v}$ [ACC]] [$_{VP}$ *consider* [t_{her} *intelligent*]]]]

If the small clause subject cannot check its case feature in this ECM-like structure, then it must raise to a higher subject position, as shown in (58)–(59).

(58) a. *She seems* [t *intelligent*].
b. *She seems* [t *to be intelligent*].
c. *She seems* [t *to have left*].

(59) a. * *It seems* [*her intelligent*].
b. * *It seems* [*her to be intelligent*].
c. * *It seems* [*her to have left*].

But movement out of the ASC is blocked by the Coordinate Structure Constraint. Therefore, the ASC is not in a structure for ECM or subject raising. Furthermore, as seen in (35) above, the verb of the first clause can be unaccusative, which precludes the possibility of ECM. This suggests that the accusative case on the ASC subject is an inherent case, not a structural case. But an inherent case can only be assigned in the specifier of a lexical category (Vainikka 1993/94), so this supposition leads to the hypothesis that the accusative subject is generated in spec-VP with inherent accusative case. The question then is why the accusative subject appears before negation and aspectual material in the ASC. To answer this, consider the features entered into the numeration of the ASC. Since tense and subject agreement features are lacking, the relevant features in an example such as *her not have recorded it* in (55b) are those given in (60) below, with their checking order; the tree derived from (60) is given in (61).[5]

(60) [EPP] < [NEG] < [$F_{V\text{-}o}$, $F_{N\text{-}o}$] < [PERF]

(61)

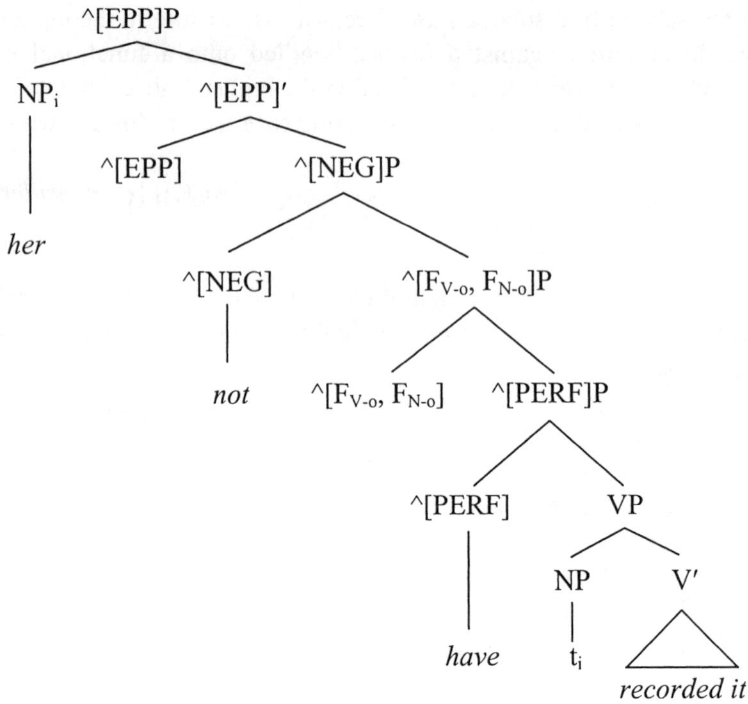

The subject raises to spec-^[EPP]P to check the EPP feature. The functional structure for (55a), is similar, except without the local negation, and with more complex aspectual projections, including ^[PROG].

The main point to emerge from this discussion is that a satisfactory account of the ASC construction in (1)–(2), (55), and other examples seen above, requires recourse to a functional category, ^[EPP], which is not part of the standard inventory. This category is automatically available on the feature-based construction of functional categories.

This account raises a couple of questions pertaining to the economy conditions formulated in previous chapters. First, in light of the Economy of Projection of Infl-Categories, repeated below, is it possible for the feature matrix [EPP] to be projected as a functional head?

(62) *Economy of Projection of Infl-Categories*
If features F_1, F_2, ..., F_n are elements of a feature matrix M projected as a functional head ^M within the Infl-system of a clause, then one of F_1, F_2, ..., F_n must be a clausal feature (such as a V/A-feature matching some $F_{V/A}$ on a verb or adjective within that clause).

But the EPP feature is a clausal feature: it is present in the numeration precisely to provide for the derivation of a clausal structure, and it is not projected to match an N-feature on some nominal within the numeration. So the projection of [EPP] as a clausal functional head in (61) does accord with the Economy of Projection of Infl-Categories.

The second question raised by this account is the following: if an inherent accusative subject can be generated in the ASC, then what prevents this from happening in a small clause complement of *seem*, which would result in examples such as (59) above? The answer to this can be discerned from the other known case in which an inherent accusative subject is generated. In child language, the inherent accusative (or genitive) subject is generated as a last resort, when the resources to check structural cases don't exist, because the child has no functional categories. If the generation of an inherent accusative subject in the ASC is a last resort, when no structural case could possibly be checked, then it will be blocked in (59) since a structural nominative case can be checked in (59) through raising of the subject.[6]

2. Small clause complements of perception verbs

2.1. The ASC-like structure of "Bare Infinitive" complements

The small clause complements of perception verbs, as in (63) below, look like ASCs of the sort seen above, even more so when they are coordinated, as in the first sentence of (64).

(63) a. *We saw him check out a book.*
b. *We heard him open a soft drink can.*
c. *We watched her get into her car.*

(64) *I saw him check out the book and her return it three hours later. I think they are working in cahoots with one another.*

The coordinate structure in (64) even has an interpretation similar to that of an ASC construction; compare the representation of (43) given in (53) above with the representation of the perception complement in (64), given in (65) below.[7]

(65) $[\exists e, e_1, e_2]\ [\ (e = e_1 + e_2) \wedge \text{check-out}\ (x_1, b, e') \wedge \text{return}\ (x_2, b, e'')\ ]$

The coordinate structure in (64) and its interpretation in (65) are suggestive of the ASC clauses seen above. But first, basic facts about the status of small clause perception complements need to be ascertained.

Note that the perception report in (66a) does not entail (66b).

(66) a. *I saw him not be counted.*
b. *I saw him.*

(66a) could be true of a situation in which I watched the working of the mechanisms of a counting process as they performed in such a way as to fail to count the referent of *him*, yet in which I did not see either him or any token of him that would make it true that "I saw him". This would be the case, for example, if I were watching barcoded pieces of paper, coded for people, feeding automatically into a machine with a barcode reader to count people who were at a large convention, and saw his paper, with his name at the top, feeding into the machine upside-down, so it would not register his presence at the convention. (66a) can be used to truthfully describe this situation, of which (66b) nevertheless is not true. This shows that *him* in (66a) is not an object of the verb *see*, a result which favors the small clause analysis of sentences like those in (63), (64), and (66a), in which the nominal following the perception verb is not an object of this verb, but rather, a subject of a (small) clausal complement of the verb. Observations of this sort underlie the semantic analysis of these structures in Higginbotham (1983).

Given the small clause status of the perception verb complement, it would be natural to think that this complement is in an ECM environment, with its accusative subject checking case against a feature projected on *v* (or Agr_O) of the higher clause. But if this were so, we would expect the subject of the perception complement to raise under passivization of the higher clause, as in other ECM examples, such as (67).

(67) a. *We consider* [*her intelligent*].
b. *She$_i$ is considered* [t$_i$ *intelligent*].

But, as is well known, this does not happen in a perception verb complement.

(68) a. *They saw* [*him leave*].
b. * *He$_i$ was seen* [t$_i$ *leave*].

(69) a. *They are watching* [*him leave*].
b. * *He$_i$ is being watched* [t$_i$ *leave*].

The main implication of these facts is that the subject of the small clause perception complement does not check case against a case feature in the higher clause by Exceptional Case Marking.

Further evidence for this conclusion comes from the c-command behavior of an ECM subject versus the subject of a small clause perception complement with respect to material in the higher clause. An ECM subject behaves as if it c-commands elements in the higher clause; see Postal (1974: 120–124) and Lasnik (1999: 137–140).

(70) *The DA proved* [*two men to have been at the scene of the crime*] *during each other's trials.*

(71) *The DA proved* [*nobody to have been at the scene of the alleged crime*] *during any of the trials.*

(72) * *Joan believes* [*him$_i$ to be a genius*] *even more than Bill$_i$ does.*

In (70), the ECM subject *two men* binds the anaphor *each other* in the adjunct phrase modifying the higher clause. In (71), the ECM subject *nobody* licenses the negative polarity item *any*, which also occurs in an adjunct phrase modifying the higher clause. Finally, in (72), the ECM subject *him$_i$* binds the r-expression *Bill$_i$* (which occurs in a phrase modifying the higher clause VP), producing the effects of a violation of Binding Theory Condition C, which states that r-expressions such as proper names should not be bound. These relationships result from the ECM subject c-commanding the associated anaphoric or negative polarity expression. This c-command configuration would not hold if the ECM subject remained in subject position of the infinitival complement, but it results from raising of the ECM subject to check its accusative case feature against the matching feature in the higher clause. Verb raising of the higher verb (Koizumi 1993, 1995) preserves the surface word order between the higher verb and the ECM subject. These examples contrast with ones in which the subject of a finite clause fails to bind corresponding elements within modifiers of the higher clause.

(73) * *The DA proved* [*that two men were at the scene of the crime*] *during each other's trials.*

(74) * *The DA proved* [*that nobody was at the scene of the alleged crime*] *during any of the trials.*

(75) *Joan believes* [*that he$_i$ is a genius*] *even more than Bill$_i$ does.*

In (73)–(75), the finite clause subject checks its case feature against a nominative case feature associated with finite Tense within the local clause. Thus, it does not raise to a position within the higher clause, where it would c-command the anaphor, NPI, or r-expression in the adjunct phrase which follows the complement clause and modifies the higher clause. Thus, the anaphor in (73) is not bound, a violation of Binding Theory Condition A; the NPI in (74) is not licensed by a negative or affective element; and the r-expression in (75) is free.

In contrast to this behavior of ECM subjects, subjects of small clause perception complements do not show evidence of c-commanding an element in comparable adjunct phrases. This can be seen in (76)–(78) below, where the detective is understood to do the staking out and monitoring in (76) and (77), and the unavailable reading marked by the asterisk in (76) is the one on which the DP *two men* binds the anaphor *each other*, meaning that the detective saw each man leave while the detective was staking out the other's house, and the detective heard each man confess while the detective was monitoring the other's phone calls. Likewise, the asterisk in (77) marks the unavailability of an NPI reading for the polarity item *any* in *anyone's house* and *any phone calls.*

(76) a. * *The detective saw [two men leave] while staking out each other's houses.*
b. * *The detective heard [two men confess] while monitoring each other's phone calls.*

(77) a. * *The detective saw [nobody leave] while staking out any one's house.*
b. * *The detective heard [nobody speak] while monitoring any phone calls.*

(78) a. *Joan saw [him$_i$ fall] even before Bill$_i$ realized what was happening.*
b. *Joan heard [him$_i$ cough] while Bill$_i$ was sneaking around the house trying to keep quiet.*

As a result, the anaphor in (76a,b) is unbound, *anyone* in (77a,b) is not licensed as an NPI, and the r-expression in (78a,b) is free, and therefore licit.

Thus, the subject of a small clause perception complement does not raise to a position within the higher clause. But there is evidence that the subject of a small clause perception complement raises internally to the complement clause, since it appears before aspectual auxiliaries and clausal negation. In making this observation, it has to be noted that the perfect cannot appear in small clause perception reports; see Higginbotham (1983) for discussion. Thus, the case for subject raising rests on progressive and passive forms, as in (79) below.

(79) a. *I saw [him being followed].*
b. *I saw [him not being followed].*
c. *I saw [him be observed from the balcony].*
d. *I saw [him [slip into the conference room] and [not be observed]].*

The ASC coordinated under an overt auxiliary verb, observed in the previous section, and the small clause complements of perception verbs, discussed above, clearly appear in different constructions. But from what has been observed above, it seems evident that they have the same structure. In both, the subject appears with accusative case; in both, the subject undergoes clause-internal raising; and in both, the accusative case is not checked by ECM; in fact, it does not seem to be a structural case at all.

On the basis of these considerations, the small clause complement in perception reports seems to have the same internal structure as the ASCs seen in the previous section. On this hypothesis, the functional categories involved in the derivation of (79b) are those given in (80), and the structure of the perception complement is as given in (81).

(80) $[\mathrm{EPP}] < [\mathrm{NEG}] < [F_{\mathrm{V\text{-}o}}, F_{\mathrm{N\text{-}o}}] < [\mathrm{PROG, PASS}]$

(81)

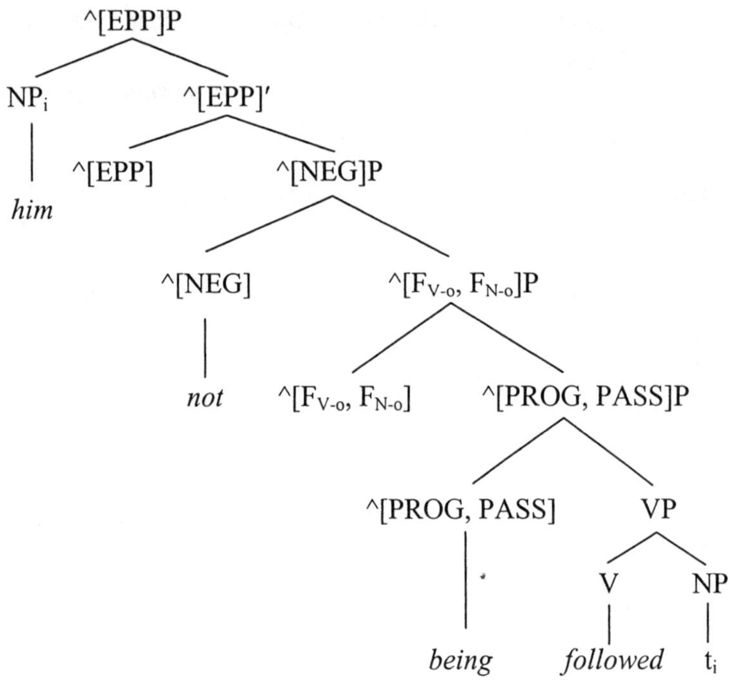

This explains why the subject raises within the small clause, but not to a position outside the small clause, either ordinarily, or under passivization of the higher clause.

2.2. Higginbotham's (1983) account

Higginbotham (1983) proposes that significant properties of perception reports with small clause complements follow from raising of the small clause at LF, as in (83) for (82), allowing for a straightforward mapping to the interpretation with restricted quantification represented in (84).

(82) *John sees [Mary enter].*
(83) [*Mary enter*]$_i$ [*John sees* t_i]
(84) [$\exists e'$: enter (m, e')] [$\exists e$: see (j, e', e)]

According to Higginbotham, this derivation, and the resulting representation in (84), confers referential transparency on the perception complement with respect to the main verb. Furthermore, it blocks raising of the small clause subject under passivization of the main clause, in line with the observations in (68)–(69) above. Such raising under passivization in (82) would produce the structure in (85) below, and then, upon raising of the perception complement after Spell-Out, the LF structure in (86), in which the trace t_j is not bound.

(85) *Mary*$_j$ *was seen* [t_j *enter*].

(86) [t_j *enter*]$_i$ [*Mary*$_j$ *was seen* t_i]

Finally, note that this account would also prevent the small clause subject from c-commanding material in adjuncts modifying the main clause, in line with (76)–(78) above.

Higginbotham's account was consistent with other points of the theory of grammar at the state of development it had at the time. Higginbotham assimilated the raised perception complement in (83) to the status of an indefinite nominal, raised at LF to an A′-position adjoined to S in the same way that quantified NPs were assumed to undergo Quantifier Raising at LF. This predicts that *wh*-extraction of arguments out of the perception complement should be possible along the lines of comparable extraction out of quantified NPs, as in (87) below.

(87) *What did you see* [*every picture of* t_{wh}]?

This result is correct since, as Higginbotham noticed, *wh*-extraction of arguments is possible out of small clause perception complements.

(88) a. *What did John see* [*Max give* t_{wh} *to Bill*]?
b. *Which poem did Maria hear* [*Max recite* t_{wh}]?

(89) a. *Who did John see* [t_{wh} *enter the room*]?
b. *Who did you see* [t_{wh} *leave in the middle of the meeting*]?

However, the proposal holds up less well in light of more recent insights into the behavior of quantificational nominals. To begin with, quantificational nominals such as that involved in (87) are no longer thought to be uniformly subject to an operation of Quantifier Raising realized as A′-movement to a position adjoined to S. Quantifier scope effects are more accurately attributed to movement to A-positions, specifiers of functional categories within the clause (cf. Hornstein 1995, 1999). Furthermore, indefinite nominals, to which Higginbotham assimilates small clause perception complements, are the least inclined to undergo LF movement. LF scrambling of definite nominals is what renders them islands for movement; indefinites stay in-situ, where they are bound by existential closure. (See Diesing 1991.)

Next, if the unbound trace t_j in (86) is responsible for the failure of raising of the small clause subject under passivization of the higher clause in (85), then VP-fronting in the context of object-to-subject raising in the passive, as in (90), with the structure in (91), should also be impossible.

(90) *Given to Mary, the book was.*

(91) [$_{IP}$ [$_{VP}$ *given* t_j *to Mary*]$_i$ [$_{IP}$ [*the book*]$_j$ *was* t_i]].

To derive (91), the object *the book* is first promoted to subject position, then the VP overtly fronts. The result is an LF in which t_j is unbound, just as in (86). (Note that *the book in* (90) can be replaced with an indefinite NP, which is not subject to any kind of raising, so the existence of (90) cannot be accommodated by assuming that the DP *the book* raises and adjoins above the fronted VP in (91), to a position c-commanding its trace within the VP.) The LFs in (86) and (91) have the same status with respect to the binding of movement traces.

In fact, if the small clause perception complement undergoes movement to an A′-position, adjoined to S, as in Higginbotham's analysis, then a more accurate point of comparison for (88)–(89) would be *wh*-extraction of arguments out of topicalized constituents, which overtly adjoin to S, or out of in-situ *wh*-phrases, which covertly adjoin to S. The former are shown in (92) below; and the latter in (93) with the associated LF in (94).

(92) a. * *Who did* $[_{IP}$ *[pictures of* t_{wh} $]_i$ $[_{IP}$ *you* t_{Aux} *buy* $t_i]]$?
b. * *Which book will* $[_{IP}$ *[copies of* $t_{wh}]_i$ $[_{IP}$ *we* t_{Aux} *distribute* $t_i]]$?
c. * *Which room will* $[_{IP}$ *[enter* t_{wh} $]_i$ $[_{IP}$ *she* t_{Aux} $t_i]]$?
(cf. *(She said she would enter this room, and) Enter this room, she will.*)

(93) * *What should she see [whose pictures of* $t_{wh}]$?

(94) $[_{CP}$ *What [whose pictures of* t_{wh} $]_i$ $[_{C}$ *should]* $[_{IP}$ *she* t_{Aux} *see* $t_i]]$?

Thus, Higginbotham's account is not sustainable within the light of current insights into quantification and movement, though it successfully explained various properties of perception reports with small clause complements within the context of grammatical theory of the time, and though it supports the derivation of a suitable semantic representation.

Notes

1. The ASC clause in (5a), taken in isolation, looks like an ACC-ing gerund. But an ACC-ing gerund would have to be an argument of a predicate or an adjunct clause, either by itself or in coordination with the first clause. And it is clear that the ASC clause in (5a) is not an argument or adjunct, whether on its own, or in coordination with the first clause. Rather, in coordination with the first clause, it forms a root clause.
2. The tree in (40) is a slight simplification. Johannessen proposes a less orthodox structure with [C′ and C′] coordination. The CP nodes dominating each C′, as well as the specifier of the first CP, containing the wh-phrase, lie outside the coordinate structure in a nonlinear fashion. It will fully serve the present purposes to use the [CP and CP] coordinate structure in (40) without invoking nonlinear structures.
3. On Johannessen's formulation, there is, in fact, no change in the syntactic category of the coordinated constituents since it is C′ in both the input tree and the output tree; see her examples (37) and (39) on her pp.229–230.
4. See Postal (1974: 120–124) for delineation of the empirical basis for this claim. The outlines of the analysis were suggested by Chomsky and Lasnik (1995) (originally published in 1993), and developed by Johnson (1991) and Koizumi (1993). See Lasnik (1999: 137–140) for further discussion.

5. The accusative case of the direct object pronoun in *her not have recorded it* is checked against the light verb *v*, not shown here.
6. In the derivation of (59), if the determination of last resort for the assignment of an inherent accusative case to the subject of the small clause complement were made after expletive insertion, then the last resort condition would be met, and the examples in (59) would be derived as grammatical. Thus, the need for the assignment of this case must be determined before expletive insertion, when the last resort condition is not met. This suggests that last resort operations apply cyclically.
7. For discussion of the semantic properties of perception complements, see Higginbotham (1983).

Chapter 6
The acquisition of functional features

1. Introduction

This chapter is the first step of an investigation of child language acquisition of functional categories in light of the feature-based theory of functional categories developed in Chapter 2. On the feature-based theory, clausal functional categories are just matrices of features matching or instantiating features on lexical items in the numeration.[1] According to this theory, the child must acquire the system of functional features, the checking order defined on them, and the distribution of features into feature matrices projected as functional heads, in addition to acquiring the functional morphemes and their relationships to the features expressed. The features, their checking order, and the distribution of features into feature matrices, can be extracted from the alternations among functional morphemes, their merge order into clausal structure, and the effects of matching features which condition movement by attracting their copies. We focus here on the development of the functional categories and their merger into phrase structure since on this point the feature-based theory creates possibilities and makes predictions which differ from those of other theories of functional category acquisition. This chapter looks into the acquisition of the features themselves, and their manifestations in early child language. The next chapter investigates the profile of acquisition of the adult functional categories, and shows that aspects of the growth of the adult functional system can be better explained in terms of the feature-based construction of functional categories than in terms of standard accounts in the literature on the acquisition of functional categories.

On the feature-based theory, it is possible that, in the process of mastering the system of functional features, and the checking order defined on them, children might create feature matrices which don't exist in the adult target. A predictable instance of this arises in the early stages of child language acquisition when the child does not have command of the full system of functional features, or, for whatever reason, cannot project adult functional categories with their complete complements of features.[2] In this circumstance, it is to be expected that the child might project an individual feature F by itself, as a category ^[F], where F is normally projected with other features in the adult system. For example, [WH] might be projected without [Q], resulting in *wh*-fronting without subject-Aux inversion. Or nominative case might be acquired before tense, and projected by itself onto a head ^[NOM], without finite tense features. Many instances of this will be observed in the present chapter. Another scenario for the projection of non-adult feature matrices would be obtained if the number of feature matrices which the child can project as functional heads is limited in early child language, forcing features which are separated out in the adult grammar to "double up" in the child grammar. Instances of this will be observed in the next chapter (including some reanalyzed examples from this chapter).

Some theories dismiss the structures expressing functional elements in early child language as ad hoc adjunction structures, thus invoking different processes of phrase structure construction for early child language functional categories and later ones. The present results demonstrate the potential of the feature-based theory of functional categories to explain early child language functional category structure as a product of the ordinary mechanisms of functional category construction under the rather special conditions of child language.

The features examined here are listed in (1) below.

(1) [NEG]
[Q], [WH], [DECL], [COND], [PRESUPP]
[$F_{N\text{-}s}$, $F_{V\text{-}s}$], [EPP], Tns, [NOM]
(values of Tns include $F_{V\text{-}T}$[fin] and $F_{V\text{-}T}$[inf])

For ease of reference, these features are separated into classes according to whether they are verbal-inflectional features, complementizer features, or negation. The feature-based theory allows that, under exceptional circumstances in child language, a selection of features from two different classes, or from all three, might be projected together as a single functional category, a result which is not provided for by other theories of functional category acquisition. This will be discussed in the next chapter.

2. Preliminaries

2.1. Feature projection versus functional category adjunction

The possibility of projecting functional features individually rather than as part of the normal feature complement of an adult functional head is more of a live option under the feature-based theory than under a theory based on the standard fixed stock of functional categories. This raises a question concerning the status of some functional elements in early child language. Hoekstra and Jordens (1994) and Radford (1990, 1996) argue that early functional elements in child language are generated in a position adjoined to a maximal projection, not as the head of a functional projection. Arguments for this position include quite general and methodological ones. Hoekstra and Jordens (1994: 123) note that the status of X as a functional head selecting a complement YP is more specialized and restricted than that when X is adjoined to YP, and therefore requires stronger evidence in its favor, including that instances of X occur in complementary distribution with one another. This argument has some force if the functional element is identified as an instance of a standard functional head; for example, an early complementizer element should exhibit alternations with other complementizer elements in order to be considered an exemplification of C^o. However, the alternation set may be smaller, and therefore the criteria of alternation may be weaker, if an early functional element is regarded as an instantiation of a single feature rather than of a standard functional head. For example, in order to be considered an exemplification of [WH], a *wh*-element should show alternation with other *wh*-elements, but not necessarily with a full set of complementizer elements. Thus, the alternation condition can be considerably weaker for exemplifications of individual features than for full functional categories.

Other arguments turn on more particular theoretical principles. Radford (1996: 56–61) argues for adjunction of early *wh*-elements to VP, by noting that the alternative structure in (2) for a typical early child *wh*-question would violate the *wh*-criterion (see May 1985 and Rizzi 1996), since the *wh*-element in spec-CP is not in a spec-head relation with a [+wh]-head.

(2) $[_{CP}$ *what*$_i$ $[_{VP}$ *kitty doing* $e_i]]$

Furthermore, Radford notes that if early child *wh*-questions have a full CP structure such as that in (2), then the questions in (3) would have a null subject which is not a root specifier (the specifier of the highest functional category in the sentence), contrary to generalizations concerning the licensing of null subjects in English proposed by Rizzi (1994).

(3) *Where put?*
Where go?
What say?

But the *wh*-criterion is formulated for (what in the terms of the present study would be) a full interrogative C with feature specification [WH, Q]. There is no reason to expect the *wh*-criterion to be in force if a child is projecting [WH] without [Q], whether because the child has not yet acquired [Q], or because some limitation (whether of memory, processing capacity, or specifically representational resources) prevents the child from projecting [Q] along with [WH] in the example at issue. Thus the form in (2) is an expected result at a certain point of grammatical development, on the feature-based theory of functional categories, when [WH] is being projected without [Q], and in these circumstances the *wh*-criterion should not be considered applicable to examples like (2). It is also not clear that the conditions on the licensing of null subjects in English proposed by Rizzi (1994) should hold for a stage of child language when [WH] is projected without [Q]. The import of the licensing condition is that the null subject should occupy the highest specifier (the specifier of the root category) in the sentence. But if the examples in (3) are obtained by projecting [WH] by itself above the lexical VP, it is not clear that ^[WH], without V-features, qualifies as a higher root category, as a full complementizer system would. Since the root category is the root of the clausal structure, it is plausible that the root category is defined by the highest V-feature in the clause. An N-feature such as [WH] would therefore not constitute the root category of the clause.

Other researchers have argued that early instances of functional elements should count as instantiating the associated functional category; cf. Roeper and Rohrbacher (1995, 2000). This proposal is also not particularly germane to the circumstances examined here under the feature-based theory since we specifically don't want to consider, say, [WH] projected by itself, as an instance of C^{o}. [WH] projected by itself is just ^[WH], and is distinct from the projection of any other feature or subset of features of a full complementizer head.

2.2. The present study

This chapter traces the development of functional features in child language and their projection into functional category structure by examining data from longitudinal studies of three children, posted on the CHILDES website.

Children were selected for the study based on the period of child development spanned by the on-line data, and based on the frequency of data collection. It was essential that the production data cover the period of acquisition of functional structure, typically beginning sometime after 1;10 (one year and ten months) and proceeding to full complexity of functional systems sometime in the fourth year (3;1 to 3;6). A recording frequency of twice per month was considered desirable. Data for Peter (Bloom 1970), Nina (Suppes 1973), and Naomi (Sachs 1983) were selected on this basis. The data for Peter begin at 1;9-8 (one year, nine months, and eight days) and proceed through 3;1-20, with recordings typically every 2 to 3 weeks. (But the last recording was made after a delay of 3 months.) The data for Nina begin at 1;11-16 and proceed with recordings spaced every few days to every couple of weeks, with a couple of longer gaps, to 3;3-21. The data for Naomi begin at 1;9-10 and proceed in intervals of every few days to every couple of weeks, becoming more sparse towards the end, up to 3;5-7.

This study focuses on functional features which are projected in the higher and middle levels of clausal phrase structure. Aspectual features, [ACC], object agreement features [$F_{N\text{-}o}$, $F_{V\text{-}o}$], and *v*, will be ignored here. The main reason for this is that the literature contains less discussion of the clarity of the manifestations of these features in child language than the features projected higher in the clause, concerning issues such as whether expression by morphology is as indicative of the presence of a feature as expression by a lexical item, how much of a paradigm is required for a feature to be manifested, and the like.

3. Results

3.1. Peter

Early recording files capture Peter at the lexical stage, with no functional features in evidence. In a recording file at age 1;11-5, Peter has a number of 'I' subjects, but there are no pronominal subjects with nominative case in any other person or number, so there is no evidence that the 'I' subjects aren't simply an unanalyzed form of first person singular subject, rather than an expression of [NOM]. However, with that understood, the data in (4) show evidence of tense inflection on both auxiliaries and main verbs, with alternations between past, present or root infinitive, and periphrastic future.

(4) a. *I'll fix it.* (1;11-5)
  b. *I did it.* (1;11-5)
  c. *I get them.* (1;11-5)
  d. *I got it.* (1;11-5)
  e. *That's good.* (1;11-5)

This will result from the projection of a tense feature, Tns, as a functional category. In (4b,c,d), Tns is the only functional feature expressed, and is therefore evidently projected by itself, as a non-adult category ^[Tns]. There may also be subject agreement features, [$F_{N\text{-}s}$, $F_{V\text{-}s}$], expressed by inflection of the cliticized auxiliary in (4e), but this is less certain since alternations in such inflections are not in evidence, and do not show up until a couple of months later, at 2;0-10, with a better paradigm at 2;2-13. Thus, the functional category system in the example in (4e) is also probably just ^[Tns].

By age 2;0-10, Peter has other nominative subjects, as shown by (5a,b,c), and therefore is projecting [NOM], possibly by itself in (5a).

(5) a. *They go round.* (2;0-10)
  b. *He's upside down.* (2;0-10)
  c. *What she doing?* (2;0-10)
  d. *What I do?* (2;1-18)
  e. *What you do with this?* (2;1-18)

Example (5c) is particularly interesting since it shows a *wh*-expression fronting a clause with a nominative subject; this pattern is solidified by the examples in (5d,e) from the recording at age 2;1-18. These involve the projection of [WH] by itself, as ^[WH], projected above the lexical and inflectional structure of the clause. There is also greater evidence for the expression of subject-verb agreement, the projection of [$F_{N\text{-}s}$, $F_{V\text{-}s}$], at 2;0-10, in the examples in (6).

(6) a. *It goes in the front.* (2;0-10)
b. *They go round.* (2;0-10)
c. *I have to put the pen back in my pocket.* (2;0-10)

In these examples, [$F_{N\text{-}s}$, $F_{V\text{-}s}$] may be projected by itself, or in combination with Tns and/or [NOM], possibly even as an adult I-category, ^[[$F_{N\text{-}s}$, $F_{V\text{-}s}$], Tns, [NOM]]. Finally, the examples in (7) occur at 2;0-10 and 2;1-18, showing evidence of [NEG] by itself and in combination with Tns.

(7) a. *Don't take a wheels off.* (2;0-10)
b. *Don't like it.* (2;0-10)
c. *Can't open.* (2;0-10)
d. *Not finished yet.* (2;1-18)
e. *No me take it off.* (2;1-18)

Thus, by age 2;0-10 to 2;1-18, Peter shows evidence of projecting [WH], [$F_{N\text{-}s}$, $F_{V\text{-}s}$], Tns, [NOM], and [NEG], individually or in combinations. In particular, the individual feature projection ^[WH], or possibly the non-adult category ^[WH, [NOM]], is evident in (5c,d,e), and ^[NEG] is evident in (7d,e). In (7a,c), Tns and [NEG] might be projected separately, as two functional categories, or in a non-adult combination, as ^[Tns, [NEG]].

Next, at 2;1-18 and again at 2;2-13, Peter exhibits Aux-fronting in questions.

(8) a. *Would you look at these?* (2;1-18)
b. *Did you get up Jenny?* (2;2-13)

These result from the projection of [Q] by itself at the top of the clausal structure, as a head ^[Q], with [$F_{N\text{-}s}$, $F_{V\text{-}s}$], Tns and [NOM] projected (separately or together) below ^[Q].

Also at 2;2-13, Peter shows the first prospective example of *wh*-fronting together with subject-auxiliary inversion, the result of projecting ^[WH, Q], with the example in (9a) below; however, this particular utterance is performed rather often, and earlier than other instances of its kind, and so may be formulaic.

(9) a. *What're you doing?* (2;2-13)
b. *What color is this one?* (2;3-24)
c. *What is this boy doing?* (2;5-22)

d. *Now what should we do with em?* (2;8-12)
e. *Know what I'm gonna do.* (2;8-12)

But the pattern appears again at 2;3-24, in the example in (9b), and seems more securely established with the example in (9c), at 2;5-22. It is fully productive by 2;8-12, with examples such as (9d). These are produced by projecting ^[WH, Q] above all Infl projections, which in the examples in (9) include [$F_{N\text{-}s}$, $F_{V\text{-}s}$], Tns and [NOM], whether projected separately or together. In (9e), occurring at 2;8-12, [WH, Q] is projected in an interrogative complement clause, but, as in the adult grammar, [Q] is not checked by overt movement of Aux in embedded interrogatives. (In interrogative complements, [Q] is made visible under selection by the higher predicate.)

More productive examples including [NEG] are those in (10), at 2;3-24.

(10) a. *They're not supposed to be eaten anyway.* (2;3-24)
b. *They don't go in your mouth anyway.* (2;3-24)

These evidence [NEG] in combination with [$F_{N\text{-}s}$, $F_{V\text{-}s}$], Tns and [NOM]. By this time, Peter's functional category system is becoming distinctly more adult in form. Complementizer elements in contexts of clausal embedding (or implicit clausal embedding) appear at age 2;5-22 and become more common thereafter, as shown in (11).

(11) a. *See if it's finished.* (2;5-22)
b. *If you're gonna hit people.* (2;7-13)
c. *Cause Jenny's gonna get the crayon.* (2;8-12)
d. *Cause I'm taking the wrench off.* (2;9-15)
e. *Cause it'll fall down.* (2;9-15)

The complementizer element *if* instantiates a conditional mood feature, [COND], while *(be)cause* instantiates a feature of causal dependence.

Finally, starting at 2;9-15, and continuing thereafter, Peter combines complementizer features with a full suite of inflectional features and [NEG], producing the most complex combinations of the features in (1) possible within a clause.

(12) a. *Cause you don't like that sound.* (2;9-15)
b. *Cause dog cannot get out.* (2;10-19)
c. *Know why the dogs can't get out?* (2;10-19)

d. *Cause I didn't buy one.* (2;10-19)
e. *Cause they don't belong in school.* (2;10-19)
f. *Cause they're not special.* (2;10-19)
g. *If we don't have one a these.* (3;1-20)
h. *So that I won't get any holes.* (3;1-20)

Interestingly, the example in (13) may reflect the projection of a non-adult combination of features [CAUS, WH].

(13) *Cause why I'm not playing with them anymore.* (3;1-20)

Through the course of the development of his functional category system, Peter exhibits the individual feature projections displayed in the first row of Table 1; these are culled from examples in which Peter expresses only the individual feature or feature matrix indicated. ([$F_{N\text{-}s}$, $F_{V\text{-}s}$] will always be regarded as a single matrix here, since there is no evidence that one of [$F_{N\text{-}s}$, $F_{V\text{-}s}$], is projected without the other.) The second row of Table 1 lists features which Peter co-expresses within a clause, in possible combinations as larger feature matrices.

Table 1. Peter's functional projections

Individual features	^[Tns], ^[NOM], ^[WH], ^[Q], ^[$F_{N\text{-}s}$, $F_{V\text{-}s}$], ^[NEG], ^[COND], ^[CAUS]
Possible feature combinations	^[WH, Q], ^[Tns, [NOM]], ^[Tns, [$F_{N\text{-}s}$, $F_{V\text{-}s}$], [NOM]], ^[Tns, [NEG]], ^[WH, Tns, [NOM]], ^[CAUS, WH]

In the early stages of Peter's development, it is possible that the combinations in the second row of Table 1 are actually split up, and the features projected individually, as separate features, or as submatrices of the given matrices. But as Peter's development proceeds, it is progressively more likely that he is projecting the features in the larger matrices (including many adult matrices) given in the second row of Table 1. It is possible that Peter projects even larger combinations of features, but rather unlikely since at the stage when large collections of features are expressed, the results are more adult-like than in early stages of acquisition, and are therefore more likely to reflect the adult forms of functional categories. The projection of adult combinations of features as adult functional categories by Peter and the other children examined here will be explored in the next chapter.

3.2. Nina

With Nina, as with Peter, 'I' subjects appear initially without any nominative pronouns in any other person or number, and so are regarded as not reflecting nominative case. At this same time (age 1;11-29), a very limited alternation of tense elements appears, as in (14), reflecting the projection of Tns by itself, as ^[Tns].

(14) a. *Girl's holding the balloons.* (1;11-29)
b. *Duck ate my food.*

The first hint of subject-verb agreement, and further indication of Tns, is exhibited at age 2;0-10.

(15) a. *I'm eating carrots.* (2;0-10)
b. *Ari's swinging.*

By age 2;1-6, third singular nominative case pronouns appear alongside first singular, marking the presence of the nominative case feature, [NOM]. In some examples (such as, *I tell you.*) [NOM] seems to be projected by itself, without tense or subject-verb agreement.

Whereas Peter first manifested [WH] at 2;0-10 and [Q] five weeks later at 2;1-18, Nina exhibits only very formulaic *wh*-fronting with *where* and *where's* before, at 2;1-15, she shows subject-Aux inversion resulting from the presence of [Q] in the example in (16a); since subject-verb agreement is better established by this time, as evidenced by the examples in (16b,c), [Q] is apparently projected in (16a) along with Tns and [$F_{N\text{-}s}$, $F_{V\text{-}s}$]; Tns and subject agreement features may be projected separately or together.

(16) a. *Is this my lamp?* (2;1-15)
b. *You're drinking.* (2;1-15)
c. *He's climbing in the window.* (2;1-15)

Not until a month later, at 2;2-12, does Nina show any alternation in *wh*-fronting, clearly indicating the presence of [WH]; in Nina's case, unlike with Peter, some of these involve subject-Aux inversion, since Nina is already using [Q]. Further exemplification of the pattern at 2;2-28 is also given.

(17) a. *What happened to zoo?* (2;2-12)
b. *What is daddy holding?* (2;2-12)
c. *Where does that go?* (2;2-28)
d. *What's that girl doing?* (2;2-28)
e. *What is that girl doing?* (2;2-28)

Complementizers make their first appearance earlier with Nina than with Peter, as shown

(18) a. *Cause him open him eyes.* (2;2-12)
b. *Cause they're sleeping.* (2;2-12)
c. *Cause he loves Nina.* (2;2-28)

Interestingly, the subject is accusative in (18a), which is normally taken to indicate that it has remained within VP; thus, ^[CAUS] is the only functional projection in the clause. In (18b,c), ^[CAUS] is projected above projection(s) of other functional features, including [$F_{N\text{-}s}$, $F_{V\text{-}s}$], Tns, and [NOM], whether these are projected separately or in a complex I node.

Nina's first expressions of negation are monotonous repetitions of injunctions or reports beginning with *don't*. The first indication of a minimal alternation is at age 2;1-6, where Nina uses the forms with clause-initial negation in (19), although it is not clear whether these are imperative or declarative.

(19) a. *No hop Mommy kangaroo.* (2;1-6)
b. *No talk Mommy.* (2;1-6)

Clear alternations of forms of negation are not exhibited until a couple of weeks later, with the examples in (20).

(20) a. *No Leila have a turn.* (2;1-22)
b. *I can't take that off.* (2;1-22)
c. *I don't break them.* (2;1-22)

In (20a), [NEG] is possibly the only functional feature projected. In (20b,c), it is accompanied by at least Tns and [NOM], and probably by subject-agreement, which we know is expressed by this time; see (15)–(16) above.

Thus, Nina's early development of functional features differs somewhat from Peter's in the sequence of acquisition of functional features, but the same forms are produced in only a slightly different age sequence.

In Nina's subsequent development, the features introduced so far increase their frequency and the variety of their paradigms of co-occurrence; this matters for the attribution of adult functional categories to Nina's grammar, as discussed in the next chapter, but during this period little happens from the perspective of functional feature acquisition. By age 2;10-21, Nina begins to combine use of C-elements with negation and inflection elements, and these examples become more frequent and progressively more adult-like in form, as shown in (21).

(21) a. *Why can't he walk?* (2;10-21)
b. *So don't wake my baby up*. (2;11-6)
c. *Cause doesn't stand up very well.* (3;0-3)
d. *That what he doesn't like*. (3;0-3)
e. *I can't because I don't know the words*. (3;0-10)
f. *Cause he can't get out of his room.* (3;0-16)

In these, [CAUS] or [WH, Q] are projected above full clausal projections with inflection and [NEG].

The features and possible feature combinations exhibited by Nina over time are exactly as those for Peter given in Table 1.

3.3. Naomi

Naomi exhibits Tns before any other functional features (1;10-25), as Peter and Nina did. Interestingly, less than a month later, Naomi produced examples projecting Tns, subject agreement features, and [Q], all together in one clause, as in (22) below; in (23), [WH] is projected along with these other features.

(22) a. *Is it raining?* (1;11-6)
b. *Is it going to work?* (1;11-6)

c. *Are sheep running?* (1;11-6)
d. *Is kangaroo sleeping*? (1;11-21)
e. *Do you want some?* (1;11-21)

(23) a. *Where did it go?* (1;11-6)
b. *Where'd it go?*

In (22), ^[Q] is projected by itself above projections of inflectional features. In (23), [WH, Q] is projected above projections of inflectional features, with subsequent *wh*-movement and movement of Aux to ^[Q].

In other respects, the development of Naomi's system of functional features is similar to that of Peter and Nina.

4. Discussion and conclusion

The forms of early clauses produced by Peter, Nina and Naomi are readily accounted for by assuming that they can project individual features as functional categories, including ones such as [WH] and Tns, which do not project by themselves in the adult system. As will be discussed in the next chapter, standard theories of functional category acquisition invoke a fixed stock of adult functional categories. One way such theories accommodate the forms of functional material in early child clauses is to assume that functional elements initially adjoin to a lexical projection; this invokes a special mode of phrase structure composition for early child language. Another way to accommodate early child forms is to assume that the initial manifestation of a standard functional category might be partial, in that only some of the adult feature content of the category is expressed by the child. For example, an I head might be present but initially manifested solely by tense inflection. Both of these approaches to early child clause forms require special pleading, either in favor of special operations of phrase structure composition, or in favor of special usage of a standard functional head to express a fraction of its normal adult content.

The feature-based theory of functional categories provides more atomistic tools with which to approach the explanation of aspects of early child clause structure. By projecting individual features such as [WH] which are not projected by themselves in the adult grammar, the feature-based theory maintains uniform operations for the construction of phrase structure across child and adult clauses. Furthermore, the feature content expressed is exactly what is projected into clausal phrase structure; there are no primitive functional categories which are projected in child language with less than their adult content.

This account of the acquisition of the child's inventory of functional features poses an issue for the Economy of Projection of Infl-Categories, formulated in Chapter 2 and invoked several times in subsequent chapters. The principle is repeated in (24) below, where clausal features include [EPP], and features matching verbal or adjectival features on a predicative head.

(24) *Economy of Projection of Infl-Categories*
If features F_1, F_2, ..., F_n are elements of a feature matrix M projected as a functional head ^M within the Infl-system of a clause, then at least one of F_1, F_2, ..., F_n must be a clausal (verbal, adjectival, or EPP) feature.

The projection of features such as [WH] or [NOM] by themselves violates this constraint since [WH] and [NOM] are N-features, not clausal features. In Chapter 2, it was argued that the projection of N-features should be tied to the projection of associated V-features in order to prevent overgeneration of functional material.

It may be the case that the Economy of Projection of Infl-Categories is not in force in the early child grammar, that it is subject to maturation through the period of acquisition of functional features. Alternatively, it may be that the Economy of Projection of Infl-Categories is always in force in the child grammar, but that it can be over-ridden in early stages of language acquisition when the child has acquired a functional N-feature, F_N, but has not acquired a corresponding V-feature which invariably accompanies F_N in the adult grammar. In this stage, if the child wants to project F_N in order to express a simple *wh*-question, or in order to express nominative case on a subject, the child may simply choose to over-ride the Economy of Projection of Infl-Categories under the pressure of communicative needs.

Grounds for distinguishing these two explanations of the non-observance of the principle may be available in the data examined here. After [Q] is acquired, a child sometimes continues for a while to project [WH] without [Q] in a few root interrogatives; such instances of *wh*-fronting without subject-Aux inversion soon give way to the adult pattern, which results from the projection of [WH, Q]. For example, Nina shows evidence of projecting [WH, Q] at 2;2-12, with further evidence at 2;2-28 and thereafter. Yet at 2;2-28, Nina produces the example in (25).

(25) *Why those blocks on there?*

This results from the projection of [WH] by itself, without [Q], two weeks after she has acquired [Q] and shown the ability to project it together with [WH] to form *wh*-interrogatives with subject-Aux inversion. Furthermore, Nina has *do*-support at this stage, as evidenced by (17c) above (*Where does that go?*), so there is no evident impediment to Nina producing a form with subject-Aux inversion instead of (25). Nina violates the Economy of Projection of Infl-Categories in this instance even though she has all the resources to abide by it. This suggests that the principle is subject to maturation. This might be a form of biological maturation, or a form of maturation keyed to the changing practices of the child, who suspends the economy constraint in order to project functional features in a period of limited resources, as suggested above, but exhibits some delay in fixing on the constraint and abiding by it once the necessary resources are available.

The differences between the functional systems of child and adult grammars on the view developed here reflect two factors: (1.) the acquisition of the individual features, so that the child inventory of functional features is initially empty in the lexical stage, and grows steadily, as detailed in the profiles of Peter and Nina above; and (2.) the acquisition of the adult combinations of features which are projected together as a functional category. The nature of the acquisition of individual features was explored in this chapter. The acquisition of the adult combinations of features as adult functional categories involves acquiring the adult distribution of features into feature matrices, to be projected as functional heads, which requires that the child acquire the correct ordering of features, and any co-occurrence restrictions which the language imposes on the features. The next chapter shows that the acquisition of adult functional category systems also involves a further constraint, reflecting the growth of basic representational resources, which determine the number of adult functional categories which can be projected together within a clause.

Notes

1. Verbal features, such as tense and agreement features, match features on the verb. Lexical complementizers and negation elements instantiate mood features and [NEG], respectively. Lexical complementizers and negation could be counted as checking their own features, if the operation of the functional category system is to be formulated uniformly as feature checking, but this distinction does not make any evident empirical difference in how the functional category system operates. Whether or not lexical complementizers and negation are viewed as checking, or merely instantiating, their respective features, the structure of the functional category system is determined by the ordering of functional features and their distribution into feature matrices.
2. Constraints on processing capacity or verbal working memory impose plausible limitations on the capacity of the child to project adult functional categories with their complete feature contents in early child language. In the next chapter, it will be shown that a further representational constraint is in play, over and above limitations of processing capacity or working memory.

Chapter 7
The acquisition of adult functional categories

In the previous chapter, it was observed that it is possible in early child language for a feature which is projected in concert with others in the adult grammar to be projected by itself as a functional category in the child grammar. For example, it was seen that tense features, Tns, can be acquired before nominative case and expressed through the projection of a feature matrix, ^[Tns]. In theories with a fixed category T, this would be interpreted as a situation in which the tense content of T is acquired before its nominative case assigning property. But another kind of divergence in feature distribution between the child and adult grammar, involving combinations of features which don't occur in the adult grammar, is more distinctively revealing of the construction of feature matrices under the feature-based theory of functional categories. For example, based on data examined in this chapter, there is reason to believe that in early child language [NOM] and [NEG] are projected together on a single functional head, ^[[NOM], [NEG]], at a stage where the child is capable of projecting only one functional category within the verbal system of a clause. Similarly, there is evidence of heads ^[[WH], [NOM]], and a head ^[[Q], [$F_{N\text{-}s}$, $F_{V\text{-}s}$], Tns] combining the interrogative feature [Q] with tense and subject agreement features, among others. This sort of result is expected on the feature-based theory if the child has not yet learned the ordering of features in (1) below and the resulting distribution into feature matrices, or if, along the lines discussed below, the number of feature matrices which the child can project as functional heads is limited at this stage of acquisition, forcing features which are separated out in the adult grammar to "double up" in the child grammar.

(1) [Q, WH] < [$F_{N\text{-}s}$, $F_{V\text{-}s}$] < [Tns, [NOM]] < [NEG]

Many examples of these non-target (non-adult) combinations of features in child grammar will be observed in the present study, providing further support for the feature-based theory of functional categories. Systematic investigation of such divergences across languages, examining the various ways in which features can be distributed into feature matrices differently at different stages of child development, is a large, open area of research for a feature-based theory of functional categories, but the present results demonstrate the potential of this theory to explain aspects of child language data which theories in the literature write off as exceptional structures produced by ad hoc adjunction operations, rather than by the ordinary mechanisms of functional category construction.

Whereas the previous chapter investigated the development of the child's inventory of functional features, the present chapter investigates the development of the child's inventory of adult functional categories, that is, functional categories with the feature content specified for them in the adult grammar. In addition to accounting for divergences between child and adult language in the distribution of features onto functional heads, the feature-based theory of functional categories has the capacity to explain fundamental facts about the development of the adult functional category system revealed by the data examined here, concerning global constraints on the development of the functional category system. These constraints determine the number of adult functional categories which can be present within the verbal system of a clause during successive developmental stages. On an account of functional category acquisition formulated in terms of the feature-based theory of functional categories, these constraints reflect the growth of basic representational and computational resources of the child's grammar. Since they do not follow from any other theory of functional category acquisition in the literature, the existence of these constraints provides strong support for the feature-based theory.

The chapter proceeds as follows. Theories of functional category acquisition are examined in order to determine their predictions regarding the number of clausal functional categories (those in the verbal system) which should occur together within a clause, and the combinations in which they might occur. These predictions are then compared to results obtained from longitudinal data available on-line (CHILDES) for three different children acquiring English as a first language. Once the profile of the acquisition of adult functional categories is established, the data are examined for effects of instances in which (according to the feature-based theory) a feature matrix projected as a functional head in the child grammar has a combination of features which doesn't occur in the adult grammar. Among theories in the literature, bottom-up structure-building accounts (Guilfoyle and Noonan 1992, Vainikka 1993/94) are found to offer predictions most in accord with the results of the present study, but these accounts are not fully adequate to the data examined here. A new account of child language acquisition of functional categories is formulated in terms of the feature-based theory of functional categories developed in Chapter 2. The new account exploits the conception of functional categories as matrices of features, matching or instantiating features on lexical items in the numeration, projected as functional heads in accord with a partial linear order defined on the features. It posits growth in the number of feature matrices which can be projected into syntactic structure, rather than development of a fixed stock of functional categories conceived as primitives. This account allows for non-adult combinations of features to be projected as functional categories in early stages of language acquisition, and it accounts for the observed constraints on the number of adult functional categories which can be present within the verbal system of a clause during successive developmental stages.

In order for the results of the present study to be relevant regardless of the number of functional categories which are actually present in the adult English grammar, and in order not to prejudice the study in favor of the feature-based theory from the outset, comparisons among different theories of functional category acquisition will be discussed in relation to a three-category system consisting of I, Neg, and C. Furthermore, the counts of functional categories per clause undertaken in this study counted only these three functional categories. This was done so that the results would err, if they must, in the direction of understating episodes in the growth of the functional category system, rather than overstating them. Results showing growth in the functional category system of the sort made possible by the feature-based theory which understate episodes of such growth by delineating fewer functional categories than actually exist in the grammar of English will only be strengthened when interpreted in light of a larger number of functional categories; understated results should scale up, with further inquiry, to any larger number of functional categories which might actually obtain in the grammar of English. Results which overstated episodes of growth in the functional categories of English by delineating more categories than actually exist would be compromised, and the results of the study would not scale downward smoothly with further inquiry based on a smaller number of functional categories. The decision to count exactly three functional categories, therefore, was taken in order to maintain the relevance of this study, regardless of how many functional categories are actually present in the grammar of English. When we turn to the feature-based theory, these category labels will always be understood to be mere labels for their feature-based instantiations; functional heads projected from adult feature combinations include those given in (2), where [NULL] is the case checked against PRO subjects of infinitives.

(2) Neg = ^[NEG]
C ∈ { ^[Q], ^[Q, WH], ^[DECL], ^[COND], ^[CAUS], ^[PRESUPP] }
I ∈ { ^[[$F_{N\text{-}s}$, $F_{V\text{-}s}$], [EPP], [$F_{V\text{-}T}$[fin], [NOM]], ^[[EPP], [$F_{V\text{-}T}$[inf], [NULL]]] }

Of course, when the child produces non-adult combinations of features such as [[WH], [NOM]] or [[NOM], [NEG]], as described above, this cannot be expressed at all in terms of the fixed category labels, and resort must then be made to the descriptive apparatus of the feature-based theory.

1. Theories and predictions

1.1. Strong continuity accounts

One approach to the acquisition of functional categories is to suppose that functional categories and their projections are innate, that the entire system is specified in the genome for pre-natal, ontogenetic development, and as a result, is present at birth. Then the use of functional categories does not depend on any post-natal increase in basic representations of the child's grammar. This is the strong continuity view of Boser et al. (1992), Poeppel and Wexler (1993), Lust (1994), and others.

But even on this view, the productive use of a functional category is dependent on exposure to appropriate linguistic input: it would take exposure to data for the child to learn the elements that fall under a functional head, and to learn that they fall together as a class instantiating this functional head at a particular position within the clause. Other factors potentially influencing the increase in use of functional categories include the increase in length and overall complexity of child utterances, and, for certain constructions, the setting of relevant parameters. On this view, a functional projection is available and should be exhibited as soon as lexical items are acquired to mark its presence, by filling its head or specifier. If movement dependent on parameter settings is required for a lexical item to fill the head or specifier of a functional category, the relevant parameters must be set in order for such movement to make the presence of the functional category manifest.

The role of learning, as opposed to innate structure, can be further refined in the context of strong continuity accounts. As noted above, it would take exposure to data for the child to learn the elements that fall under a functional head X, and to learn that they fall together as a class instantiating X at a particular position within the clause. When a few elements of the functional class have been learned, the child may not at first perceive that these are instantiations of the functional head X, and so may simply adjoin them, in line with proposals by Hoekstra and Jordens (1994) and Radford (1990, 1996). But once the child acquires a number of elements that fall under X and categorizes them together as instances of X, then the child has fully "acquired X" by learning how to use the innate structure consisting of X and its phrasal projection. Having acquired X, the child should be able to use elements within the X-system in conjunction with other functional elements provided the child's memory and computational facility permit the required degree of phrase structure complexity.

On this view, the presence of the I-system would be exhibited as soon as a child demonstrated productive use of some auxiliary verbs and infinitival *to*, to appear in I^{o}, independently of the status of other functional categories. The C-system would be exhibited as soon as the child demonstrated productive use of complementizers and was capable of producing utterances of sufficient length to accommodate clausal subordination, independently of other functional categories. The C-system might be exhibited earlier, in monoclausal utterances, in interrogative forms with an auxiliary in C following I-to-C movement, accompanied, in *wh*-interrogatives, by a *wh*-element in spec-CP. Neg has been acquired when the child uses the negative elements *not* and *no* productively (including clause-medial uses; before Neg is acquired, negative elements might be adjoined utterance-initially).

Strong continuity accounts predict that examples exhibiting one, two, or a full complement of functional categories within a single clause should appear regularly in the child's production data from the earliest point from which it is clear that the functional categories can appear singly in productive use, and the requisite MLU and phrasal complexity of utterance is attained. If we plot the number of functional categories exhibited within the verbal system of a clause in child language productions over time, the strong continuity view would predict that this number should begin at zero, and that it should grow from zero to three (counting I, Neg, and C) as functional elements are acquired and phrasal complexity increases, and that the maximum of three should be attained, and maintained, once each of the functional categories is productively manifested in its own right, and the phrasal complexity of utterances permits their co-occurrence.

As a matter of fact, in the child language that will be examined here, these three functional categories are exhibited singly quite early on in the child's development, and utterances of sufficient length to accommodate all three of them within a clause appear relatively early as well. Therefore, the prediction of the strong continuity approach for these children is that full functional structure will be exhibited early and quite regularly in the production data.

The assumptions of strong continuity do not allow in any evident way for the existence of stages in functional category acquisition exhibiting effects which would be produced in the feature-based theory by non-adult feature combinations, such as the matrices [[NOM], [NEG]], [Tns, [NEG]], or [[WH], Tns, [NOM]].

In summary, the strong continuity approach predicts that functional structure, innately specified, should exhibit itself in full complexity within a clause as soon as the functional categories are acquired singly, and the requisite phrasal complexity is attained. Furthermore, the effects of feature matrices with certain non-adult combinations of features are not readily accommodated under assumptions of strong continuity.

1.2. Radford's maturational theory

If functional categories are not innate, then they may be acquired through development realized as a form of biological growth or maturation. Radford (1990, 1996) proposes that functional categories are initially absent, and then emerge gradually, in parallel. The initial step, in which child utterances involve only lexical projections, is the lexical stage or "VP-stage"; during this period, child utterances are bare VPs or APs, including some with overt lexical subjects and some without overt subjects. Following the lexical stage, according to Radford, the functional system matures, with parallel development of the various functional categories essentially independently of one another.

Based on this view, we would expect that a given functional category should be instantiated across examples with increasing frequency by an increasing variety of head and specifier elements. Radford's view leads to the determinate prediction that once each of the functional categories I, Neg, and C has become firmly established in the child's productions, exemplified by a representative sample of appropriate elements, then the child should be capable of producing all three functional categories within a single clause to the extent permitted by the phrasal complexity of the child's grammar. As under the strong continuity hypothesis, clauses exhibiting one, two, or all three of these functional categories should appear regularly once each functional category has become established singly and the phrasal complexity of the child grammar is sufficient to accommodate all three functional categories. As under the strong continuity approach, a plot of the number of clauses with a specified number of functional categories co-present within the clause should include a substantial number of clauses with three functional categories (counting I, Neg, and C) once these conditions are satisfied. Again, in the child data examined here, there are fairly determinate early points in child development when these conditions hold, at which we can check the prediction that all functional categories should then be able to appear together within a single clause.

On this theory, there is no evident reason for the existence of data in early stages of functional category acquisition manifesting effects which in the feature-based theory would arise from non-adult feature combinations, such as the matrices [[NOM], [NEG]], [Tns, [NEG]], or [[WH], Tns, [NOM]].

1.3. Induction

Contrary to the proposal that functional categories are innate, or biologically scheduled for development, is the view that the acquisition of functional categories is primarily the result of induction on the data, using an innate endowment consisting of general learning abilities, but no articulated innate linguistic structure, and with no role for maturation or biological growth that is particular to the syntactic structures involved. On this view, the role of articulated data structures such as syntactic trees is up for reconceptualization relative to the accounts considered above, which directly attribute these structures to an appropriate level of description of the language user's cognition. An eliminativist approach would eschew reference to such structures entirely in the account of language knowledge and use, in favor of collocations, statistical relationships, and other relations defined purely on word sequences (at the syntactic level, with similar relations defined on sound sequences at the phonological level). In this event, we cannot refer to the acquisition of a functional category per se, but only to the acquisition (defined as suitable command of use) of the associated class of functional elements themselves. The predictions, in this event, would depend on assumptions about whether or not the command of a given class of functional elements was independent of the command of other classes of functional elements. To the extent that they are independent, the prediction would be that once the child has attained command of complementizer, inflectional, and negative functional elements, and has acquired the requisite MLU and phrasal complexity to combine three different functional elements, one from each of these classes, within a single clause, we should expect to see clauses with elements from one, two, or all three classes in the production data of the child.

On this view, the effects of functional heads defined by non-adult combinations of features, while not definable as such, could be the result of alternate patterns for the realization of sets of functional elements which have been abducted from primary linguistic data. But since these alternate patterns are not in any obvious atheoretic sense simpler than the target pattern – since they clearly amount to simplifications in the context of hierarchical phrase structure, but not necessarily in any atheoretical statistical sense – it is unclear whether they are predicted by accounts of language acquisition as purely inductive over patterns of observable morphemes.

Alternatively, under an account of language acquisition using associationist mechanisms, it might be admitted that the data structures underlying a generative linguistic account of the language user's knowledge of language constitute an allowable characterization of that knowledge at an appropriate level of description, but that such structure emerges in a way that is not dependent on biological growth and which is not in any nontrivial sense a manifestation of genetic endowment (no more than any other learning capacity is). In this case, the acquisition of syntax can be usefully characterized (in part) in terms of the presence of functional categories, and the predictions are similar to those for the strong continuity and maturational approaches: effects of non-adult combinations of features are not expected, and once the child has acquired each of the functional categories C, Neg, and I, and has acquired the requisite phrasal complexity to support all three of these functional categories in a single clausal structure, we should expect to see clauses with one, two, or all three different types of functional element exhibited in the child production data. Since this condition is reached at fairly determinate points in the longitudinal studies examined here, we can check this prediction against the experimental data.

1.4. Bottom-up structure building accounts

If functional categories are not present at birth and merely waiting to be triggered or lexically instantiated, and if they do not develop in parallel, through maturation or inductive inference, there remains the possibility that they mature or develop in a particular sequence. Guilfoyle and Noonan (1992) and Vainikka (1993/94) present versions of this view on which the lexical stage of Radford is followed by a stage in which the I-system is present, but not the C-system, followed finally by attainment of the full, adult complement of functional categories. This view, called the bottom-up structure building hypothesis, is maturational in that the functional systems develop or mature one-by-one, from the bottom of the tree structure to the top. But each functional system conforms to innate restrictions on phrase structure and never, at any stage, violates principles of Universal Grammar; the resulting view thus has a component of continuity, and so is characterized as the weak continuity hypothesis.

Guilfoyle and Noonan propose that the I-system is acquired immediately after the lexical stage, and that the C-system is acquired subsequently. On this basis, they identify several different stages in the acquisition of various constructions across several different languages: a lexical stage with only VP present; a stage in which the I-system is present, but not the C-system; and a stage in which the I-system and C-system are both present. They claim that some C-elements appear in the second stage, when only the I-system is present, but the C-elements appearing in this stage do not occupy their ordinary positions in clausal phrase structure, and their appearance induces some compensatory readjustments in the position of other clausal elements. For example, in English *yes/no*-questions during this stage, subject-auxiliary inversion is obtained as a result of Aux moving to a [+wh] I^0, while the subject (exceptionally for this stage of development) remains in spec-VP. See section 5.1 below for further discussion.

This predicts an initial lexical stage with no functional elements, followed by a stage (the I-system stage) in which I-elements occur freely, occasionally accompanied by a *wh*-element adjoined to IP. Complementizers should not appear during this stage.

Vainikka (1993/94) traces the acquisition of functional elements through the longitudinal data of four different children (Nina, Eve, Sarah, Adam), with data drawn from previous studies (Suppes 1973, Brown 1973), posted on the CHILDES database. Vainikka delineates a lexical stage with no functional elements, which she identifies as a VP-stage for clausal structure. Nominative subjects are generally absent in this stage (although Vainikka notes some inexplicable examples in the data for Eve and Sarah), and Vainikka proposes that the genitive and accusative subjects which occur commonly in this stage appear in spec-VP. Next, Vainikka delineates a stage in which I-elements occur (Aux, *to*, nominative subjects), but no productive C-elements. (The incipient *wh*-NPs which occur at this stage seem to be adjoined.) Following this IP-stage, Vainikka delineates a stage (Pre-CP) in which productive *wh*-elements appear, but they never appear with nominative subjects, only with genitive or accusative. Vainikka analyzes such examples as using the I-system to express C-elements, with the subject reverting to spec-VP. This stage results in the acquisition of some true C-elements before the C-system has developed to accommodate them. They must then be accommodated with the available resources of the grammar at that stage, in the I-system, forcing compensatory adjustments in the placement of normal I-system elements. Next, the C-system develops, permitting full expression of I-elements and C-elements together within a single clause, with everything in its normal, adult, position. See section 5.2 below for further discussion.

Both Guilfoyle and Noonan and Vainikka posit a stage in which the I-system has developed but the C-system is still absent, and both note that some interrogatives can be formed in this stage. Both accommodate early question formation during the IP-stage by having the subject revert to spec-VP in interrogative forms. Essentially, the appearance of typical C-structures at this stage, before a C-system has developed, is accommodated by having the I-system partly take on the role of the C-system, with compensatory loss of its capacity to support the full inventory of I-elements. The result is a trade-off in this stage between the expression of I-elements and the expression of C-elements. This trade-off disappears with the maturation of a full-fledged, independent C-system. On these accounts, C-elements can "double up" on the I-system, but when they do, they displace I-elements, rather than co-occur with them. Thus, the effects of non-adult combinations of Infl and Comp features are not predicted by these accounts.

Turning to the overall profile of functional category development, the bottom-up structure-building accounts predict a lexical stage with no functional elements, followed by a stage fully exhibiting I-elements, and expressing certain C-elements at the expense of I-elements, followed by a stage in which all clausal functional categories can be expressed together. Counting the functional categories of the verbal system which can occur together within a single clause, we get 0 for the lexical stage, followed by 1 for the IP-stage (I, sometimes with the function of C), followed by 2. Adding the expression of negation (which Vainikka and Guilfoyle and Noonan don't explicitly address), these predictions can be revised as follows: 0 functional categories for the lexical stage; 1 for the IP-stage exemplified without negation, and 2 for exemplifications of the IP-stage with negation; 2 for the CP-stage exemplified without negation, and 3 with negation. Crucially, the full complexity of instances of all three functional elements occurring together within the verbal system of a single clause is not predicted to appear until the onset of the CP-stage, which happens a considerable period of time after C-elements, I-elements, and negation have singly made their independent appearances in the clausal phrase structure of the child. On the bottom-up structure building view, if we plot the number of clauses with a specified number of functional categories present within the verbal system of a clause in child language productions over time, we should find that even when I-elements, negation, and C-elements have independently manifested themselves, their co-occurrence together is blocked during the IP-stage (Guilfoyle and Noonan) or the Pre-CP stage (Vainikka), even though utterances are otherwise quite long and complex, because there is a structural constraint on their co-occurrence. The graph should exhibit a substantial number of clauses with two functional elements, including combinations of Infl+Neg, and Comp+Neg, but no clauses with Comp+Infl or Comp+Infl+Neg. In particular, clauses with all three functional categories do not appear automatically once the relevant functional elements manifest themselves productively and the child has attained the requisite phrasal complexity to represent all three functional categories within a single clause.

This prediction is quite distinct from that made under the strong continuity view, the maturation in-parallel account of Radford (1990), or the view of functional category acquisition as pure induction on the data. All of these lead to the expectation that exemplifications of the full suite of functional categories should appear once each one of them has clearly established itself and the phrasal complexity of the child grammar permits their co-occurrence. These comparisons beg a definition or characterization of phrasal complexity. A measure of phrasal complexity appropriate for this purpose will be defined in section 2.3.

1.5. Feature-based theory of functional categories

Next, implications of the feature-based theory of functional categories presented in Chapter 2 will be taken up with regard to the acquisition of functional categories. On the feature-based theory, one necessary condition for the acquisition of clausal functional heads X_1, …, X_n is that the child has to acquire elements which instantiate or carry features checked against each of these heads. Another necessary condition is that the child must have the capacity to represent *n* matrices of features (with their component features and submatrices) in order to represent these *n* clausal functional categories together within a single clause. This representational capacity might be innate and fixed, or it might mature. If the representational capacity is innate and fixed, then predictions for acquisition of functional categories match those of strong continuity approaches described in section 1.1 above. If it matures, then predictions depend on hypotheses regarding the nature of this maturation.

On the feature-based theory, clausal functional categories are just matrices of features matching or instantiating features on lexical items. If this system matures, it would not be surprising if the capacity to support adult feature matrices, and to project them in syntax as functional projections, were to proceed in a step-wise fashion, that is, it would not be surprising if the number *n* of matrices corresponding to adult functional heads matured from 0 to 1, then to 2, and finally (for the system of English functional categories considered here) to 3. In this maturational scenario, the development of the system of functional categories would be analogous to the development of the child's inventory of functional features, observed in the previous chapter. The initial state ($n = 0$) would be the lexical stage, with only lexical projections. At the next hypothesized stage ($n = 1$), any one functional element could be supported, but not more than one. C-elements would be expected to occur, hosting a raised auxiliary (under I-to-C movement) and moved *wh*-expressions, unless clausal and derivational complexity did not support subordinate clauses and adult-style question formation. At the next hypothesized stage ($n = 2$), any two functional elements could be supported: I+Neg, as well as C+Neg and C+I. At the final hypothesized stage ($n = 3$), any three functional elements should be supported, producing clauses with C, I, and Neg all together.

Note that on this account, C-elements should appear without I elements as soon as clausal and (if necessary) derivational complexity allow, predicting effects which the bottom-up structure building accounts accommodate by re-analyzing the role of the I-system. Furthermore, non-adult feature matrices are possible on this theory; for example [[WH], [NOM]] could be constructed and projected as ^[[WH], [NOM]] if the child has not yet learned that [WH] and [NOM] are projected on distinct heads, or if the resources are not available to project ^[WH] as a separate head from ^[NOM]. This prediction is not shared by the other theories surveyed here.

As expressed above, the hypothesis at issue is that the number of adult clausal functional categories which can be represented together within a clause increases incrementally. The hypothesis, formulated in this way, defines the relevant count of functional categories to be those which can occur together within a single clause, rather than spilling across clausal boundaries in a complex sentence, and also excludes from this count any nominal functional categories, such as a determiner system. These restrictions reflect properties of the theory of phrase structure composition outlined in Chapter 2. On that theory, clauses are constructed by different operations than those which effect clausal subordination, the attachment of adjunct clauses, or the insertion of complex nominals. The construction of phrase structure for a clause is a modular operation, a derivational phase in the terminology of Chomsky (2001), producing a Complete Functional Complex for the main predicate of the clause, and providing matches for all or most of the morpho-syntactic features introduced by lexical items within the numeration for the clause. (The clause formation operations are formulated as standard merge operations in Minimalist syntax, and the resulting clause structure roughly corresponds to an elementary tree in Tree Adjoining Grammar.) As a result, the construction of the set of functional categories for a clause is taken to be a computational episode, distinct from the combination of clauses with other clauses and the insertion of complex nominals (which involve other types of operations, tree adjunction or tree substitution in Tree Adjoining Grammar). The present hypothesis is thus that the operations of clause formation exhibit resource-based constraints on the number of adult clausal functional categories which can be represented together within a single clause.

1.6. Processing capacity, working memory, and phrase structure complexity

A child cannot exhibit a structural functional category until it has acquired at least some functional elements instantiating that category. And a child cannot exhibit a given number, say n, of functional categories within a single clause unless the child has the working memory and processing capacity to produce and process the relevant morphemes in the context of phrase structure trees of sufficient complexity to permit the representation of n functional categories on top of a suitable lexical (verbal or adjectival) projection. Thus, an investigation of particular, domain-specific maturational or resource-based constraints on functional category acquisition must control for limitations of working memory and general language processing ability. More to the point, we cannot claim that certain facts about child language are evidence for domain-specific maturational or resource-based constraints on functional category acquisition unless we show that the cited facts cannot be attributed to limitations of working memory and general language processing capacity. To show this directly might be quite difficult. The present study will use a measure of phrase structure complexity as a control for limitations of working memory and general language processing ability. The facts D_i cited here as evidence of domain-specific maturational or resource-based constraints on functional category acquisition for child i are all produced after the child has produced phrase structures with large selectional chains involving a mixture of lexical and functional heads. The formation of these chains should require working memory for a sequence of categorially diverse lexical and functional syntactic heads, and the ability to generate and process hierarchical syntactic structure, and nested semantic relationships, well in excess of what is required to produce a clausal structure with three functional categories on top of a lexical projection. For this reason, it is concluded that limitations of working memory and general language processing ability would not prevent the expression of three functional categories together within a clause in the data D_i. The effects of working memory and processing limitations on the aspects of functional category development examined here are thus effectively controlled for by phrase structure complexity.

In adopting this approach, it is essential not to oversimplify the claims which could be made on behalf of the effects of processing requirements. For example, McKee and Iwasaki (2001) argue that the use of a functional element relies on a link established in late processing between the functional element and its associated lemma, "a lexical unit containing both semantic and syntactic information" (McKee and Iwasaki 2001: 130).[1] They argue that instances of missing functional elements could reflect not missing functional category structure (an explanation in terms of linguistic competence), but a failure to commit the late processing required for access of the functional element, and crucially, they argue that children do this even when the functional element has been already acquired, that is, the child has already exhibited an ability to link the functional element to its lemma.[2] The missing functional element results from a failure to access it on a given occasion of use, possibly as a result of processing pressure. On the basis of this view, the transition to a state of consistent expression of functional elements, and their co-expression with one another, would mark a development in processing ability, not necessarily a growth in representational resources.

However, even this appeal to processing, as specific to functional categories as it is, can be controlled for by citing selectional chains of appropriate length and composition in the child data. Specifically, if there are selectional chains containing *n* functional categories ($n = 1, 2, 3$), whether or not *n* functional categories occur together within a single clause, then, on the proposals of McKee and Iwasaki (2001), this should demonstrate the capacity to put *n* functional categories together in a single clause, since there is no distinction on their account between the late processing required to link functional elements to their associated lemmas when they occur within a clause, or across clausal boundaries. A systematic delay in the production of *n* functional categories per clause across the longitudinal data for a child should therefore not be attributed to the processing constraints proposed by McKee and Iwasaki. Some further constraint seems to be implicated in such a case.

In summary, the best way to show that there are particular, domain-specific maturational or resource-based constraints limiting the number of functional categories which a child can express within a clause at a given point in development is to show that the number of functional categories which can appear together within a single clause at that time is limited to a value below that which we would expect the child to have attained given the inventories of functional elements available to the child and the state of general linguistic and cognitive development of the child. This is accomplished in the present study by using a measure of phrase structure complexity as a control for working memory and general processing capacity. The measure used is defined in section 2.3 below.

2. Procedures

2.1. Counting functional categories

In order to explore the general profile of the acquisition of functional categories, the objective of the present study was to examine child production data in several longitudinal studies fully spanning the period of acquisition of functional elements, and to count and record the number of functional elements which co-occur within the verbal system of a single clause. At the end of the counting process for each child studied, the number of clauses with one functional category was plotted alongside the number of clauses with two functional categories and the number of clauses with three functional categories in a three-line graph, plotted against time, marked by the age of the child at the time of the recording session. The predictions made by the theories of functional category acquisition reviewed above were then evaluated in light of the resulting graphs. Evidence of non-adult combinations of features was then sought at appropriate points in the development of the functional category system.

The children studied were the three featured in the previous chapter, selected for the reasons given there. They were, with the ages covered by the study, Peter (1;9-8 to 3;1-20), Nina (1;11-16 through 3;3-21), and Naomi (1;9-10 through 3;5-7).

The data presented various challenges for the task of obtaining an accurate count of functional categories used in the child utterances. These included child imitations of caretaker and researcher utterances, incomplete child utterances, and occasions when the child would repeat an utterance, sometimes as many as ten or more times in a row. In order to address these difficulties directly, and to assess the significance of a given child utterance for the count, a quite laborious hand count was conducted, rather than one using automatic frequency counters available for use with the on-line data. With the hand count, child imitations of caretaker and researcher utterances could be discarded on the spot. Incomplete utterances were examined individually and a judgment made as to the number of functional categories exhibited, using a conservative standard that required exemplification of functional material in order to count the associated functional category as present; see below for more on this. Back-to-back repetitions of child utterances were counted as a single utterance for the purpose of contributing to the count of clauses exemplifying a given number of functional categories. Near repetitions, with some variation in lexical content and some separation by intervening utterances, were judged on an individual basis according to whether or not they should be regarded as distinct utterances. Lines from songs and nursery rhymes were excluded from the count, as were expressions which seemed formulaic. As an example of the latter, utterances of *(Be)cause why?* seemed to be formulaic rather than productive, and so were not counted as exhibiting a complementizer *because*. Likewise, as in Vainikka's (1993/94) study, instances of questions such as *What's that?*, which were ubiquitous in some files, were regarded as formulaic, and not as exemplifying Infl or Comp. Finally, the hand count made it possible for notes to be taken concerning the variety of functional elements which occurred within a given recording session, and the contexts in which they occurred.

In the previous chapter, a functional feature was not recorded as definitively present in the child grammar until a minimal alternation in the expression of the feature was observed consisting of at least two different values of the feature. In the present chapter, an adult functional category will not be regarded as definitively present in the child grammar until a partial paradigm of values of features composing the category is observed. For this reason, the counts conducted here will be self-consciously conservative, not counting an adult functional category as present in the child's grammar until several different occurrences of the category have been recorded with different feature values.

A clause was counted as one exhibiting a given number of functional categories whether it was a main or subordinate clause. Although copular *BE* is clearly in I in the adult grammar, since it occurs before negation and undergoes raising to C in interrogatives, it was counted as a main verb in the present study since its presence in I in simple clauses (declaratives without negation) is not manifested by word order. Furthermore, since early instances of fronting of copular *BE* in interrogatives appear to be formulaic (*What's this?* repeated ad infinitum, for example), they were also not counted as evidence of I. Only in later, more complex, instances of fronting were copular verbs counted as evidence of I.

A more theoretical issue is whether the presence of a functional category is indicated by lexical content, by morphological content, or both. If we count lexical content, then the presence of the I-system is indicated by an overt auxiliary verb and by the infinitival marker, *to*; the presence of the C system is indicated by an overt complementizer or by Aux-fronting, and the presence of Neg is indicated by *not* or cliticized *n't*. If we count associated morphological content, then I could be indicated by tense alternations, subject agreement alternations, or nominative case on preverbal subjects. In the present study, lexical content was counted, and was considered the preferred indicator of the presence of a functional category. Among other things, this permits a neutral stance on the issue of whether the Optional Infinitive phenomenon (see Wexler 1994) involves a missing functional category, or just unspecified tense features. Nominative case on subjects was counted, but the count of instances of nominative case was kept separate so that its contribution could be assessed separately and, if necessary, subtracted out for comparison if it turned out to diverge from the evidence provided by lexical heads.

If we stick with the most conservative counting technique, according to which a functional category is indicated when its lexical content is present, we will not be able to separate Agr_S and T; apart from existential sentences on the accounts of Chomsky (1995a) and others, only subject agreement and tense morphology would do that. But for the purposes of the present study, it does no harm to bundle Agr_S and T into one category, I(nfl). As discussed in the previous section, the major difference in predictions of different theories of the development of functional categories in child language lies in the way in which the number of functional categories grows. The profile of growth of the functional system is therefore the main object of interest here; the number of functional categories present at a given time is merely a means for determining how the count of functional categories changes over time. By bundling Agr_S and T into I, we just obtain a slightly more coarse-grained profile of the growth in the functional system, from which we can still determine the nature of that growth. These results should scale up smoothly to studies assuming a split Infl since counts of I in the present study should systematically divide up into contributions from the component categories in a more refined study. Furthermore, the choice between split Infl and unitary Infl should not matter to the search for non-adult combinations of features. In that search, the objective is to find feature combinations which would not be produced by the adult grammar. An instance in which any Infl-features are projected together with mood features or [NEG] is a non-adult combination, regardless of whether Infl is split or unitary.

As discussed in the previous chapter, Hoekstra and Jordens (1994) and Radford (1990, 1996) have argued that early functional elements in child language are generated in a position adjoined to a maximal projection, not as the head of a functional projection. On the feature-based account, the functional elements which Hoekstra and Jordens and Radford consider adjoined are ones which express an individual feature of the child grammar projected by itself, which is normally part of a larger suite of features projected as an adult functional category (e.g., [WH] projected without [Q]). Although we continue to adopt the feature-based account of these functional elements, we will not count them as manifestations of the adult functional category since they do not exemplify its full feature content. For convenience, such functional elements will be identified here as sub-adult functional categories.[3] They are projected from perfectly licit feature matrices, and form perfectly legitimate functional categories of the child grammar, but they are not adult functional categories, and are therefore not to be counted in the study of this chapter.

When we turn to examine evidence for non-adult combinations of features projected as functional categories, we will find that some of the instances analyzed by others as involving adjunction can be interpreted as evidence of a non-adult combination of features. However, the plausibility of the claim that the features are projected together in a non-adult combination in these instances, and not projected individually, hinges on knowing how many functional categories are present at a given stage of acquisition, and in order to determine this in a fashion which doesn't beg questions, we will follow conservative counting techniques to first establish the overall profile of acquisition.

In order to have some measure of the effects of the stringency of counting techniques, the present study will employ two different standards, one more stringent than the other, to count functional categories which occur together within a clause. The data for each of the three children will be analyzed twice over, once according to each standard, and the results compared.

The first standard is a liberal one of first mention, on which it is assumed that the number of functional categories exhibited within the data for a child increases from n–1 to n at the first appearance of a few examples with n functional categories which cannot be dismissed as imitations or as formulaic, nonproductive expressions. On this standard, the appearance of elements which would occupy a functional category X in the adult grammar is taken to be evidence for the presence of X in the child grammar.

The second, more stringent, standard responds to the observation of Hoekstra and Jordens (1994: 123) that a functional element occupying a functional head "must be in complementary distribution with other members of its category." Accordingly, the more stringent standard requires evidence of a paradigm, or partial paradigm, of elements instantiating a functional category, at least a minimal set of alternations to be exhibited across the set of elements which exemplify the head or specifier of a functional projection. Early functional elements which don't exhibit such a paradigm or partial paradigm are assumed to be sub-adult categories.[4]

The data for Peter, Nina, and Naomi will first be examined using the more liberal "first mention" standard for counting functional categories. Then the more stringent standard will be applied to the data for each of the three children, and any changes in the interpretation of the data will be noted.

At the end of the counting process for each child studied, the number of clauses with n functional categories, for each $n = 1, 2$ and 3, was plotted in a 3-line graph against time, realized as the age of the child at the time of the recording session.

We expect, in general, that clauses with one functional category will become established before clauses with multiple functional categories. However, the different theories make different predictions regarding the shape of this graph. The strong continuity view predicts that once all three functional categories (I, Neg, C) have become established singly, and once the MLU and phrasal complexity of child clauses are sufficient to support all three functional categories at once, then all three should be able to co-occur within a single clause. Radford's (1990) view of in-parallel maturation, and a view of acquisition as based on pure induction from the data, predict roughly this same result. The bottom-up structure building view, in contrast, predicts that in the IP (or Pre-CP) stage, each of the functional elements (I-elements, Neg, C-elements) should have become independently established, at a point when the child utterances already exhibit considerable complexity, but I-elements and C-elements should not appear together within a single clause until the C-system is acquired. Hence, there should be a stage in which two functional categories can appear (I+Neg, or C+Neg), but such that clauses with three functional categories do not appear until later, when the full CP-structure is attained. Finally, on the feature-based theory of functional categories, if the capacity to project matrices of functional features as functional heads matures, there should be a stage at which any two functional categories can co-occur, but not all three.[5]

2.2. Size normalization and nominative subject filtering

The number of child utterances typically varies somewhat across files of recording sessions. In some cases, recording sessions are very regular in length, and interaction with the child produces a consistent rate of child utterances, with the result that the number of child utterances varies little across files of recording sessions. But with some children, there are periods during which the recording sessions are distinctly shorter than those established as the norm for recordings of that child, or during which the rate of child utterances produced is lower than the norm for that child.

It is therefore worthwhile normalizing the counts of functional categories per clause with respect to the size of the file, or number of child utterances in the file, in order to see if such normalization reveals any patterns over time obscured by the absolute count. The CHILDES transcripts separate out child conversational turns, and within each turn, utterances are delimited by a hash mark, '#'. This provides two different standards of normalization: one based on conversational turns, and one based on utterances delimited by the hash mark. Taking utterances to be delimited by the hash mark drastically overcounts child utterances relevant for the present study, since the utterances, thus delimited, often consist merely of sound effects, isolated noun phrases, or other non-clausal material, sometimes repeated many times in succession, as in the examples in (3)-(4) from the data for Peter.

(3) [Peter, a single conversational turn at 2;1-0]
egg # egg # egg # egg # egg # egg # egg # egg # egg # egg.

(4) [Peter, three separate conversational turns at 2;1-18]
a. *choo choo # choo choo # choo choo # choo choo #*
b. *too big # too big # too big # too big # too big # too big # am too #*
c. *choo choo # choo choo # woo woo woo woo*

If we count conversational turns as utterances, this undercounts utterances, since a single conversational turn can have more than one child utterance. But the undercount is not as drastic as the overcount described above since conversational turns often contain just one utterance with clausal structure, and rarely contain more than two or three. Thus, when this technique undercounts, it does so by one or two; in contrast, counting utterances delimited by '#' overcounts more often, and by much larger margins. In this study, a file contains the transcript of a single recording session, or of two or three sessions recorded within a couple of days of one another. The size of a file will be taken to be the number of conversational turns by the child in that file. Normalization results are obtained as follows, but kept separate from the raw (unnormalized) counts: a count $C_{i,k,n}$ of the number of clauses with exactly n functional categories, $n = 1, 2, 3$, in file k for child i, is normalized for file size by multiplying $C_{i,k,n}$ by the average file size for child i, and dividing this result by the size of file k. Thus, counts for larger than average files are normalized downward, and counts for smaller than average files are normalized upward.

Another concern that arises regarding the absolute count of functional categories per clause is the role of examples in which the presence of a nominative subject contributes to the count of the number of functional categories in a clause. This is a concern for a strategy which would count functional categories as revealed only by the presence of lexical, not morphological, content. It is also a concern for practical reasons since first person singular nominative subjects typically predominate in the early files, and such repetition tends to be pervasive in these files. For example, of the initial 29 instances of nominative subjects in Peter's file at 2;1-18, all but one is first person singular, 16 of the remaining 28 are all self-reports about Peter writing and drawing on a pad, and 9 of these 16 are repetitions of the utterance *I writing*, and several of the remainder are the variants *I write* and *I'm writing*. It's not clear how many of these should count as independent instances of the use of a nominative subject. A couple were nearly immediate repetitions, as in (5).

(5) Child: *I writing.*
Researcher: *You're writing?*
Child: *I writing.*

In such cases, a judgment had to be made as to how many instances of Infl were being exhibited. These considerations do not rule out counting nominative subjects as exemplifications of Infl. For example, Peter's file at 2;1-18 contains a greater variety of nominative subjects elsewhere than in the sequence mentioned above. But, for the reasons just given, there remain questions about the exact accuracy of counts of Infl as exemplified by nominative case.

In order to gauge the effects of counting nominative case as an exemplification of Infl, we will produce a new, alternate, plot from the plot of functional categories per clause counted according to the "first mention" standard by systematically subtracting away the count of clauses in which the presence of Infl was inferred solely from the presence of a nominative subject. If comparison of the two graphs suggests that nominative subjects were merely one component of the totality of Infl elements in the child's production data, then the original graph of functional categories over time will stand unquestioned, including nominative subjects as evidence of Infl. If, on the contrary, comparison of the two graphs suggests that nominative subjects are being produced at some points of the child's development independently of other manifestations of Infl, then the alternate graph, obtained by subtracting away the count of clauses in which Infl was inferred from a nominative subject alone, will be used as the preferred graph of the count of functional categories per clause over time.

2.3. A measure of phrase structure complexity

The notion of phrase structure complexity at issue is not one limited to the count of verbal and functional projections within a single clause, for only the feature-based theory sketched in section 1.5 invokes this distinction; the contending theories do not invoke it. Therefore, in deciding whether or not a child has sufficient phrase structure complexity to support the representation of a given number of functional categories per clause, it is legitimate to cite examples of phrase structure complexity across clausal boundaries, and across the boundary of a nominal argument as examples of overall phrase structure complexity which the child can wield at a given point in development.

For this reason, phrase structure complexity will be measured in terms of the complexity of selectional chains involved, including chains across clausal and argument boundaries. A head X selects a category Y if Y is a complement of X, regardless of whether X is lexical or functional. If a head X_1 selects X_2P, and X_2 selects X_3P, and, in general, X_i selects $X_{i+1}P$ (for $i = 1, 2, \ldots, n-1$), we will say that $(X_1, X_2, \ldots, X_n)$ is a selectional chain of n heads. This does not capture the complexity of specifiers or adjoined elements, so this complexity measure is a minimal measure.

For example, in the sentence in (6) below, with the intransitive verb *sneeze*, I selects VP, headed by V; thus (6) exhibits a selectional chain (I, V) of two heads within the clause.

(6) *Max* [$_{I}$ *has*] [$_{VP}$ [$_{V}$ *sneezed*]]

In (7), with the transitive verb *catch*, I selects VP, headed by V, and V selects its object NP, headed by N; this sentence therefore exhibits a selectional chain of length three within the clause, namely, (I, V, N).

(7) *Max* [$_{I}$ *has*] [$_{VP}$ [$_{V}$ *caught*] [$_{NP}$ [$_{N}$ *fish*]]]

The selectional relationships in the above examples were all within the presented clause, and counted towards the complexity of this clause. With more complex DP or CP objects, larger selectional chains are produced, but these would span the clausal structure of the main clause and the structure of the DP or CP complement of the main verb; the object-internal part of this chain would then not contribute to the measure of the complexity of the main clause. However, it would still count towards the overall complexity of phrase structure produced by the speaker.

With additional functional structure, longer selectional chains are produced. In the subordinate clause of the sentence in (8) below, C selects IP, I selects NegP, Neg selects VP, and V selects NP, producing a selectional chain (C, I, Neg, V, N), of length five.

(8) *Bill believes* [$_{CP}$ *that* [$_{IP}$ *Max* [$_{I}$ *is*] [$_{NegP}$ [$_{Neg}$ *not*] [$_{VP}$ [$_{V}$ *catching*] [$_{NP}$ [$_{N}$ *fish*]]]]]]

Furthermore, since the higher clause contains I and V heads, with I selecting VP headed by the main clause verb *believe*, and *believe* selecting CP, the total selectional chain in (8), spanning the main and subordinate clauses, is (I, V, C, I, Neg, V, N), of length seven. And note that four of the heads in this chain are functional heads. The measure of the complexity of the subordinate clause in (8) calculated above is based on a minimal system of functional categories. If the gerundive form *catching fish* has an associated aspectual projection headed by a functional category Prog or Asp (see, for example, Borer 1994 and Tunstall 1994), then the selectional chain for the subordinate clause would be (C, I, Neg, Asp, V, N), of length six. And if I is factored into Agr_S, T, and Agr_O, the selectional chain would be still more complex.

For purposes below, phrase structure complexity will be computed counting only one inflectional head (I), along with C, Neg, V, D, and N.

2.4. Reliability

There are features of the present study which impose intrinsic limitations on the degree of interrater reliability which can be expected between two people independently performing the counts involved. In passing through a file and deciding for each child utterance whether it provides an example of *n* functional categories appearing together within a clause ($n = 1, 2$, or 3), one must make many decisions pertaining to the issues discussed in section 2.1 above. If a child has a string of ten very similar, but not identical, utterances, one must decide how many to classify as repetitions, which are not to be counted. As discussed in section 2.1, I employed conservative counting techniques which classified many early instances of functional elements as instances of sub-adult functional categories. For example, many utterance-initial instances of negation (e.g. in *no lie down*, Nina 2;1-29) were regarded as sub-adult categories. Furthermore, when the counts of *n* functional categories per clause in a file are very small, say five or less, a decision of the sort just mentioned concerning a single data item can cause a difference in outcomes of 20% or greater. Such small numbers were the norm for counts of examples with three functional categories per clause, and they were also obtained for counts of examples with one and two functional categories per clause in the periods when the child first began to exhibit functional categories, and later, to exhibit two functional categories per clause.

The counts presented in this study were obtained by the author. A research assistant was employed for a semester to provide independent counts on a subset of the files for each of the three children studied. During a training session using four transcript files for Nina, it was found that the research assistant was overcounting functional categories in early child utterances relative to the counting methods employed by the author, and instructions to the research assistant were refined. The research assistant then performed counts for 29 files, eleven of the Nina files, four from Peter, and fourteen from Naomi. The results for one functional category per clause turned out to be incommensurable with the author's: the research assistant counted far more instances of nominative case as productive than the author did, and therefore obtained consistently higher counts than the author. The counts of examples with three functional categories per clause were too small for percentage differences to be meaningful, for reasons discussed in the previous paragraph; they ranged from 0% (1 example counted versus 0) to 100%. Only in counts of examples with two functional categories per clause were the counting criteria similar enough, and the numbers large enough, to permit meaningful comparisons. The interrater reliability of these counts was 90.0%, with a range of 76.7–100% over individual files.[6]

3. Results

Imitations, immediate repetitions, and clearly formulaic utterances, including lyrics from songs and nursery rhymes, were not counted at all. With this minimal amount of filtering, all functional elements within the clausal system were counted to obtain a result for the number of functional categories per clause under the loose standard. The initial instances were then examined further and selectively filtered out if they did not exhibit at least a partial paradigm for the functional system in question, to obtain a result under the more stringent standard. Since the results are absolute numbers, they will depend on the number of child utterances in the recording session; this is controlled for by normalizing the results for file size. The effects of counting nominative subjects as exemplifying I are then examined.

In section 4, once the basic pattern of development of the functional category system has been ascertained for a child, the files are examined for evidence of the effects of feature matrices containing non-adult combinations of features, projected as functional categories.

3.1. Peter

According to the "first mention" criterion, a functional category is counted as present in child language if it is exemplified by a functional element which would occupy a position (head or spec) within the associated functional system in an adult grammar. The count of clauses containing a specified number of functional categories according to this criterion in Peter's production data is given in Figure 2.[7] (Figures 2–12 are in the Appendix.)

Not pictured in Figure 2 are counts of clauses consisting of a lexical projection only, without functional elements. A handful of clauses with a single functional category appeared at 1;11-5, and within a month the number of such examples began exhibiting a pattern of fast monotonic growth. Clauses with exactly two functional categories were absent until 2;1-18, and then began a pattern of low, variable occurrence, until making a sudden jump to a more substantial level of 43 at 2;6-16 and thereafter. Clauses with three functional categories appear at the end of the period in which recordings were made, on a trajectory of apparent growth, although the data end too soon for the growth trend to be definitively established.

But the number of child utterances varies somewhat across recording sessions. Normalizing the results in Figure 2 with respect to the number of child conversational turns, as discussed in section 2.2 above, yields the results illustrated in Figure 3 in the appendix. The normalized results present the same overall pattern as those in Figure 2. The numbers are slightly different, but in both cases we have low initial counts of clauses with a specified number (1, 2, or 3) of functional categories, followed by a sudden onset of substantially higher counts. In both cases, the initial examples require closer examination in order to determine how variable they are, whether some of them are plausibly formulaic, and whether they are good candidates for exhibiting sub-adult functional categories, which are not counted. Since the normalized results do not differ substantially from the absolute counts, the analysis hereafter will be based on the absolute counts.

Next, we address concerns that arise from taking nominative subjects as the basis for counting Infl, even in the absence of other Infl-elements in a clause. Systematically subtracting away the count of clauses in which the presence of Infl was inferred solely from the presence of a nominative subject, we obtain the results shown in Figure 4. This has no effect on the count of clauses with three functional categories; and it has little effect on the count of clauses with two functional categories, which still exhibit a sudden increase at 2;6-16. But subtracting away the contribution of nominative subjects lowers the number of examples of clauses with one functional category. This doesn't change the basic result from 2;3-3 onwards, where there remain a substantial number of clauses with one functional category. At most, the effect of subtracting away the count of clauses in which Infl is revealed solely by a nominative subject is to shift the sudden increase in the count of clauses with one functional category a month or two back, from 2;1-0 to 2;2-13 or 2;3-3. Thus, here too, nothing is clearly revealed until we undertake further screening of the early examples in order to see which of these examples will survive the more stringent standard of counting that requires a paradigm, or partial paradigm, of instantiating elements in order to count a functional category as present. We now turn to this task.

Returning to Figure 2, at 1;11-5, the examples with one functional category include only one with an auxiliary (*I'll fix it*), and a handful of examples with first person singular nominative subject (*I see it*, *I do it*, *I get them*, *I put them back*). Thus, there is no paradigm of auxiliaries or of nominative subjects, and no paradigm of Infl elements overall in this file. The same is true at 1;11-17. The nine examples at 2;0-10 include only one with an auxiliary (*I'll open that*), and otherwise consist of first person singular nominative subjects; again, no paradigm. But at 2;1-0, the clauses with one functional category include three different auxiliary forms in a total of four forms (*I'll*, *I'm*, *am*, *could*), as well as nominative subjects *she*, and *he*, as well as *I*. These are grounds to assert that a partial paradigm of Infl elements is exhibited at this stage of Peter's development, allowing the count of clauses with one functional category in this file to stand in the more stringent count.

Turning to examples with two functional categories, the notable feature of Figure 2 is the extensive shelf of low values, from 2;3-3 to 2;5-22, before the sudden increase to more substantial values at 2;6-16. What should we make of these? Are they incipient instances of clauses with two functional categories, or do they have a different status from the more numerous examples later? Note that the normalized results in Figure 3, and the results subtracting away effects of nominative case in Figure 4, also exhibit this shelf of low values for counts of two functional elements.

The following observations can be made about these early examples of clauses with two functional elements. All involve an auxiliary, either in a combination of Aux and negation, or with Aux-fronting. Almost all of the auxiliaries are instances of *can* or *do*, or their variants with negation, *can't* and *don't*. The remainder seem to be delivered formulaically, including *What're you doing?* at 2;3-3 and elsewhere, and *This is not working*, at 2;4-15. There are two examples which do not involve *can* or *do*, and do not seem to be delivered formulaically; they are *Will you do it?* at 2;3-24, and *Could # I have a pencil?* at 2;5-3. The presence of '#' in the latter indicates that it was not delivered as a single utterance. Finally, although *can't* and *don't* occur clause-medially in these early instances about as often as *can* and *do*, only *can* and *do* are fronted in questions in these files. In contrast, the file at age 2;6-16, the first with a substantial number (forty-three) of clauses with two functional elements, contains the examples in (9) which fall outside the limitations mentioned above (along with 37 other examples which adhere to them):

(9) a. *Have you got a present for me?*
b. *Would you like a pretzel?*
c. *I'm not crying down there.*
d. *Will you put it back?*
e. *I'm not gonna let go with it.*
f. *Are we going on the choo-choo train?*

This constitutes a substantial and quite varied inventory of clauses with two functional categories at 2;6-16 and thereafter. In contrast, the very limited inventory from 2;3-3 to 2;5-22 seems to be a different, more restricted, phenomenon. It is plausible to suppose that any two of Infl, Neg and Comp can occur productively together from 2;6-16 onward, and that the more restricted combinations up through 2;5-22 involve sub-adult categories.

Turning to examples with three functional elements in Figure 2, four of the five examples at 2;10-19 are introduced by the complementizer *(be)cause*. The remaining example is *Know why the dogs can't get out*. In contrast, the 17 examples at 3;1-20 involve three different complementizers, *(be)cause*, *so* and *if*, and a variety of I+Neg combinations. It is therefore plausible to say that *(be)cause* and *why* are sub-adult categories at 2;10-19, but that C, I, and Neg are being productively combined as adult categories in clauses with three functional categories at 3;1-20.

Thus, a more stringent count of clauses with functional elements begins counting clauses with one productive functional category at 2;1-0, clauses with productive combinations of two functional categories at 2;6-16, and clauses with productive combinations of three functional categories at 3;1-20. The results of this more stringent count are represented in Figure 5.

In order to assess the import of these results, it is important to know when the phrasal complexity is achieved to support multiple functional categories, and at what point productive Comp elements appear, occupying positions within a complementizer system. The requisite phrasal complexity is attained at a surprisingly early age. As early as 2;1-18, Peter has a selectional chain of at least five heads in the example in (10).

(10) *I wan(t) (t)a put the toys away.*

Since, under either of the counting standards of Figure 2 or Figure 5, Infl is present at this point, we assume that the nominative subject occupies spec-IP in (10) and that the infinitival marker *to* occupies the infinitival I node. Thus, (10) exemplifies the selectional chain (I_{fin}, V_{fin}, I_{inf}, V_{inf}, (D), N), which includes six heads if D is present at this stage, and five heads otherwise. This file exhibits a selectional chain of at least three lexical heads in *Take it to the living room*. The next file, at 2;2-13, exhibits the example in (11), with a selectional chain containing at least five heads:

(11) *S(u)pposed to go on the inside.*

However, there are no signs of productive Comp until 2;6-16. At this age, which supports two functional categories, there are a number of examples with selectional chains containing five or six heads. The combinations of two functional categories include, along with productive Aux+Neg and I+Neg combinations, the C+I combinations shown in (12).

(12) a. *Is this part of the train?*
b. *Have you got a present for me?*
c. *Would you like a pretzel?*
d. *Are they people feet?*
e. *Does that make you sick?*
f. *Will you put it back?*
g. *Where are you going?*

These examples exhibit productive use of Comp and Infl together. So at this point, Peter has productive Neg, Infl and Comp occurring separately, or two at a time, and he has sufficient phrasal complexity to permit examples in which Neg, Infl, and Comp all occur together. But he has, in fact, no examples with Neg, Infl and Comp all occurring together, and won't exhibit such examples until many months later (2;10-19 at the earliest, and 3;1-20 for fully productive examples).

Thus, the overall pattern of acquisition of functional categories for Peter is the successive growth in the number of functional categories which can co-occur together illustrated in Figure 5, with the quite sudden appearance of substantial numbers of clauses which make productive use of one functional category, followed later by the quite sudden increase in that number to two, apparently followed, at the end, by the quite sudden increase in that number to three. Both Infl and Neg elements are used productively (one at a time) by the onset of the productive use of a single functional category, at 2;1-0. Comp elements do not come into productive use until later, at 2;6-16, where they combine productively with Infl elements in clauses with two functional categories. Since Infl, Neg and Comp elements are all being used separately, or in combinations of two, by 2;6-16, but never appear in combinations of all three, despite Peter's demonstrated ability at this time to produce the requisite phrasal complexity, there seems to be a structural constraint against the productive use of three functional categories until months later, at 3;1-20.

3.2. Nina

Counting clauses with specified numbers of functional categories using the first mention criterion, which counts functional elements as present whether or not they exhibit a paradigm of any sort, yields the results in Figure 6. For reasons of space, the first two recording sessions, which have zero functional elements, and the third and fourth, which have two elements each, are not represented in Figure 6.[8] Tacking these onto the beginning of Figure 6 yields an initial, nearly flat, segment with very few functional elements of any kind. This ends at 2;1-15, where Nina suddenly exhibits 29 clauses with one functional element, and continues at this pace until 2;2-6, at which point this number takes another discrete jump to 47. The profile of clauses with two functional elements exhibits a similar pattern, but with somewhat less dramatic numbers. There are few (typically no) examples with two functional elements, until 2;2-28, at which point the number jumps to 14, and it continues at roughly this magnitude (with the curious exception of a session at 2;3-5), until it takes another discrete jump to 22 (at 2;9-13), and then to 42 (at 2;9-21). Examples with three functional elements appear in modest numbers from around age 3 onward, but do not grow to a substantial level during any of the recorded sessions.

The recording sessions with Nina did not vary tremendously in the number of child utterances, measured as conversational turns. A couple of sessions which were exceptionally short were among those exempted from representation in Figure 6. The remaining files, which range from 394 to 798 child utterances, mostly contained around 700. In Figure 7, the results in Figure 6 are normalized with respect to the number of child utterances. As is evident, the normalized results present the same profile of acquisition as the results in Figure 6, with discrete increases in the numbers of clauses with one functional element, and clauses with two functional elements, occurring at the same points as in Figure 6.

If we disregard the contribution of nominative subjects to the counts in Figure 6, by subtracting away all sentences which exhibit Infl exclusively as a nominative case subject, we obtain the results in Figure 8. The totals in Figure 8 are reduced in relation to the corresponding totals in Figure 6, but the overall pattern is the same, except for the initial examples with substantial numbers of clauses with one functional element. If we disregard nominative case, then the onset of examples with one functional element is less sudden, and such examples begin to reach substantial levels later, at 2;3-5 instead of at 2;1-22. But we will continue to assume that finite Infl is implicated in the appearance of a nominative subject (the checking of a feature for nominative case on the subject), and therefore to include the instances of nominative subjects in the counts of functional elements, as in Figure 6.

It remains to examine the data for Nina under the more stringent standard of counting functional elements, which counts them only when they exhibit a paradigm, or partial paradigm. The initial examples of clauses with one functional element, before 2;1-15 are not sufficiently numerous to exhibit a paradigm until possibly at 2;1-6, but the examples in this file, given in (13), are very limited:

(13) a. *He's eating his cereal.*
b. *It's raining.*
c. *It's cooking.*
d. *He's cooking.*
e. *He's sleeping.*

The examples at 2;1-15 and beyond are distinctly more varied, including nominative subjects other than first person singular, and auxiliary elements other than cliticized *is*. Turning to clauses with two functional elements, the five examples at 2;1-29 include only instances of *can't* and *don't*, which is not much of a paradigm. The 14 examples of clauses with two functional elements at 2;2-28, in contrast, include complementizers, fronted *wh*-expressions, as well as *won't* and *don't*, as do the 12 examples at 2;3-14. These seem to be varied enough to exhibit productive use of two functional categories. If not, the 22 examples at 2;9-13, with varied combinations of Comp+Infl, Comp+Neg, and Infl+Neg, would have to count as productive. But we will count the earlier examples, beginning at 2;2-28 here since Nina's combinations of auxiliaries, nominative subjects, complementizers, and negation are already quite varied; they include examples such as, *Cause he loves Nina*, *What is that girl doing?*, and, *I won't need that blanket*. The onset of three functional categories is less clear, as is evident in Figure 6, and Figures 7 and 8 do not shed any light on the onset of clauses at this level of complexity. The six examples at 3;0-16 all involve the complementizers *'cause* (5 examples) or *so* (1 example). The 9 examples at 3;3-1 likewise all involve the complementizer *'cause*, except for one which has *so*. The six examples at 3;3-21 include a *that*-relative as well as complementizers *(be)cause* and *so*, and thus provide a better paradigm despite the smaller number of examples. Thus, 3;3-21 presents the best case for the onset of three functional categories. Nevertheless, in light of the notable consistency of examples with three functional categories, which are essentially absent until Nina turns 3, and very persistent thereafter, and in light of the fact that the recording sessions for Nina typically contain only about four-tenths the number of child utterances as the sessions charted for Peter in Figures 2 and 5, one might take the onset of three functional categories for Nina to be somewhat earlier. In recognition of these points, we will extend the onset back to 3;3-1, but no earlier for the stringent count, recognizing that there is some arbitrariness in this choice. With these observations (and choices), the results of the more stringent count are shown in Figure 9. Under slightly different choices, with even more stringent counting standards, as discussed above, the onset of one functional category could be put off until 2;2-6, the onset of two functional categories until 2;9-13, and the onset of three functional categories until 3;3-21. However, under this even more stringent count, the onset of clauses with one functional category would be even more abrupt, with an initial value of 47 instead of 29, as would the onset of clauses with two functional categories, with an initial value of 22 instead of 12. Thus, this even more stringent count would just strengthen the conclusion arrived at here, that the number of functional categories exhibits a pattern of growth characterized by sudden, discrete jumps from zero, to one, to two, to three.

As early as 2;4-26, Nina has achieved the phrasal complexity that would be required to represent three different functional categories, C, I, and Neg, together in a clause. At this stage, she utters sentences with selectional chains containing as many as five heads, as in, *I want to pull it up* (I_{fin}, V, I_{inf}, V_{inf}, N), and, *You gonna steps on the monkeys*, which has a selectional chain of five heads counting the determiner *the*, and four heads otherwise. In this same file, Nina produces clauses with a number of different Comp+Infl combinations, such as, *Cause Teddy Bear's crying*, and *Cause he go on sidewalk*, but the range of Comp+Infl examples is not yet very productive.

At 2;9-21, Nina has everything that would be required to represent three functional categories in a single clause. Included among many examples with selectional chains of five or more heads were the following:

(14) a. *I will try to put a bottle in his mouth.*
(I$_{fin}$, V, I$_{inf}$, V$_{inf}$, P, (D), N)
b. *It's more fun to not be sad.*
(A, I$_{inf}$, Neg, V$_{inf}$, A)

Furthermore, at this stage she has productive examples of Comp+Infl and Infl+Neg. Examples of her Comp+Infl combinations are given in (15) below.

(15) a. *So you will see my tummy better.*
b. *It open # so the horsie could get out.*
c. *I wanna pull this out # ... so she could go up high.*
d. *(Be)cause he's getting out of his crib.*
e. *Do you see a big plate and a little plate?*
f. *How can we open it now?*
g. *Can he sit on the couch?*

Thus, at this point, Nina has three functional categories, which she can produce independently or in combinations of two, and she has sentences with sufficient phrasal complexity to support three functional categories. Yet she does not produce clauses with three functional categories at this point, and doesn't begin to until 2;11-16, and she doesn't begin to produce even partial paradigms of such examples until 3;3-1 and 3;3-21.[9] Thus, there seems to be a further structural constraint on Nina's capacity to produce clauses with three functional categories at this point, a constraint which is finally lifted by about age 3;3-1.

3.3. Naomi

Figure 10 presents the counts of clauses with different numbers of functional categories in the production data for Naomi. The files for Naomi vary greatly in size, measured as the number of child utterances. A version of Figure 10 normalized with respect to the number of child utterances is given in Figure 11.

The initial examples of clauses with one functional category are notably nonproductive. The 15 instances of nominative subjects at 1;10-18 are all first person singular, and sometimes occur in repetitive blocks such as those in (16)–(17) (counted as only two distinct instances of the use of a nominative subject), each of which presents four successive conversational turns by Naomi.

(16) *I want coffee.*
I want coffee.
I want coffee.
I want coffee.

(17) *I want banana.*
I want banana.
I want apple.
I want apple.

As late as 1;11-2, Naomi exhibits only one form of Aux element (*I'm singing down. I'm trying.*), and nominative subjects only in the first person singular. These seem to be formulaic constructions rather than productive use of an I node. But at 1;11-6, examples surface with Aux elements *'s*, *is*, *are*, *did*, and *can*, and the nominative subjects include third person singular as well as first person singular; altogether, this constitutes a partial paradigm of Infl elements. At this point, even though the number of examples with candidate I elements is not vastly greater than in earlier files, Naomi could be said to exhibit productive use of I.

There is a handful of early, isolated, and presumably formulaic, instances of clauses with two functional elements. Turning to files with multiple instances, the four examples at 2;0-18 all involve *can*, *do*, and non-fronted instances of *can't* and *don't*, a pattern which was argued above to be not productive in the discussion of Peter's data. The four examples at 2;1-1 and the five at 2;1-9 consist almost entirely of examples with sentence-initial *what's* and *where's*, which are considered adjoined by Radford (1990) and others; but see section 4.2 below, where these *wh*-elements are interpreted as the result of projecting a non-adult combination of features. The five examples at 2;1-17 and subsequent files, though not initially more numerous, include fronted *wh*+Aux, and (by 2;2-25) the complementizer *'cause* as well. These are the first recording sessions which could be argued to exhibit productive use of two functional categories by Naomi, and such use is well established by 2;4-30. The onset of productive use of two functional categories will be taken to be at 2;1-17.

There is an isolated example of a clause with three functional categories at 2;3-17, shown in (18).

(18) Mother: *Why do you think Kristen's crying?*
Naomi: *Cause she's not crying.*

Since *(be)cause* does not make sense in this context, it might be mistakenly used as a coordinator across discourse, to mean "But she's not crying." As a result, this is not a compelling example of three functional categories. The examples with three functional elements beginning at 3;2-10 vary across a number of different combinations of Comp, Infl, and negation, although these examples are not numerous in any one recording session. They include the following:

(19)
a. *Why are we not getting it anymore?* (3;2-10)
b. *Because I don't want them to happen.* (3;2-10)
c. *Doesn't she look funny?* (3;3-27)
d. *I'm gonna cover these up because I don't like them.* (3;3-27)
e. *Aren't they pretty?* (3;4-0)
f. *Would you tear it off so I won't see it?* (3;4-0)
g. *So you won't get water in your eyes.* (3;5-7)
h. *She can't have anything because she didn't say anything.* (3;5-7)

If high numbers are required within a single recording session, then Naomi's sessions are not long enough for her to demonstrate productive use of three functional categories within a single clause. But we might take the variety and lack of formulaic patterns in the instances of clauses with three functional categories over the different recording sessions from 3;2-10 onward as evidence that Naomi has productive use of three functional categories during this period.

With these observations and choices, Naomi's productive use of functional categories, exhibiting at least partial paradigms, is represented in Figure 12.[10]

At 2;3-17, Naomi produces sentences with selectional chains consisting of five heads, and the example in (20), which has seven (tracing the chain down into the PP object of *put*), not counting the determiner on the final nominal, and eight counting that determiner.

(20) *I don't want to put it back on the table.*
(I$_{fin}$, Neg, V, I$_{inf}$, V, P, (D), N)

In this same file, Naomi produces Comp+Infl and Infl+Neg combinations, including those in (21), as well as the example in (20).

(21) a. *What are you doing with it?*
b. *Do you want some bread?*
c. *Cause she's tired.*
d. *She's not crying.*
e. *I don't like sugar.*

Thus, it appears that at 2;3-17, Naomi has the resources to represent and produce clauses with three functional categories. Yet, she does not produce such clauses at all until the period from 3;2-10 onward.

3.4. Summary

The same basic results were obtained for all three of the children whose production data was examined here. The onset of clauses with a particular number *n* (= 1, 2, or 3) of clausal functional categories (C, I, Neg) was typically marked by a period in which *n* functional elements are used in very limited combinations, with a very limited selection of lexical items, a nonproductive pattern assumed (initially) to involve sub-adult categories. The onset of this period was soon, or immediately, followed by sessions in which *n* functional elements appear in more productive combinations, taken as evidence for the presence of *n* functional categories. Disregarding the counts of nonproductive instances, the maximum number of clausal functional categories present in the child's clauses exhibits an overall pattern of discrete growth, from 0, to 1, to 2, to 3. For all three children, it is possible to identify a stage at which they exhibit productive use of all three clausal functional categories in isolation, or in combinations of two, and at which they exhibit the phrasal complexity to represent all three clausal functional categories, but at which they are still some time away from producing all three functional categories together. This lag is recorded in Table 2.

Table 2. The emergence of three functional categories per clause

	Phrasal complexity sufficient for 3 FC's	C, I, Neg used 1 and 2 at a time	C, I, Neg together: 3 FC's
Peter	2;1-18	2;6-16	3;1-20
Nina	2;4-26	2;9-13	3;3-1
Naomi	2;3-17	2;3-17	3;2-10

The first column of ages in Table 2 records the age at which each child has attained a phrasal complexity of utterance sufficient to accommodate three functional categories together within a single clause, and the second column records the (greater or equal) age at which the child exhibits productive use of each of the three clausal functional categories, C, I, Neg, and, indeed, productive combinations of C+I and I+Neg. The last column gives the age at which productive use of three functional categories in a single clause is first clearly manifest.

Likewise, for Peter and Nina, it is possible to identify a stage at which they exhibit productive use of two clausal functional categories in isolation, one at a time, and at which they exhibit the phrasal complexity to represent two clausal functional categories, but at which they do not yet produce two functional categories together. This is shown in the appropriate lines of Table 3 below.

Table 3. The emergence of two functional categories per clause

	Phrasal complexity sufficient for 2 FC's	2 FC's, used 1 at a time	2 FC's together
Peter	2;1-18	2;3-24	2;6-16
Nina	2;1-15	2;1-19	2;2-28
Naomi	1;11-2	2;2-25	2;1-17

Naomi doesn't fully exhibit this pattern since she has clauses with two functional categories ([I+Neg] and [C+I]) as early as 2;1-17, but it is not until 2;2-25 that she exhibits either of C or Neg by itself, rather than in combination with I. But this is probably an artifact of the relatively small sizes of Naomi's recording files, which typically range around 200 utterances, as opposed to 800–1400 for Peter and 500–800 for Nina.

4. Discussion of results

4.1. The development of the adult functional category system

The graphs in Figures 5, 9, and 12 exhibit a step-wise increase in the complexity of the functional systems in the children's grammars. Tables 2 and 3 provide an essential point of detail regarding this step-wise growth. Table 2 shows that Peter produces clausal phrase structures of sufficient complexity to represent all three functional categories together in a single clause by 2;1-18, and he exhibits each of the three clausal functional categories C, I, and Neg individually by 2;6-16, yet he does not productively combine all three functional categories in a single clause until half a year later, at 3;1-20. By 2;9-13, Nina has acquired all three clausal functional categories, and uses them independently and in productive combinations of two, and exhibits sufficient phrasal complexity to support examples with all three functional categories, yet she does not begin to regularly produce examples with three functional elements until two and a half months later (3;0-3), and does not produce anything close to a partial paradigm of such examples until several further months (3;3-1). Likewise with Naomi. It appears that at 2;3-17, Naomi has the resources to represent and produce clauses with three functional categories. Yet, she does not produce such clauses at all until the period from 3;2-10 onward, nearly eleven months later. Turning to Table 3, Peter exhibits command of at least two functional categories which he can use singly in a clause and he demonstrates phrase structure complexity sufficient to combine those two functional categories within a single clause well before he actually produces examples with two functional categories per clause. Nina exhibits a similar pattern, though in her case the time lag is smaller.

Tables 2 and 3 show that the growth in complexity of the functional systems cannot be reduced to growth in the general phrase structure complexity of the children's utterances. Furthermore, to the extent that the production of phrase structure complexity on the measure used here, the length of selectional chains of both functional and lexical heads, requires working memory and processing capacity roughly in proportion to the length of the chain, or to the number of functional heads in the chain, the results in Tables 2 and 3 show more indirectly that the representation of multiple functional categories within a clause lags behind acquisition of the requisite working memory and processing capacity.[11]

These results can now be evaluated in light of the theories of functional category acquisition surveyed in section 1 above. On any theory, a child cannot exhibit functional heads X_1, …, X_n together within a clause until the child has acquired a suitable inventory of functional elements, consisting of subsets of morphemes or lexical items associated with each of X_1, …, X_n, and has achieved the working memory and processing capacity to compute representations of X_1, …, X_n together within a clause. Any further limitation would have to follow from the details of the acquisitional process which the theory proposes, which in turn depend on the nature of the functional categories posited by the theory. On the strong continuity account, functional structure is innately specified, and is available for use by the child once it has been triggered by appropriate linguistic input. It follows that, once a suitable inventory of functional elements is on hand, and the child has sufficient working memory and processing capacity, then any functional category, or combination of functional categories, should occur in the child's grammar. On Radford's (1990) maturational account, all functional categories mature in parallel. Thus, on this theory too, once a suitable inventory of functional elements is on hand, and the child has sufficient working memory and processing capacity, any functional category, or combination of functional categories, should occur. Therefore, these theories do not provide grounds to expect the step-wise growth of the functional category system revealed in Figures 5, 9, and 12, with the lags in the representation of multiple functional categories per clause exhibited by Tables 2 and 3.

The bottom-up structure building accounts are more on the mark since each of the children studied exhibits many Infl and Neg elements, and combinations of the two, before s/he shows a paradigm of Comp elements. But even the bottom-up structure building account does not account for the productive occurrence of C+I combinations six to eleven months before the child achieves the adult capacity to represent all three functional elements productively within a single clause. On the bottom-up structure building accounts, there are structural constraints against the representation of C, I, and Neg together, and these accounts rule out the C+I combinations until the last stages of the acquisition of functional categories, and this prediction does not seem to be borne out.

Instead, it seems that there is a structural constraint against the representation of three functional categories together in a single clause. What we have is something close to the results predicted by the structure-building accounts, but suggesting a crucial difference: not that the child's functional systems grow from the bottom of tree structure to the top, but that the resources for the representation of functional categories undergo growth from the lexical stage (resources for zero functional categories), to the 1-category stage, at which any one functional category can be represented, to the 2-category stage, at which any two functional categories can be represented (I+Neg, C+I, or C+Neg); and finally to the capacity to represent three functional categories, the adult stage with regard to the number of categories distinguished in this study.

A question arises: if the 1-category stage really reflects the capacity to represent any one functional category, why doesn't the C-system manifest itself productively in this period? A plausible answer is that the projection of the C-system in a clause is triggered by clausal complementation (see Grimshaw 1991, 1997); on these grounds, we shouldn't expect a productive C-system until the grammar grows in other respects (including acquisition of predicates which select a clausal argument) to an extent that supports finite subordinate clauses. These make their initial appearances later on. In fact, their establishment roughly accompanies the onset of the two-functional category period. Only from this point on would we expect to find productive C-elements.

Returning to the basic profile of growth, from zero clausal functional categories, to the capacity to represent any one (limited by extraneous factors, as discussed in the previous paragraph), to the capacity to represent any two, to the capacity, finally, to represent all three, we have seen that standard theories of the development of functional categories presented in the literature do not predict, or account for, this pattern. These theories are all based on a standard clausal architecture of functional categories, as indissoluble or indivisible collections of features, including a categorial feature which defines the category of the functional head, to which all the other features associated with that category are tied.

The feature-based theory of functional categories presented in Chapter 2 makes available different representational possibilities, as seen in Chapters 3, 4, and 5, and makes different constraints on acquisition formulable, as suggested in section 1.5 above. On the feature-based theory, a functional category is an unlabelled locus for a matrix of noncategorial features. The capacity to combine a set of features together and project them at such a locus is a basic representational capability of the grammar. The results in section 3 above, and particularly the results illustrated in Tables 2 and 3, suggest that this capacity is not fixed, but rather develops. The child initially cannot project even one such matrix of features as a functional category in the syntax. Subsequently, the child is capable of projecting one such matrix in the functional structure of a clause, but not more than one. After an additional period of time, typically several months, the child acquires the ability to project two such matrices as separate functional categories in the functional phrase structure of a clause, but not more than two. Finally, the child acquires the ability to project three such matrices together as separate functional categories in the functional phrase structure of a clause.

Interpreted in this way, the capacity to project a given number of matrices of functional features in the functional phrase structure of a clause is a basic representational capacity, reflecting basic representational resources of the grammar, and the child's limitations in the number of matrices which can be projected together as separate functional categories in the functional phrase structure of a clause is a basic limitation in representational resources. The distinctive profile in the acquisition of functional categories discovered in section 3 is, on this analysis, a straightforward reflection of the growth in representational resources available to the child. The capacity to project *n* matrices of functional features lags behind the development of complex phrase structure, and thus behind the development of working memory and general processing capacities required for complex phrase structure (including phrase structure involving multiple functional categories across clausal boundaries). It is a specific capacity to project a given number of matrices of functional features, and (before the capacity has matured fully), a limitation specific to that capacity. Given its lag behind the development of complex phrase structure, it is unlikely to be an epiphenomenon of limitations of working memory or other more general capacities. We take it here at face value. The capacity to project *n* matrices of functional features is a basic representational capacity of the grammar, which matures as *n* grows through the values 0, 1, 2, and 3.

4.2. Non-adult feature matrices

In the previous chapter, it was observed that, prior to the acquisition of the adult functional category system, children project individual features in order to express functional material. The discussion there did not determine whether multiple features projected under these circumstances were projected individually, in scattered form, or aggregated into non-adult feature matrices comprised of non-adult combinations of features. The two possibilities were presented in the two rows of Table 1 in Chapter 6, and the matter was left at that.

The results of the present chapter provide some grounds on which to resolve this issue. It was found above that the projection of adult functional categories depends on a representational capacity which constrains the number of functional categories which can be projected together within a single clause. These results were obtained using conservative methods, counting a functional category as present only when a suitable partial paradigm of its manifestations is exhibited. As such, this result does not automatically apply to the examples of the projection of functional features in early child language discussed in the previous chapter, since we assumed there that a functional feature would be projected as soon as it is expressed (with a minimal alternation to assure that the feature is truly being expressed). A representational constraint on the co-occurrence of adult functional categories within a clause does not necessarily apply to the projection of features onto sub-adult functional categories of the sort observed in early child language. However, as discussed above, the constraint on the projection of adult functional categories implicates a process of maturation of underlying representational resources for the projection of functional categories. Thus, it is a sound conjecture that when multiple functional features are projected in early child language onto sub-adult functional categories, there will be representational pressure to aggregate them, and project them as one complex feature matrix, rather than to project them in scattered form, as multiple feature matrices each with one feature. The relevant examples from the data for Peter, Nina and Naomi are examined here.

The examples in (22) below occur in the first two recording sessions in which Peter is credited with one functional category on the stringent count; they can't be examples of two adult functional categories since the two functional category stage begins much later, at 2;6-16.

(22) a. *What she doing?* (2;1-0)
b. *Where's the pocketbook go?* (2;1-0)
c. *What you do with this?* (2;1-18)
d. *Where's the bolt # go in?* (2;1-18)

Peter exhibits a minimal alternation in nominative case in this period, and thus expresses [NOM]. There are no alternations indicating Aux-fronting; the contraction *where's* is common in child language before the point at which productive *wh*-fronting is acquired, and is generally regarded as monomorphemic at this stage, simply a variant pronunciation of the *wh*-word. The *wh*-forms therefore are simply manifestations of the feature [WH]. Thus, Peter projects both [WH] and [NOM] in these examples. The question is whether he projects them in scattered form, as separate heads ^[WH] and ^[NOM], or in aggregated form, as a head ^[[WH], [NOM]]. We know that Peter can represent only one adult functional category at this point: the recording lies within the one functional category stage delineated in the present chapter. This suggests representational pressure which would favor projection of fewer functional heads, thus the aggregated form. On this hypothesis, (22a) would be generated upon projection of the matrix [[WH], [NOM]], with *what* and *she* appearing in multiple specifiers of ^[[WH], [NOM]]P. Since [WH] < [NOM], the pronoun subject will move into spec-^[[WH], [NOM]]P first, checking [NOM], and the *wh*-expression will subsequently move to a higher spec-^[[WH], [NOM]]P, checking [WH]; thus the *wh*-initial word order is obtained. The examples in (22b,d) will be generated similarly if they involve expression of [NOM]; otherwise, they could be generated by projection of [WH] by itself, as ^[WH], with movement of the *wh*-word to spec-^[WH]P.

Peter also produced the example in (23) during this period.

(23) *I no want go home.* (2;1-18)

Since Peter is under representational pressure to project only one functional category at this point, this would best be generated from the non-adult matrix [[NOM], [NEG]], assuming that *no* appears in the head of this category and the subject moves to its specifier.

Also during this period, still well within the one functional category stage for adult categories, Peter produced the examples in (24), in which tense features on an auxiliary are projected in the same clause as [NEG].

(24) a. *Can't find it.* (2;1-0)
b. *Mommy don't go home.* (2;2-13)
c. *That's not my writing.* (2;2-13)
d. *Don't have top on.* (2;2-13)
e. *Don't have enough room!* (2;3-3)
f. *You can't have that scissors.* (2;3-3)

It was argued in section 3 above that these don't exhibit enough of a paradigm to count as evidence of two functional categories. In a grammar with capacity to project only one functional category then, they are best accounted for as the result of projecting the non-adult feature matrix [Tns, [NEG]] as a single head ^[Tns, [NEG]], in which a tense submatrix is combined with [NEG]. In this same period, there are some examples of this type with nominative subjects, as in (25).

(25) a. *I can't do it.* (2;2-13)
b. *I can't reach it.* (2;3-3)

Assuming representational pressure, these are best regarded as projections of the non-adult matrix, [Tns, [NOM], [NEG]].

Nina, in her stage for the projection of one adult functional category, produced the examples in (26), expressing tense features, [NOM], and [NEG] within a single clause.

(26) a. *I don't break them.* (2;1-22)
b. *I can't take that off.* (2;1-22)
c. *I don't know.* (2;1-29)
d. *He can't see.* (2;1-29)
e. *He don't use your eyes.* (2;1-29)
f. *That don't go.* (2;1-29)

There is no paradigm of Aux+*n't* yet, or any other manifestations of two adult functional categories. Assuming that the representational pressures of the one functional category stage have some force for the projection of sub-adult functional categories, the examples in (26) appearing at this stage are best regarded as resulting from the projection of a single functional head ^[Tns, [NOM], [NEG]], that is, projection of a feature matrix consisting of a tense feature submatrix, Tns, together with the individual features [NOM] and [NEG].

Finally, Naomi, during her stage for one adult functional category, produced examples projecting Tns, subject agreement features [$F_{V\text{-}s}$, $F_{N\text{-}s}$] and [Q], all together in one clause, as in (27) below; in (28), [WH] is projected along with these other features.

(27) a. *Is it raining?* (1;11-6)
b. *Is it going to work?* (1;11-6)
c. *Are sheep running?* (1;11-6)
d. *Is kangaroo sleeping?* (1;11-21)
e. *Do you want some?* (1;11-21)

(28) a. *Where did it go?* (1;11-6)
b. *Where'd it go?*

Under representational pressure, the examples in (27) are best regarded as resulting from merger of the non-adult category ^[[Q], [$F_{V\text{-}s}$, $F_{N\text{-}s}$], Tns] to VP, with the auxiliary subsequently moving to this functional head. The examples in (28) will be produced from the merger of the non-adult category ^[[Q, WH], [$F_{V\text{-}s}$, $F_{N\text{-}s}$], Tns] to VP, with the auxiliary subsequently moving to this head, and the *wh*-word to its specifier. In addition, in this period Naomi exhibits merger of ^[Tns, [NEG]] in instances of *don't*, and of ^[[WH], [NOM]] or ^[WH] in questions such as *What's Mommy doing?*, of the sort observed with Peter and Nina.

On the feature-based theory, the examples in (22)–(28) project features which are adjacent in linear order together as one feature matrix in the child grammar, whether or not they are projected together in the adult grammar. These early examples can be directly accommodated on the feature-based view of functional category composition, and need not be discarded as involving ad hoc adjunction structures, standing apart from the normal mechanisms for the expression of functional elements. As discussed below, none of the other theories of functional category acquisition surveyed in section 1 above accommodates these examples so readily, through a minor perturbation of the normal operations of functional category generation.

The non-adult functional categories in evidence are listed in (29) below.

(29) a. ^[[WH], [NOM]]
b. ^[[NOM], [NEG]]
c. ^[Tns, [NEG]]

d. ^[Tns, [NOM], [NEG]]
e. ^[WH]
f. ^[[Q], [$F_{V\text{-}s}$, $F_{N\text{-}s}$], Tns]
g. ^[[Q, WH], [$F_{V\text{-}s}$, $F_{N\text{-}s}$], Tns]

The feature-based theory of functional categories directly provides for non-adult combinations of features such as those in (29) in the acquisition of functional categories. On the feature-based theory, the projection of such categories would be the expected result if the child seeks to express multiple features which are projected onto separate functional categories in the adult grammar, but the child does not have the representational resources to project multiple functional categories as projection sites for those features. In this case, the child is free to create divergent forms from those in the adult grammar, subject only to universal constraints. The universal constraint on the projection of features is just that the partial linear order be respected, that is, a feature (or feature matrix) F_i cannot be projected lower in phrase structure and checked earlier than another feature or matrix F_j if $F_i < F_j$. The merger of the heads in (29) in the examples cited above conforms to this general constraint. Thus, although the heads in (29) involve feature combinations which do not obtain in the adult grammar of English, they are nevertheless consistent with the universal constraint on the projection of features onto functional categories. This makes them plausible candidates for the sort of divergence from the adult grammar which we expect in language acquisition, producing forms which reflect the exercise of different options than the adult grammar, but respecting universal constraints.[12]

The effects of projecting these heads are not obtained on other theories of functional category acquisition. Specifically, they are not obtained by employing the mechanisms made available by those theories, with different options from those exercised in the adult grammar, but subject to universal constraints on how the mechanisms of the theory are deployed. On accounts which appeal to a fixed stock of functional categories, the functional categories are defined by their categorial features. It is possible that a feature may occasionally be mistakenly assigned to the wrong category at an intermediate stage of child language acquisition, but to admit the wholesale reassignments exhibited in (29) would amount to an admission that the functional categories are, in effect, not defined by their categorial features, but rather, by their total feature composition, which is precisely the claim of the feature-based account. An attempt to accommodate the categories in

(29) on the basis of a fixed stock of functional categories would, in effect, mean acquiescence in the main points of the feature-based theory.

5. Structure building approaches to the acquisition of functional categories

The results of the present study lend the most support to an acquisitional scenario involving maturation of the capacity to represent functional categories, formulated in terms of the feature-based theory of functional categories, as compared to standard theories of the acquisition of functional categories available in the literature. But among those other theories, the second-best fit with the present results was with the bottom-up structure building accounts of the acquisition of functional categories. These accounts, along with the account formulated in terms of the feature-based theory of functional categories, actively predict that the number of clausal functional categories that can occur together within a single clause should undergo maturational growth in a monotonically increasing sequence from 0, to 1, 2, and finally, 3. Other accounts discussed in section 1 do not predict this result. Furthermore, the bottom-up structure building accounts are similar in spirit to the account proposed here founded on the feature-based theory of functional categories in that they propose a structure building maturation of functional categories with some sort of sequential constraint.

As noted in section 4 above, the empirical deficiency of the bottom-up structure building theories is that they do not account for the productive occurrence of C+I combinations five to eleven months before the child achieves the adult capacity to represent the full suite of functional elements productively within a single clause, as shown in Table 2. On bottom-up structure building, the C-system is the last functional system to be acquired, so C+I combinations should not appear until the final stage in the acquisition of the functional systems, contrary to the results observed here.

At a more conceptual level, the main difference between the present account and a bottom-up structure building account is in the theoretical primitives on which the theories are based. Bottom-up structure building deals with particular, identifiable functional categories, imposing a particular sequence of acquisition on them, whereas the present account proposes maturational growth of an underlying representational resource, which accommodates successively greater numbers of functional categories obtained derivatively, as bundles of functional features, not involving categorial features. The present section seeks to examine this conceptual difference. Since the bottom-up structure building accounts are the closest in spirit to the present account, and the closest in predicting the empirical results reported in section 3, it is worthwhile comparing these accounts more closely with the account proposed here.

5.1. Guilfoyle and Noonan

Guilfoyle and Noonan (1992) present one such account. They argue that various features of child language, including the lack of verbal passives, the possibility of null subjects, word order possibilities due to the presence or absence of verb-second in child German, and word order in child English *yes/no*- and *wh*-questions, can all be explained on the basis of a progression from a purely lexical system, to one with I but not C, and then to a complete suite of adult clausal functional categories. The maturation of functional categories one-by-one is a universal aspect of their account, but there is "crosslinguistic variation in the timing of the emergence of individual functional categories" [p.251] due to variation in the salience of functional elements in the input as a result of language specific factors such as the richness of morphology. In the present account, as well, language specific factors affecting the salience of a particular class of functional elements within a language can play a role in determining when that class of functional elements is learned. For the sake of comparison with results of the present study, discussion here will be confined to learning of the English I and C systems.

At the lexical stage, Guilfoyle and Noonan propose that *wh*-expressions and the negation element *no* appear adjoined to VP, in utterance-initial position. Next, Guilfoyle and Noonan identify a stage within which the child exhibits subject-auxiliary inversion (SAI) in *yes/no*-questions, but not in *wh*-questions. They propose that C is absent in this stage, since otherwise it would be hard to explain the lack of uniform SAI in all questions. Instead, Guilfoyle and Noonan propose that in this stage the child has acquired I, but not C, and that the child has chosen a parameter setting in this stage according to which questions are typed as interrogative with [+wh] marked on I^o rather than on C^o. In *yes/no*-questions, the auxiliary verb moves to I, and spec-IP, functioning as an A′-position, hosts a question operator, while the subject exercises an option under the chosen parameter setting to remain in spec-VP. In *wh*-questions, the *wh*-expression adjoins to

IP in the absence of a C-system, and the auxiliary verb does not move to I, but the subject exercises the option of moving to spec-IP, producing a pattern of *wh*-questions without SAI. Subsequently, the C-system is acquired, and both *yes/no*- and *wh*-questions take the adult structure involving SAI.

This account posits fundamental structural differences between *yes/no*-questions and *wh*-questions during the penultimate stage. Aux moves to I in *yes/no*-questions, but not in *wh*-questions; spec-IP is an A′-position in *yes/no*-questions, but an A-position in *wh*-questions. These features of the analysis raise a number of questions. Why doesn't the child conclude that spec-IP is generally an A′-position in all questions and move *wh*-expressions to spec-IP? Guilfoyle and Noonan propose that the child expects the [+wh]-IP language to have an overt question morpheme in I, but English doesn't, so the child for some reason "assumes that the subject remains *in situ* exceptionally" [p.270] in a *yes/no*-question. The child doesn't conclude this of a *wh*-question, presumably because the *wh*-operator is explicitly present, but the *wh*-expression is adjoined to IP, so it is not clear why it should lead to different expectations on the part of the child with respect to the position of the subject in a *wh*-question as opposed to a *yes/no*-question. And if the child perceives the *wh*-operator as such in a *wh*-question, it is not clear why the *wh*-expression should not appear in spec of the [+wh] IP, rather than being adjoined.

The empirical basis for these differences is the Aux-subject order in early *yes/no*-questions, versus the subject-Aux order in early *wh*-questions. Guilfoyle and Noonan capture this difference through intricate assumptions about the dispensation of the I-system in the child grammar, and by appealing to two different mechanisms for entering functional elements into phrase structure: adjunction and functional category instantiation.

The feature-based theory can capture these facts by appealing only to the mechanisms for the projection of feature matrices as functional categories. At the stage of these early child questions, the child can project at most one functional category in a clause, and has limited command of functional features. Question formation at this stage therefore has to be accomplished with very limited resources. The *yes/no*-questions cited by Guilfoyle and Noonan can be produced by merging ^[Q] with the lexical VP, resulting in Aux movement to ^[Q], which yields Aux-subject order.[13] If the fronted auxiliaries are judged to exhibit a paradigm of tense marking, then this account can be amended minimally to postulate merger of ^[[Q], Tns] with the lexical VP. The *wh*-questions cited by Guilfoyle and Noonan can be produced by merging ^[[WH], [NOM]] to a lexical VP, with (as usual) [WH] < [NOM]. The subject then moves first to spec-(^[[WH], [NOM]])P, and the *wh*-expression subsequently moves to spec-(^[[WH], [NOM]])P, producing multiple specifiers, but with the *wh*-expression preceding the subject in linear order. The auxiliary, meanwhile, remains in its base position. If nominative case is judged not to be manifested at this stage of language development, the same effects are obtained by merging ^[[WH], [EPP]] to the lexical VP.

Guilfoyle and Noonan account for differences between early *yes/no*-questions and early *wh*-questions by proposing that this stage is marked by the presence of a single functional system, the I-system, but that the I-system can host C-elements on occasion, and when it does, it does so at the expense of the child's capacity to support I-elements. Thus, in *yes/no*-questions, when the [+wh]-IP posited by Guilfoyle and Noonan behaves most like the C-system, the subject must revert to spec-VP, instead of raising to spec-IP. The discussion above suggests that we reconceptualize this account: to say that the I-system is present at a stage of acquisition, and that it can host C-elements, but only at the expense of I-elements, is just to say that the child has one functional category at this stage and can only project limited combinations of features in exercising this limited representational capacity.

5.2. Vainikka

A slightly different bottom-up structure building account, but one very similar in spirit, is proposed by Vainikka (1993/94). Vainikka addresses a range of issues concerning the case of subjects in child language, and notes, particularly, that children exhibit an increase in oblique (non-nominative) subjects in their incipient productive *wh*-questions.[14] Some children, including Nina (Suppes 1973, investigated here as well), use oblique subjects early on, and subsequently develop nominative subjects; these children participate in the pattern noted by Vainikka by returning to oblique subjects in incipient productive *wh*-questions. Vainikka proposes that oblique subjects surface in spec-VP, and that nominative subjects are reliant on use of the I-system for nominative case assignment. Like Guilfoyle and Noonan, Vainikka proposes an initial lexical VP stage, followed by a stage in which the I-system is present. The I-system is involved in the productive use of nominative subjects, and is marked by the presence of auxiliaries, tense marking, and subject agreement, but does not exhibit CP-elements. Productive *wh*-questions are developed before the development of a C-system, and are marked by an increase (in some children, a resurgence) of subjects with an oblique (accusative or genitive) case, as in the following examples from Nina.

(30) a. *Look what my got.* (2;3)
b. *Know what my making?* (2;4)

Vainikka proposes that the incipient *wh*-questions are accommodated within a [+wh]-IP, with the *wh*-expression in spec-IP; this results in a compensatory reversion of subjects to spec-VP, where they typically appear with an oblique case. This produces a distinct stage of the acquisitional process in which nominative subjects regress in favor of oblique subjects at the onset of *wh*-questions. Vainikka calls this the "Pre-CP" stage. Subsequently, the child acquires a C-system and produces *wh*-questions with nominative case subjects using the adult CP-structure.

Vainikka's account, like that of Guilfoyle and Noonan, posits an I-system between the lexical stage and the full CP-stage, and proposes that it hosts I-elements, and some incipient C-elements, but that it hosts C-elements only with compensatory loss in its capacity to host I-elements. As with Guilfoyle and Noonan, this is a rather stipulatory way to effect the claim that at a certain point in the acquisitional process there is an upper bound on the complexity of functional material that can appear in the clausal functional system, but without any restriction on the categorial status of that material. This result follows straightforwardly, indeed, automatically, on the account proposed here.

5.3. Summary

The present study found that the complexity of the clausal functional systems grows successively as the child develops. The bottom-up structure building account predicts this result, as does the account proposed here in terms of the feature-based theory of functional categories. The present study also found that C, I, and Neg elements regularly co-occurred in combinations of two at a point when children had the phrasal complexity to represent three clausal functional elements, yet the three types of functional element did not occur productively together. This result is not predicted by the bottom-up structure building accounts, although it follows straightforwardly from the proposal that there is steady growth in the number of functional feature-bundles that the child can project. Finally, in the present section we have noted that the bottom-up structure building accounts explain certain effects of an incipient C-system by superimposing them on the I-system, resulting in loss of capacity to represent I-elements, then reallocating these responsibilities to the fledgling C-system when it is finally assumed to make its appearance. The present section argued that this mode of analysis effectively acknowledges a limit to the complexity of the functional systems, but attempts to capture the effects of that representational constraint in a stipulatory fashion, focusing on shifting roles for standardly defined functional categories. The present chapter proposes that these limits in representational capacity can be formulated more directly by concentrating on more basic representational resources, specifically, from steady growth in the number of functional feature matrices which the child can project into syntactic structure. Bottom-up structure building emerges from this examination as a way of capturing the effects of the increase in representational capacity of functional feature-matrices, but hobbled by retaining a conception of functional categories as categorially fixed and indivisible, with results which are empirically less adequate and conceptually more strained than those of the account proposed here.

6. A new picture of maturation

6.1. On the maturation of representational resources

As shown in previous sections of this chapter, there is evidence that the system of verbal functional categories matures in the development of child language. But the functional categories themselves do not mature into place in a fixed sequence. Rather, the capacity to represent functional categories matures, supporting a progressively larger number of functional categories in the child grammar regardless of their categorial identity. This suggested that the maturation involved is actually the growth of a basic representational resource, rather than a growth of functional structure directly.

In addition to the growth of this basic representational resource, the child is acquiring functional features, and the checking order defined on them in the adult grammar. In early stages of acquisition, the child will project matrices with non-adult combinations of features, subject only to the universal constraint that feature matrices respect the ordering of features. The projection of matrices with non-adult combinations of features may result in part from the representational limitations imposed by the inability to represent multiple functional categories together within a clause. As the feature system is more securely acquired, and representational capacity grows, the adult functional categories in (2), or the categories in an equivalent split Infl system, eventually crystallize out and become stable.

This provides a new kind of maturational theory in the study of child language acquisition. Instead of supposing that particular syntactic structures mature, such as the fixed stock of standard functional categories, the present approach follows Minimalist syntax in reducing particular syntactic representations to more basic representational and derivational primitives. The development of child language is then characterized, in part, by development of these more basic representational and derivational resources.

This extends a trend in the conception of maturational principles which was already underway in Principles and Parameters syntax. At the most particular level, particular constructions, such as the double object construction or the passive, could be said to mature. Under Principles and Parameters syntax, the focus for claims of maturation became more abstract – basic operations or elements of syntactic structure could be said to mature, such as A-movement (Borer and Wexler 1987), X′-theory, Case theory, or Theta theory (Felix 1992), or the functional systems (Radford 1990, Guilfoyle and Noonan 1992, Vainikka 1993/94). Within Minimalist syntax, many of these modules of grammar are reduced to even more basic representational and derivational systems. A fascinating aspect of this reduction is that the resulting primitives have the character of basic resources of the grammar subject to optimization or economy constraints (shortest move, least effort, full interpretation; cf. Chomsky 1993, 1995a, 1995b). As a result, the maturational perspective can now appeal to maturation of measurable basic resources, rather than to maturation of substantive pieces of grammatical structure. The resources in question are not, as far as we can tell, fully general cognitive resources such as memory or computational power since the effects of maturation observed here are subsequent to the development of phrase structure complexity. The attainment of a high degree of phrase structure complexity would seem to exhibit a high level of development of general cognitive resources such as memory and computational power. The fact that this, by itself, is not sufficient for the representation of functional categories suggests that functional categories depend on something further, beyond the development of memory and computational power sufficient to represent complex phrase structure.

The maturational picture sketched here seems desirable to the extent that it makes maturation of linguistic structure more explicable. It is not maturation of fully articulated, dedicated linguistic structures, but of more basic, measurable resources which make those structures possible. This is more akin to other instances of biological maturation which, like evolutionary development, do not create new structures out of nothing, but by shifting or reallocating more basic resources from other uses.

6.2. Minimal functional projection and the maturation of minimal functional structure

In Chapter 2, a principle was formulated for the adult grammar regarding the projection of a minimal suite of functional categories to serve the feature-matching needs of a given numeration. This principle, the Economy of Projection of Infl-Categories, is repeated in (31), where clausal features include [EPP], and features matching verbal or adjectival features on a predicative head.

(31) *Economy of Projection of Infl-Categories*
If features F_1, F_2, ..., F_n are elements of a feature matrix M projected as a functional head ^M within the Infl-system of a clause, then at least one of F_1, F_2, ..., F_n must be a clausal (verbal, adjectival, or EPP) feature.

The present chapter demonstrated an incremental, step-by-step growth in the functional categories available to the child, regarded as basic representational resources of the grammar.

The two issues are linked or related in that they both pertain to the extent of the system of functional categories. The child acquisition account postulates growth in the capacity to represent functional categories, from 0 to a number sufficient to represent constructions in the adult grammar, but it does not in any way specify an upper bound for that growth. At this point, a number of open questions arise. Does the growth reach a universal (cross-linguistic) upper bound, or does it produce an intrinsically unbounded number of functional categories? If the growth is intrinsically unbounded, does it nevertheless stop at a language-particular value determined by the representational needs of the particular language? Could it be, for example, that the growth is, on biological grounds, potentially unbounded, but that representational capacity not needed by the language being acquired is not built, or is pruned when it turns out not to be needed? More specifically, could it be that children learning English as a sole first language acquire a handful of functional categories, and that capacity beyond this is pruned, while children learning (say) Semitic languages acquire a larger total of functional categories (according to much recent research), on the order of ten or fifteen, and that only capacity beyond this larger total is pruned for learners of these languages?

A basic idea regarding child language acquisition of functional categories can be distilled out of these considerations. It is formulated in (32) below.

(32) There is no fixed, universal limit to the number of functional categories which can be attained through the growth of the underlying representational capacities. But the number actually attained (and available for actual use) is pruned to what is required for the representational needs of the language being acquired.

This leaves open the question whether children – or adults – might be able to activate or acquire a larger number of functional categories if they subsequently acquire a language which requires a larger total of functional categories.

Now a link emerges between the syntactic analyses of Chapters 2–5 and the results obtained here on child language acquisition of functional categories: both involve a minimalist principle specific to their particular domain. In child language acquisition, the capacity to represent functional categories grows (or gets pruned) to an extent required for the language being acquired, but no more. In the developed grammar (as well as in developing grammars), the number of functional categories projected in the derivation of a particular sentence is kept minimal relative to the need to match or instantiate features on lexical items in the associated numeration.

7. Results of studies of functional category acquisition in other languages

7.1. The growth of functional categories

How well would the account of the acquisition of functional categories developed here travel across languages? Since the growth of basic representational resources in the child's grammar is a plausible aspect of biological maturation, there is reason to expect the present account to be more or less invariant across languages. There are, however, some factors to consider before drawing this conclusion. The development of a functional category, a matrix of functional features projected into syntactic structure on the theory developed here, is dependent in part on the acquisition of associated lexical items bearing these features, and dependent also on the perception that these items fall together as a class. Furthermore, in some cases, evidence for the existence of a functional category will be dependent on movement processes of the language which make the presence of the functional category manifest to the learner. These factors potentially admit some cross-linguistic variation in the acquisition of a functional category. Nevertheless, in the present study, these other conditions for the representation of a functional category were generally met before the development of the capacity to represent the functional category by projecting an associated feature matrix; thus, maturation of the capacity to project feature matrices was the determining factor. In any language for which this is the case, the development of functional categories will be controlled ultimately by biological maturation, whatever differences there might be in the acquisition of individual functional elements. To this extent, the account predicts that other languages should exhibit a roughly similar contour of growth in the functional system to that found here.

In order to pursue this issue, an extended longitudinal study of multiple children across the appropriate age range would be required for each language investigated; such an investigation is beyond the scope of the present work. Instead, some studies in the literature will be surveyed. This discussion will focus on the literature on German since the acquisition of German has been claimed to provide particularly clear evidence for the strong continuity hypothesis, that an invariant system of functional categories is innate. These claims will be addressed at the end of the this section; we begin with studies of robustly longitudinal data.

Accounts of the development of the functional category systems in children learning German are mostly based on verb movement, particularly in the verb-second (V2) construction. To review some points discussed at greater length in Chapter 3, German exhibits SOV word order in subordinate clauses with complementizers, as shown by the contrast between (33) and (34), and OV order of a verb participle with respect to the object, as shown in (34b).

(33) a. *Er sagte, daß Hans das Buch liest.*
he said that Hans the book read
b. *Er sagte, daß Hans das Buch gelesen hat.*
he said that Hans the book read has

(34) a. *Er sagte, Hans liest das Buch.*
b. *Er sagte, Hans hat das Buch gelesen.*

The positions of the verbs in (33), and of the main verb in (34b), are normally taken as evidence of underlying SOV word order (e.g. Webelhuth 1992; see Zwart 1993 for a contrary view). But in finite clauses without an overt complementizer, such as (34) above and (35) below, the finite verb appears in second position following the subject, as in (34), or following other chosen constituents, as in (35).

(35) a. *Das Buch liest Hans heute.*
the book read Hans today
b. *Das Buch hat Hans heute gelesen.*
the book has Hans today read
c. *Heute liest Hans das Buch.*
d. *Heute hat Hans das Buch gelesen.*

This is normally taken to be the result of movement of the finite verb to C (via I), with accompanying movement of a "topicalized" constituent to spec-CP, producing a verb-second structure, as depicted in (36). See den Besten (1983) and subsequent work.

(36) [$_{CP}$ [$_{AdvP}$ *heute*] [$_{C}$ C [$_{I}$ I [$_{V}$ *hat*]]] [$_{IP}$ *Hans* t_{AdvP} [$_{VP}$ [$_{VP}$ *das Buch gelesen*] t_{V}] t_{I}]]

A further characteristic of verb-second is that the finite verb originates to the right of negation and clause-medial adverbs, and raises leftward across them, emerging to their left in C. With V-movement to C in V2 structures, the movement of V through I is not directly manifested. If V-to-I movement is obligatory in general in the derivation of finite clauses in German, then the position of the finite verb in (33a,b) indicates that I is right-headed. If V-to-I is not obligatory, and if it does not take place other than in the derivation of V1 and V2 structures, then the position of the finite verb in (33a,b) is the verb-final base position, and it is then possible to maintain that I is left-headed (see Travis 1984). Verb-first (V1) constructions are exhibited in interrogatives.

Returning to child language acquisition, Meisel (1994) examines longitudinal data for three bilingual children learning German and French.[15] Meisel proposes that these longitudinal data exhibit gradual development of functional categories. An initial lexical stage, with the German merged SOV word order, is followed in sequence by the development of third person singular subject-verb agreement, then the development of first and second person singular subject-verb agreement, and then by the expression of tense. Verb movement effects (consisting of verb-second, and [V Neg] order of the main verb with respect to negation) emerge at the same time as first and second person subject-verb agreement. Meisel concludes that the appearance of verb movement effects and non-third person agreement marks the development of finiteness, structurally realized as the projection of an inflectional functional category. Meisel identifies this category as I[+F], where the feature [+F] triggers V2, which in this stage is effected within the I-system (IP-V2).

A similar structure is proposed by Clahsen, Penke, and Parodi (1993/94) in their analysis of longitudinal data from seven children learning German monolingually. They identify two developmental stages, delineated by MLU, for children learning German: Stage I (MLU $\leq$ 1.75), and Stage II (1.75 $\leq$ MLU $\leq$ 2.75). They deny the existence of a lexical (VP) stage, and propose that Stage I reflects the presence of a single functional projection, FP, headed by an inflectional category F marked by the finiteness feature [+F], which induces V2 and V1. Their proposal for the existence of FP in Stage I rests on observed verb-second and verb-first effects, and a general V-before-subject pattern; occurrences of finite verbs before negation (while infinitives followed negation); and a clear correlation between verb raising and inflection for subject-verb agreement. But these effects are achieved at a stage of short two- and three-word utterances, and in the absence of verb-second effects above a raised subject, which would implicate an additional functional category above FP. Furthermore, although the finite verb raised above negation in Stage I, producing [V Neg Subj] order, there were not instances of [V Subj Neg], which would require a higher functional projection above that hosting the raised subject. Thus, Clahsen et al. propose that Stage I is characterized by the presence of FP as a lone functional projection. The age bracket for Stage I varies across the seven children; at the lower end, the period for Stage I is 1;8–2;0 (Simone), and at the upper end, it comprises the middle weeks of 2;4 (Inga). In stage II, the children front *wh*-expressions and begin to produce [V Subj Neg] order, as well as lexical complementizers. These provide evidence for a CP projection above an existing IP. The age range for Stage II varies across the children; at the low end, the period for Stage II is 2;0–2;2 (Sabrina, Simone), and at the upper end it is 2;5–2;9 (Mathias).

Although they differ with respect to positing a purely lexical stage, these two accounts are very similar in their proposals regarding the nature and development of the functional category system. Both propose a form of bottom-up structure building, in which a single functional projection XP headed by X[+F] develops first, and exhibits some standard behavior of an inflectional head, hosting subject agreement and tense features, while also performing some of the functions of the C-system by serving as a site for verb-second effects. Both Meisel and Clahsen et al. are clear that the posited functional system at this stage does not host complementizer elements or *wh*-expressions, so it performs some, but not all, the functions of the C-system.

These results can be accommodated quite naturally on the present account. Returning to the features for V2 proposed in Chapter 3, at the stage when a single feature matrix can be projected into syntactic structure, I-features [[$F_{V\text{-}s}$, $F_{N\text{-}s}$] Tns, [NOM]] and Top = [TOP_V, TOP_N] in German will be bundled together and projected onto a single functional head, ^[Top, [$F_{V\text{-}s}$, $F_{N\text{-}s}$], Tns, [NOM]], which will consequently serve some I-system functions, while hosting the verb and a V2 topic element in a verb-second structure. Complementizers are absent at this stage since mood features are incompatible with Top.

Some apparent discrepancies between the account of Meisel versus that of Clahsen et al. can be dismissed for the present purposes. Meisel claims evidence for a lexical stage, while Clahsen et al. find no support for such a stage. But Clahsen et al. base their conclusion on aggregate data across Stage I; this leaves open the possibility that Stage I could resolve into two substages, a lexical Stage Ia, beginning with the earliest two-word utterances, and a later Stage Ib, characterized by the presence of FP (that is, on the account developed above, the presence of ^[Top, [$F_{V\text{-}s}$, $F_{N\text{-}s}$], Tns, [NOM]]). Thus, the issue of a lexical stage for the children studied by Clahsen et al. can be taken to be undetermined, pending further resolution of Stage I over time. The Meisel study, on the other hand, is sometimes criticized for its reliance on the data of children acquiring two languages bilingually. This is conceivably relevant to the contour of functional category acquisition, but the similarities between Meisel's results and those of Clahsen et al. over the range of data for which they are comparable (namely, the one functional category stage and the subsequent development of separate C- and I-systems) suggest that the bilingualism of the children in the Meisel study is not a factor that should lead us to disregard the results of that study for comparison with studies of monolingual acquisition of German.

Poeppel and Wexler (1993) examine the transcript of a 213 minute recording session with a monolingual German child, Andreas, at age 2;1. They conclude that Andreas has an adult system of IP and CP projections. Their main evidence is the existence of the word orders in (37) below with a finite verb V_{fin} occurring before a subject which has, in turn, raised above negation and clause-medial adverbs; this contrasts with SOV orders in infinitives, which reflect the merge order (or underlying order) of the German clause.

(37) a. Obj V_{fin} Subj Neg/Adv
b. Adv V_{fin} Subj Neg (Obj)

As Poeppel and Wexler note, these orders are obtained at a point when the I-system is in full evidence; the position of the subject before negation and clause-medial adverbs further attests to subject raising to spec-IP. The verb-second configuration in (37), with the finite verb preceding the subject, is therefore achieved in a functional projection above IP, which is presumably the C-system. Poeppel and Wexler note that verb-second effects could be achieved in a single functional projection XP directly above VP; but there would be no provision in such a system for the subject to raise to a position preceding negation and clause-medial (VP left-peripheral) adverbs. They note further that the straightforward prediction for a system with a single functional projection above VP would be [Neg/Adv Subj] order, with a VP-internal subject.

The data for Andreas examined by Poeppel and Wexler are properly suggestive of at least two functional projections. But in the absence of longitudinal data, the implications of this fact are unclear. If Andreas exhibited these characteristics from the earliest point at which the length and phrasal complexity of his utterances made them possible, this would support the strong continuity hypothesis. But it is possible that the data from Andreas reflect a more advanced stage of acquisition (as Clahsen, Penke and Parodi suggest) at which, in the terms of the present account, at least two bundles of functional features can be projected into syntax. It is worth noting that Andreas's age at the time of the recordings (2;1) lies within the range for Stage II in the scheme of Clahsen, Penke and Parodi (though near its lower end), during which CP and IP systems are in evidence together.

Boser, Lust, Santelmann and Whitman (1992) cite data from a large sample of children, with ages starting at 1;9, showing effects of verb raising and *wh*-movement, offered in support of the strong continuity hypothesis. They do not attempt to identify paradigms and thus to control for the possibility of adjunction of functional elements when they are initially acquired, and their earliest examples of *wh*-movement could involve adjunction of *wh*-elements. Alternatively, on the feature-based account, they could involve projection of sub-adult functional categories, permitting *wh*-fronting in the absence of a functional category with the full content of C^o, as proposed in section 5.1 above for *wh*-fronting in early child English. The extent of Clahsen, Penke and Parodi's Stage I (as early as 1;8–2;0) indicates that many of the children studied by Boser et al. will have the capacity to project only one functional category when they are first observed, and, based on the ages alone, it should be expected that many acquired the capacity to project two functional categories within a single clause during the course of the study, if not before the beginning of the data collection. Thus, the effects observed in the study conducted by Boser et al. can be plausibly attributed to the growth of functional categories, realized as the capacity to project matrices of features into syntactic structure.

7.2. Feature ordering and feature co-occurrence restrictions

Once children acquire the capacity to project multiple functional categories together within a single clause, the acquisition of functional structure is not yet necessarily complete, since the child also has to acquire the full partial linear ordering on functional features, and any co-occurrence restrictions on them, in order to attain the adult system of functional categories for a language. Schönenberger's (2001: 293–316) account of a stage in the acquisition of Swiss German provides a particularly clear and illuminating example which, in the terms of the present study, can be interpreted as the acquisition of feature co-occurrence restrictions at an age (approaching 5;0) when the capacity to represent multiple functional categories within a clause is already well developed. Her results also challenge the claims made by some researchers, discussed in section 7.1 above, that the extent of verb movement is acquired very early in the acquisition of Germanic languages, a claim which has been advanced in favor of the strong continuity hypothesis.

For finite clauses in Swiss German, Schönenberger proposes a split CP, in the tradition of Rizzi (1997), consisting of a lower head Fin°, containing tense features for the finite verb, and a higher head, Force°, expressing the mood (and for main clauses, at least, the illocutionary force) of the clause. Schönenberger notes that the complementizer introducing an embedded clause serves to mark both the finiteness of the clause and its force; she therefore proposes that, in the adult grammar, the complementizer is generated in Fin°, and raises to Force°. The finite verb in most indicative embedded clauses remains in clause-final position in the adult grammar (in-situ, or moved to a right-headed Infl, a matter on which Schönenberger makes no decision). In embedded *wh*-interrogatives and relatives, the finite verb moves into the C-domain, specifically, Schönenberger argues, to Force°. Embedded clauses can exhibit verb-second in complements to bridge verbs and in certain other contexts.[16] In these, but not all, respects, verb movement in adult Swiss German is much as it is in adult High German.

But up until approximately age 5;0, the two Swiss German children studied by Schönenberger exhibited verb movement possibilities in finite embedded clauses which the adult grammar lacks.[17] In finite complement clauses introduced by a complementizer, the verb in this stage of child Swiss German raises to a position preceding a full nominal subject (which Schönenberger assumes to occupy spec-IP); a pronominal subject can appear immediately before or after the raised verb. These possibilities are realized not only in indicative complements introduced by *dass* 'that', but also in conditional, presuppositional, and other nonindicative complement clauses introduced by complementizers such as *öb* 'whether' and *wenn* 'when'. This is illustrated in (38) below, from Schönenberger (2001: 294–295), with a preverbal pronoun in (38a), a postverbal pronoun cliticized to the raised verb under phonological adjacency in (38b), and a post-verbal DP in (38c).[18]

(38) a. ... [*öb si chunt achli ufe*]
whether she comes a bit upstairs
'whether she comes upstairs for a while'

b. *wenn hämmər ka Honig*
when have-we no honey
'when we don't have any honey'

c. *dass werdet mini Ohre au bruu*
that become my ears also brown
'that my ears become brown too'

The structure of these, according to Schönenberger, is illustrated by (39) below, for (38a).

(39)

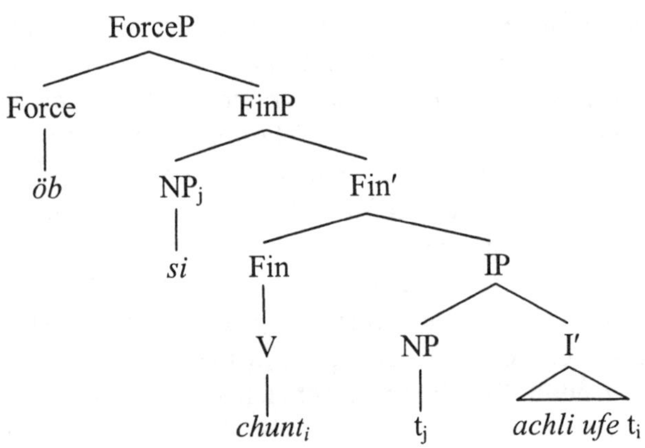

If Fin is part of a split-CP, as Schönenberger maintains, and not simply a highest inflectional category with tense features, it must have some feature content other than tense features. In child language examples of the sort given in (38), these must include a V-feature attracting the verb which, by analogy to V2 in other Germanic languages, we might identify as [TOP_V]. The possibility of the pronominal subject occupying the specifier of the category projected from this feature, indicates the presence of an N-feature, [TOP_N]. (The optionality in position of a subject pronoun will be addressed below.) On these grounds, the data in (38) indicate that non-indicative mood features such as [COND] and [PRESUPP] are compatible with the feature matrix Top = [[TOP_V], [TOP_N]] for child Swiss German up to about the age 5;0, even though, as in German and Mainland Scandinavian, they are not generally compatible in the adult grammar. That is, child Swiss German at this stage exhibits the feature ordering given in (40), realized in complement clauses, where M can be a feature matrix with mood features other than just indicative, and F_I is the matrix of verbal inflectional features.[19]

(40) M < Top < F_I

Within the context of a feature-based syntax of functional categories, in finite embedded clauses in child Swiss German, the finite verb moves to ^Top, which corresponds to Schönenberger's head 'Fin'. A subject pronoun will move to spec-^[Top]P if it is grammatically designated as a topic element, and will otherwise remain in spec-IP. Around age 5;0, the child learns the feature co-occurrence restriction that nonindicative M features are incompatible with Top features. From that point onward, a nonindicative finite complement cannot have Top, and therefore lacks verb raising to the position Schönenberger identifies as Fin°, or to any other supra-Infl position.

Schönenberger's analysis of this stage in the acquisition of Swiss German, formulated here within a feature-based syntax, is a clear and explicit demonstration of the fact that feature orderings and feature co-occurrence restrictions can be acquired independently of the acquisition of the representational resources required to project multiple functional categories. This provides justification of the approach of this chapter and the previous one in separating out the ability to project feature matrices as functional heads in syntactic structure, from the acquisition of the features themselves, along with their correct ordering and co-occurrence restrictions for the language at hand, which are required in order for matrices with the correct feature composition to be projected as functional heads in the correct order for the language.

Notes

1. See Garrett (1988) and Levelt (1989) for use of lemmas in processing theory, particularly in the explanation of the differences between word substitution errors based on sound similarity versus ones based on affinities of meaning.

2. Thanks to Matthew Rispoli for discussion of these issues, but he would not necessarily agree with my conclusions.
3. Negation expressed as utterance-initial *no*, as in, *No me take it off* (Peter, 2;1-18), are also considered to be adjoined by Radford and Hoekstra and Jordens, and are regarded here as instances of a sub-adult category
4. A precedent for this, in a slightly different domain, is Rohrbacher's (1993) proposal that a verbal functional category X is projected in the grammar of an adult language just in case the language exhibits a sufficiently robust paradigm of lexical items (words or affixes) which would appear in X.
5. One advantage of employing conservative counting techniques is that evidence of I-elements and C-elements co-occurring during the stage when two functional categories are present but bottom-up structure building would deny that the C-system is present, cannot be easily dismissed; such evidence should then count against the bottom-up structure building theories, and in favor of the feature-based theory.
6. Again, only files with five or more instances (according to both counts) were included since percentage reliability numbers are too unstable for small files. The reliability of all counts of two functional categories per clause, including small files, was 82.5%, with a range of 0–100% over individual files.
7. Most of the files for Peter actually contain transcripts of two recording sessions – one on the date given in Figure 2, and a second a day or two later. These were kept in their combined format for the sake of rough parity in file size and to maintain a pattern of sampling points at roughly two-week intervals.
8. There is a large time gap (2;5-28 to 2;9-13) in the on-line data for Nina. Also, a handful of the available recording sessions were left out of Figure 6 due to length and frequency considerations. The recording sessions which were left out are from months in which there is a surplus of available sessions (four altogether in the month), and their exclusion from Figure 6 thus helps to keep the sampling points in Figure 6 more uniform over time. Furthermore, three of the recording sessions left out of Figure 6 were grossly undersized relative to the others (one-third to one-half the size); their exclusion thus contributes to size-uniformity in Figure 6.
9. Nina produces a lone example with three functional categories at 2;9-21, namely, *Why can't we open this piano?*. However, there are no other examples of this sort at 2;9-21.
10. As with Peter and Nina, we can draw an additional graph by subtracting away from Figure 10 all examples in which the presence of a Nominative subject contributes to the count. But as with Peter and Nina, this graph does not add any insight into the issues under consideration here, and therefore will not be presented here.

11. The number of functional heads in the chain, as opposed to syntactic heads in general, is relevant to controlling for limitations of working memory and processing capacity particular to the use of functional elements on proposals such as that of McKee and Iwasaki (2001), reviewed in section 1.6.
12. On the analysis presented here, the child grammar does not observe the Economy of Projection of Infl-Categories in projecting the heads in (29a,e) since neither [WH] nor [NOM] is a clausal feature – they are both N-features. The implications of this fact are discussed in Chapter 6, section 4, and in section 6.2 of the present chapter.
13. This yields the effects of subject-Aux inversion, although in fact, Aux-subject order was generated within the auxiliary VP, and is merely maintained upon Aux movement to ^[Q].
14. The focus on productive *wh*-questions, in line with procedures undertaken in the present study, dismisses formulaic questions such as *What about XP?*, *What's that?*, and *Where's XP?*.
15. The data were drawn from the DUFDE project (Deutsch and Französisch – Doppelter Erstspracherwerb) at the University of Hamburg. The ages of the three children examined in Meisel's study of the acquisition of functional categories begin in the range 1;2 to 1;6 and proceed through ending dates in the range 4;7 to 5;10.
16. The set of contexts for verb-second in embedded clauses in adult Swiss German seems to be somewhat larger than for German examples discussed in Chapter 3, and includes complements introduced by *wil* 'because', and certain relative clauses, depending on the discourse or presuppositional status of the clausal content. Nevertheless, the contexts of embedded verb-second in the Swiss German child language examined by Schönenberger are much broader still, providing a firm foundation for the contrasts between adult and child Swiss German which Schönenberger attests.
17. The children studied by Schönenberger lived near Lucerne, and so were classified as speakers of the Lucernese variety of Swiss German.
18. Schönenberger marks all of these examples with '%' to indicate that they are child-specific, that is, obtained in child Swiss German, but not in adult Swiss German.
19. As discussed in Chapter 3, V2 structures in which the subject is the topic element are actually produced by Top = $F_{N\text{-}s}$, with Top features combined with subject N-features in a feature matrix projected as a single functional head. The ordering in (40) should be revised accordingly, splitting the matrix of Infl-features, F_I, at least into separate components for subject N-features and tense features. The resulting structure for (38a) is then no longer strictly isomorphic to the tree in (39).

Chapter 8
The representation of functional categories as a factor in Specific Language Impairment

Children with Specific Language Impairment (SLI) are ones who exhibit "significant limitations in language ability that cannot be attributed to problems of hearing, neurological status, nonverbal intelligence, or other known factors" relevant to language performance, including oral function and social interaction skills (Leonard 1998: 25). The limitations in language ability are indicated by poor performance (at least 1.25 standard deviations below the mean, on a widely used criterion) on comprehensive tests of language competence, including production tests and, in some diagnoses, comprehension tests. The exclusion of factors which are not language specific, and thus the diagnosis of impairment specific to language, is based on performance at or above the lower bound of normal ranges on standard screenings and tests for nonverbal intelligence, where the lower bound of the normal range is commonly taken to be one standard deviation below the mean.[1]

The limitations in language ability exhibited by children with SLI include a lag in the growth of MLU relative to age, compared to normally developing (ND) children, as well as certain deficits in morphology and syntactic productivity. Some researchers have argued that deficits exhibited in specific language impairment can be attributed to limitations in verbal working memory, which interferes with the identification of functional elements in the speech stream, and thereby delays their acquisition; see Baddeley (2003) for a summary and references to work on this topic. Research into the inventories of functional elements for children with SLI has found deficiencies in the expression of tense and/or subject agreement (see Clahsen 1989, 1991; Leonard et al. 1992; Rice and Oetting 1993; Wexler 1994; Rice, Wexler, and Cleave 1995; Rice and Wexler 1996; Oetting and Horohov 1997; Wexler 1999; among others), or deficiencies in the expression of other elements associated with Infl, such as nominative case (see Loeb and Leonard 1991). Moreover, each functional category tends to be less robustly exemplified in the speech of children with SLI than in that of suitably matched normal children (see Morehead and Ingram 1973; Leonard 1995.) However, on most of these proposals (except Wexler 1999;

see also Schütze and Wexler 1996), the functional projections are not assumed to be absent in the grammars of such children, and the observed differences are attributed essentially to differences in the rate of development or extent of use of functional elements (see Eyer and Leonard 1995; Leonard 1995, 1998). So it has been widely concluded that children with SLI don't have any general representational deficiency in their functional category systems; they just don't acquire these systems as early, or use these systems (especially Infl) as robustly, as normally developing children.

But there are possible forms of representational deficiency in functional categories which would not be detected by the examinations carried out in the studies cited above. The previous chapter showed that, in child language acquisition of the clausal functional elements (C, I, Neg), there is a developmental pattern in general representational capacities which is superimposed on the acquisition of particular lexical items involved. Children initially have the capacity to represent no clausal functional elements at all (a stage proposed by other researchers). This is followed by a stage in which, within a given clause, the child can use any one clausal functional element which they happen to have lexically acquired, but not more than one. And this is followed by a stage in which, within a clause, the child can use elements from any two clausal functional categories, (e.g., tense and negation), but not from more than two categories. This is followed, finally, by a stage in which the child can represent any three clausal functional categories together within a clause.

The feature-based theory of functional categories is uniquely well-suited to explain a particular consequence of this developmental scenario. At a stage when the child is not yet capable of forming and projecting a feature matrix with the feature composition of an adult functional category X, the child can project a feature matrix consisting of a subset $\{F_1, \ldots, F_n\}$ of features of X as a functional category $\hat{}[F_1, \ldots, F_n]$ (including the important special case when $n = 1$), producing effects which have been analyzed by other researchers (Radford 1996, Hoekstra and Jordens 1994) as adjunction of negation or of a *wh*-expression to a lexical structure. Furthermore, when a child is not yet capable of forming and projecting the feature matrices for two adult functional categories, X and Y, the child can nevertheless project a single feature matrix containing a subset of the features occurring within X, together with a subset of the features occurring within Y. Examples of such non-adult categories seen in Chapter 7 were ^[[NOM], [NEG]] and ^[[WH], [NOM]].

These considerations present a new way in which children with SLI might, in fact, have a general deficit in their representation of functional categories: the maturational development in the number of functional categories which can occur together within a clause might lag with respect to a normally developing (ND) peer, so that, at an appropriate point of comparison, the child with SLI will represent fewer functional categories per clause than the ND counterpart. Due to an overall slower linguistic development by children with SLI, the appropriate ND counterpart for this comparison is not an age-matched child, but a child matched in mean length of utterance (MLU) and other measures of general language development. If children with SLI have any *specific* deficit in their capacity to represent functional categories, then this should show up in comparison to ND children with the same MLU and overall syntactic complexity, and roughly the same inventory of functional elements acquired and in use. Children who lag in this respect relative to ND peers should be expected to project non-adult combinations of features at points when their (otherwise) language-matched ND peers no longer do so.

The present chapter investigates this issue by analyzing transcripts of the speech of children who meet the criteria for SLI. For each file of a child with SLI examined, the MLU is computed, the phrase structure complexity of the child's utterances is observed and recorded, the inventory of functional elements exhibited by the child is noted, and finally, the number of clausal functional categories which can be represented within a clause is determined, as was done for ND children in Chapter 7. The development of the functional category system of children with SLI is then compared to that of ND children who are language-matched in all other respects (including ones new to this study, such as phrase structure complexity). Implications for previous studies of the status of functional categories in the language of children with SLI will then be discussed.

1. Theories and predictions

This section reviews some of the most established and widely discussed accounts of SLI as a grammatical or structural deficit or impairment, as well as work which might reduce many or all such effects to deficits in working memory. These accounts are not entirely mutually exclusive: SLI does not seem to be a univocal phenomenon, or at least it does not have univocal grammatical manifestations. The multiple accounts offered in the literature therefore could account for different aspects of SLI (or at least some of them could). Furthermore, some of these accounts seem to be at least partially overlapping in scope.

The interest here in examining the accounts available in the literature is to formulate the predictions of each account, and then later in this chapter to determine whether the results obtained here could be subsumed under any of them. For surveys of these and other accounts, see Leonard (1998), Guasti (2002), and Montgomery (2003).

1.1. Deficits in agreement

One theory pertaining to the expression of functional elements by children with SLI is that these children have trouble establishing structural agreement relations, with resulting deficits in the expression of subject-verb agreement, determiner-noun agreement, and case marking on determiners and adjectives (as in German). See Clahsen (1989, 1991) for development of this view. The subject-verb agreement deficit can be realized as a lack of agreement inflection on a main verb or auxiliary, or as a failure to use an auxiliary. Clahsen, Bartke and Göllner (1997) report that tense is quite accurately expressed by German-speaking children with SLI, and also that tense is more accurately expressed than agreement for English-speaking children with SLI. Thus, the problem is taken to be with the representation and expression of agreement relations, not with tense or with I(nfl) generally.

It is worth asking whether the deficit at issue is primarily a relational or a structural deficit. Clahsen (1989) formulates it as a deficit in computing the structural relationship in which agreement is established, given the syntactic structures on which these relations are defined, commonly taken to be the spec-head configuration of a functional projection. If so, then the functional projections are fully present, and so on this supposition there is no deficit in functional category structure. But, suspending judgment on this point, we might ask whether the deficit in establishing agreement relations might indeed follow from a structural deficit. The sources cited above present evidence that agreement is problematic, but not the expression of other functional elements. But this doesn't unambiguously show that the problem is with the expression of agreement relations and not with structures required for the expression of those relations. If the problem were structural, it couldn't be absence of the I-system since tense is not observed to be affected, according to Clahsen, Bartke and Göllner (1997). But in a split Infl clause structure, in which Agr_S and T are separate functional categories, the failure to express subject-verb agreement could result from the absence of Agr_S. An absence of corresponding categories within the nominal system could account for trouble with determiner-noun agreement and with the expression of case on determiners.

In the formulation of Clahsen and associates, the deficit in agreement lies in the expression of functional relationships, not in the projection of functional category structure, so on this formulation, the hypothesis of deficient agreement is not relevant to the concern of this chapter, which is the inventory of functional categories available to the child with SLI. However, if the low rate of expression of agreement in children with SLI is due to the absence (or late development) of an Agr_S category, then it could be a consequence of a limit on the number of functional categories which can be expressed within a single clause, an idea which will be taken up later in this chapter.

1.2. Extended optional infinitives

Normal children exhibit a root infinitive phenomenon in which infinitive clauses are sometimes used as main clauses. In English, the root infinitive is typically realized as a bare, uninflected, verb stem, as in, *He go*. Wexler (1994) analyzes root infinitives as optional infinitives, in which the tense feature is optionally underspecified in an otherwise full clausal structure. This has consequences for phenomena which rely on the distinction between finite and nonfinite clauses, such as verb raising in languages with overt V-to-I movement of finite verbs.

Hoekstra and Hyams (1996) propose a variant of Wexler's (1994) account in which the T-system is present in a full clausal structure, but in which features for finiteness are not specified. Wexler (1999) formulates the condition in somewhat more intricate terms: the D-feature on the subject is assumed to be available for checking only once, hence, available for checking against only one of T and Agr_S; as a result, one of T and Agr_S must be missing from the clausal structure, with concomitant results for the representation of tense, subject agreement, and nominative case on the subject.

SLI deficits in the expression of functional elements (in the clausal system) have been approached on the supposition that the Optional Infinitive

(OI) phase persists longer for children with SLI. This is the Extended Optional Infinitive (EOI) hypothesis of Rice and Wexler (1995, 1996) and Rice, Wexler and Cleave (1995). This account has the virtue of explaining why the expression of finiteness is inconsistent by children with SLI: since the Tense feature is optionally underspecified (or one of T and Agr_S is optionally absent), the deficiency is a matter of lower frequency of representation of finiteness, not a complete lack of it. It also explains why the associated errors consist of a failure to express finiteness, rather than the expression of erroneous tense or agreement features.

An immediate consequence pertinent to the present study, if any formulation of the EOI hypothesis is correct, is that functional categories other than I (or Agr_S + T) should manifest themselves normally, once the requisite functional elements are acquired. Further consequences depend on the exact formulation of the EOI hypothesis. If the tense feature is underspecified, but T is present in phrase structure, then the EOI hypothesis does not posit any structural deficiency in the projection of functional categories; differences between children with SLI and ND children depend on the status of the Tense feature across invariant phrase structure at appropriate comparison points between the two populations. But if, instead, EOI is realized as absence of the I-system (or the T-system, or T or Agr_S), then the EOI condition is marked by one less functional category in the clausal system for children with SLI than their ND counterparts during time frames when the two diverge in their expression of finiteness.

1.3. Deficits in implicit rules

Gopnik (1990a,b), Gopnik and Crago (1991), and Gopnik and Goad (1997) propose that specific language impairment in the expression of functional elements stems from a deficiency in the application of the implicit rules of regular morphological analysis. As a result, inflected forms are learned in the same way as irregulars, as morphologically unanalyzed wholes. (Rice and Oetting 1993, Oetting and Rice 1993, and Oetting and Horohov 1997 provide evidence that not all children with SLI fit this mold.)

This account predicts difficulties in representing tense and subject agreement morphologically, as inflection. It predicts no effects on the representation of categories such as C in English, which is represented syntactically, not morphologically. Furthermore, even in the domain of I-elements, the theory predicts deficiencies only in morphological expression. It doesn't predict deficiencies in the syntactic representation of I-elements by modals, which are not inflected in English, or by other auxiliaries, although it does predict a lack of inflection on other auxiliaries. This account of SLI has little impact on an investigation involving counts of functional categories exemplified within a single clause, such as that in the previous chapter and that undertaken for SLI below, in which presence of the I-system is inferred primarily from the presence of an auxiliary verb.

1.4. Impoverished inventories of functional elements

According to some other theories, children with SLI have no deficit in structures or rules pertaining to the representation of functional categories, but their inventories of functional elements are more restricted than those of normally developing peers, language-matched in other respects.

Morehead and Ingram (1973) propose that the grammatical systems of children with SLI are similar to those of ND children, involving the same syntactic representations and rules (so the same syntactic derivations, in the context of more current theory). The child with SLI differs from the ND child in not using the representations of the grammar, and not applying its rules, as widely or as creatively as the ND child. The result is a more restricted, less grammatically varied body of utterances by the child with SLI.

Leonard (1995), examining transcripts of the speech of ten children with SLI, and explicitly looking for evidence of functional category deficits relative to ND peers, obtained results along the same lines. Leonard found that there was no functional category which failed to be exemplified by the children with SLI he examined. But the functional elements instantiating a functional category were used less frequently than by ND counterparts, and in some cases the class of functional elements instantiating a functional category was more restricted than for a ND counterpart.

We will return to these issues in section 4 below in discussion of the results of the present study. It will be worthwhile to ask what characteristics of the SLI data are due to deficits in the syntactic representation of functional categories, and what characteristics might result from restricted application or instantiation of those representations. How do we distinguish restricted application of grammatical resources from the application of a deficient grammar? This question is especially pertinent in a study such as the present one, where, as in the previous chapter, evidence of at least a partial paradigm of functional elements instantiating a functional category X is required in order to conclude that X is present. For a child with SLI, an impoverished paradigm of functional elements instantiating X might indicate that X is not present, or, alternatively, as Morehead and Ingram and Leonard interpreted their results, it might simply indicate that the use of X is restricted – that the child has acquired X, but has not acquired (or at least does not use) very many elements instantiating X.

Accounts of SLI deficits as resulting from limitations in working memory are much more general in application than just to the acquisition of functional elements. However, deficits in working memory are generally credited with difficulty or delay in the acquisition of lexical items and morphology, and this should lead to impoverished or missing inventories of functional elements. Baddeley (1986) delineated components of working memory, including a central executive, an articulatory loop system (or phonological loop), and a visual-spatial store. The articulatory loop system includes a phonological store, which stores phonological input and an articulatory control process, which helps refresh or maintain the stored material. Results of a number of studies showing differences between children with SLI and normally developing children have been attributed to working memory limitations. These studies involve memory of words or novel phonological forms under various conditions, with and without distractions which compete for working memory, and are therefore thought to show that working memory limitations can delay or impair the acquisition of lexical items and morphology. A more dynamic role for working memory could be hypothesized if the articulatory control process primes production of functional elements. This will be kept in mind along with the role of limitations in working memory on the inventory of functional elements in children with SLI.

1.5. Feature-based theory

The feature-based theory of functional categories developed in Chapter 2 distributes functional features into matrices which must be merged into phrase structure as functional heads. The projection of the functional systems thus depends not on the availability of distinct, labelled functional categories, but rather, on the availability of more basic syntactic resources, including the semantic and morpho-syntactic verbal and nominal features which define the clausal domain, the partial linear order defined on them, and the capacity to construct feature matrices.

Among the possible deficits in this system would be the absence of some of the functional features defining the clause. An absence of φ-features on the subject and matching features projected on a node playing the role of Agr_S, or a lack of Agr_S V-features, could produce deficits in agreement. However, to produce the effects observed in the studies cited above, which is a lower than normal frequency of agreement, not a total absence across utterances, these features would have to be absent only in some utterances of the child with SLI, and present in others. An occasional or frequent, but not invariable, absence of the tense feature could produce effects observed under the Extended Optional Infinitives hypothesis. Such feature deficits would match the predictions made by some of the published theories surveyed above.

But the feature-based theory makes another sort of deficit possible. The expression of functional categories depends on the capacity to construct matrices of features and to project them into syntax as individual units, to be merged into the phrase structure. The number of feature matrices which can be constructed at a given time is a basic property of the computational system of the child's grammar at that time. It is possible that a child at a given time might be able to project fewer matrices of features than children who are, in most or all other respects, language-matched. This particular computational or representational deficit would have predictable consequences. The child with this deficit would be able to represent fewer functional categories per clause than ND peers. As a result, in utterances for which the number of functional categories required is beyond the child's capacity, one or more functional categories would have to remain unexpressed. This means that utterances of the child would exhibit a deficiency overall in the expression of functional elements, but no single functional category would be invariably affected by this deficiency. Some functional elements, such as those expressing the tense feature, might turn out to be affected more often simply because they would normally be expressed more often, in a greater proportion of the child's utterances, than other elements, such as complementizers.

The primary reflex of this deficit would be that the count of the number of functional categories exhibited per clause would be less than that for a ND peer who was language-matched in other respects, including MLU and phrase structure complexity. Furthermore, a child without the representational resources to project a set of adult functional categories containing the features which the child wants to express in a clause might project a subset of the features which normally compose a functional category, or might project non-adult combinations of features as a way of adapting to the representational limitations.

This deficit might take the form of an absolute limit, with the capacity to represent functional categories topping out at a number less than that of the mature adult system, or it might be merely a developmental lag relative to ND children. On the latter scenario, at any given time, the child with SLI is capable of representing fewer functional categories than a language-matched peer, but this is due to a slower rate of maturation in the number of feature matrices which the child can project into the syntax. But on this scenario, there is no fixed limit to this capacity over time since the child with SLI eventually attains the same abilities for representing functional categories as a ND child.

If a pattern emerges in which children with SLI consistently have fewer functional categories than language-matched normal children, then we have support for the hypothesis that at least one distinguishing feature of SLI is diminished representational resources, or slower growth of the representational resources, relevant to projecting matrices of functional features as functional categories to match features on lexical items.

If this turns out not to be the case, that is, if it turns out that the number of clausal functional categories per clause for children with SLI keeps up with their language development in other respects, then we can conclude that children with SLI do not suffer from a lack of the representational or computational resources of the grammar that we have looked at here. Since these are the resources most relevant for representing tense and subject-verb agreement, the real force of the conclusion would be that the problems children with SLI have with clausal inflection – tense and agreement – are not problems with general grammatical resources pertaining to phrase structure representations; they are problems with particularities, such as acquiring and/or using particular inflectional markings or particular inflected items.

2. Method

The purpose of this study is to determine whether SLI is characterized, at least in part, by a diminished capacity to project matrices of functional features as functional categories, or a slower growth of that capacity, with projection of non-adult combinations of features as a means of partially compensating for this deficit. If this is the case, then we expect that, at comparable levels of language complexity, the child with SLI will have fewer adult functional categories per clause than a normally developing child. The objective is therefore to count adult functional categories per clause for children with SLI and compare with similar counts obtained for language-matched peers. For this purpose, language-matching will be taken to be a match in MLU and in phrase structure complexity as defined in Chapter 7, section 2.3.

The SLI data examined in this study were posted by Laurence Leonard on the CHILDES website. They consist of transcripts of recording sessions for 11 children with SLI, ranging in age from 3;8 to 5;7, posted as 11 files, one transcript per file. The children had been tested for hearing, motor skills, IQ, emotional disorders and obvious neurological disorder, and found to be within normal bounds on all these points, but all 11 of them fell more than one standard deviation below age level in performance on tests of language development; correspondingly, all 11 were diagnosed as specifically language impaired (MacWhinney 1995).

For each transcript, the MLU was calculated across all the child utterances in the file, and a lower bound for the maximal phrase structure complexity attained by the child at the time of the recording was established by determining the phrase structure complexity of some of the longer, more complex utterances in the file.

Then, for each file, a count was made of the functional categories exemplified in each clause of the file, and the maximal number of functional categories per clause was determined. The count was carried out as in the study of normal children in Chapter 7. Specifically, the count included functional categories occurring in both main and subordinate clauses; likely imitations, incomplete child utterances, and repetitions were not counted. The count was conducted by hand in order to allow judgment regarding repetition and the completeness of child utterances on a case-by-case basis. The types of elements contributing to the count were recorded, as follows. The I-system elements counted included overt auxiliaries (modals, and *have/be* in participial constructions), infinitival *to*, and nominative subjects. Overt complementizers (*that*, *if*, *whether*, *so*, *[be]cause*) and fronted auxiliaries were counted as instances of the C-system. And instances of *not* and cliticized *n't* were counted as Neg. Evidence of productivity consisting of at least a partial paradigm was required for functional elements to count as instantiating a functional category, rather than as being adjoined in the manner identified by Hoekstra and Jordens (1994) and Radford (1996), or as being a projection of a non-adult combination of features.

Since the study in this case was cross-sectional, not longitudinal as in Chapter 7, there was no issue of size normalization across recording sessions. There was also no way to record a first-use count since there is no way of knowing, given one file for each child, whether a use is a first use or not. A single count was conducted for each file, under moderately conservative criteria, requiring some evidence of a paradigm in functional elements instantiating a given functional category.

The conservative counting techniques were chosen to yield counts of functional categories with adult feature compositions. Once this was established for a file, the file was examined for evidence of non-adult combinations of features projected as a functional category. At this point, some of the instances classified as adjunction in the conservative count were up for possible reinterpretation as projections of non-adult combinations of features. If such examples were found, the possibility was considered of pushing the onset of the one functional category stage, as revealed by the conservative count, forward to an earlier age.

At this point, comparison with the normally developing children studied in Chapter 7 was undertaken. For each file for a child with SLI, the starting point for this comparison was the MLU value, which was compared with MLU values at which ND children exhibited n functional categories ($n = 1, 2, 3$), given in Table 4 below. The first column of numbers in Table 4 gives the MLU range of the files in which the child exhibited at most one functional category; the other two columns give corresponding figures for two and three functional categories. In order to assure that the children compared were truly matched in language abilities not specific to the representation of functional categories, the phrase structure complexity figures were consulted to make sure that the child with SLI had the phrase structure complexity to match expression of functional categories with MLU-matched peers. Given language-matching in these two factors, comparison was undertaken with attention to two points: the inventory of functional elements exhibited, and the maximum number of functional categories per clause.[2]

Table 4. ND children: MLU ranges for functional category stages

	MLU range for max of 1 FC	MLU range for max of 2 FC	MLU range for max of 3 FC
Peter	2.24 – 3.15	3.15 – 3.60	3.60 →
Nina	2.69 – 3.14	3.14 – 4.42	4.42 →
Naomi	2.56 – 2.53	2.53 – 3.97	3.97 →

Deficiencies in functional element inventories relative to ND peers were noted. Finally, when the children were language-matched in MLU and phrase structure complexity, and the inventories of functional elements were sufficient to constitute at least partial paradigms, the child with SLI was taken to be fully language-matched for the representation of *n* functional categories per clause (*n* = 1, 2, or 3). At this point, the functional category per clause counts were consulted to determine how the child with SLI compared to ND children at comparable MLUs, comparable phrase structure complexity, and comparable inventories of adult functional elements.

The point of proceeding in the stages described above was to separate out any deficiency in the use of functional elements, which could stem from weaknesses in morphological analysis or the command of lexical items (which in turn could stem from limitations in working memory), and distinguish it from deficiency in the structural representation of functional categories, given the acquisition of suitable functional elements to instantiate these categories.

3. Results

Using the alphabetic scheme of the CHILDES file designations, the children will be designated as children a through k.

3.1. Results for children with SLI

MLU values for the children with SLI in the study ranged from 3.06 to 4.78, and showed no strong correlation ($r = .41$, $p > .05$) in linear order with the ages, which ranged from 3;8 to 5;7.

Table 5. Children with SLI studied

Child	Age	MLU
i	5;7	3.06
k	3;9	3.07
h	3;8	3.39
b	4;3	3.51
f	4;6	3.64
a	5;0	4.00
e	4;6	4.14
d	4;4	4.14
j	4;11	4.26
c	5;0	4.40
g	5;3	4.78

Recall from Chapter 7 (section 2.3) that phrase structure complexity is measured in terms of the lengths of selectional chains exhibited in a sentence. Recall, also, that a simple clause with three functional categories might have a phrase structure complexity value as small as 4, as in (1) below (not a sentence from the study), with the sequence of heads (C, I, Neg, V) in the *if*-clause.

(1) $[_{CP}$ $[_{C}$ *if*] $[_{IP}$ *they* $[_{I}$ *have*] $[_{NegP}$ $[_{Neg}$ *not*] $[_{VP}$ $[_{V}$ *left*]]]]], *call us*.

Results for a selection of these children will now be examined in order from lowest to highest MLU. Examining a selection of the children individually in this way will permit a more careful comparison of resources available for the projection of functional categories for a child with the production data for that child. Later, in this section, some aggregate results will be compiled, before we turn to comparison of the aggregate results with those for normally developing children in section 3.2 below.

Child i, MLU 3.06, produced the utterances in (2), among others.

(2) a. *I want to play that.*
b. *He is closing his eyes.*
c. *I wanna say that word testtesttestonetwothree.*

Assuming that (2a) has an I node in the main clause, supporting the nominative subject, (2a) involves a selectional chain (I-V-I-V-N) of length 5.

Even if (2a) has no I node in the main clause, which could be the case if nominative subjects are not productive for child i at the time of the recording, the selectional chain in (2a) would still be of length 4, sufficient to support the representation of three functional categories within a clause. The utterance in (2b) involves a selectional chain (I-V-D-N) of length 4. And the phrase structure complexity associated with the selectional chain involved in (2c) could be as high as 6 (I-V-I-V-D-N), if I nodes are represented in both the main clause and the infinitival subordinate clause, and is no lower than 4, if I nodes are not present. Thus, regardless of whether or not I is actually present in (2c), child i produces utterances with phrase structure complexity at least 4, adequate for the representation of three functional categories per clause.

The file for child i contained 70 utterances with evidence of exactly one functional category. Of these, 48 evidenced I(nfl) solely by a nominative subject, but all but 4 of these were first person singular subjects, so the evidence from nominative subjects is not particularly strong for child i. The case for the presence of examples with one functional category thus rests primarily with the 22 examples which gave evidence of one functional category apart from nominative case, by displaying an overt I element (Aux or infinitival *to*). These consisted of two instances of infinitival *to*, two instances of a modal auxiliary (*can*), and 18 examples of the simple present progressive [*BE* V-*ing*], where *BE* is an appropriately inflected form of *be*. Altogether, this amounts to rather scant evidence for I, with some hints of a paradigm, but without a very solid paradigm. Remarkably, there were no instances of *not* or cliticized *n't* functioning as clausal negation, except in combination with an auxiliary (apparently unproductively; see below), and there were no complementizer elements which could be considered manifestations of an adult C.[3] Thus, the inventory of functional elements displayed by child i seems to be just {I}.

Child i produced a class of examples which contain candidates for clauses with two functional categories, including the examples in (3).

(3)
- a. *Don't look.*
- b. *No, don't fit there.*
- c. *I don't see stickers.*
- d. *Don't have horns.*
- e. *Can't see eyes.*
- f. *Won't get out.*
- g. *And it didn't hit me.*

h. *I don't know.* (multiple instances)

But the examples in (3) exhaust the patterns and lexical items involved. The form *I don't know* is used monotonously enough to be formulaic, and the [Aux+Neg] combinations do not seem to be productive enough to count as evidence of separate I and Neg categories; their occurrences in (3) would be attributed to adjunction on conservative counting standards.

However, the examples in (3) can be viewed differently in light of the feature-based theory of functional categories. Child i exhibits the capacity to project only one adult functional category at the time of the recording, yet, on the occasion of utterance of (3d), evidently wanted to express something which in the adult grammar would require two. The projection of ^[Tns, [[NEG]] would be a plausible strategy to meet the communicative needs with the limited representational resources available.

Child k, with the next lowest MLU, at 3.07, produced the utterances in (4), with the indicated selectional chains of length 5.

(4) a. *The doggie is standing on the table.* (I-V-P-D-N)
b. *I'm gonna make more cowboys.* (I-V-V-D-N)
c. *I'm playing with the choo-choo.* (I-V-P-D-N)
d. *I have to stir it.* (I-V-I-V-N)

In (4d), if *to stir it* is an infinitival complement to *have*, then the selectional chain is as given, with two functional elements, but not within the same clause. If, instead, *have to* is a complex modal in (4d), then the selectional chain is simply (I-V-N).

Instances of one functional category for child k include16 instances of *BE* V-*ing*, and 23 of infinitival *to*. This constitutes at most a very sparse paradigm for the projection of one functional category. Child k has the following examples with clausal Neg, in clauses which are candidates for having two functional categories.

(5) a. *I not take it back.*
b. *I not draw the horse.*
c. *I not like dolls.*
d. *Does not open.*

But the restrictiveness of this pattern suggests that this is not an adult Neg category, but rather, what conservative techniques would count as a negation element adjoined to a lexical VP. In the feature-based theory, these are best analyzed as the projection of ^[NEG] or ^[[NOM], [NEG]], and, in (5d), of ^[Tns, [NEG]], or of ^[[$F_{V\text{-}s}$, $F_{N\text{-}s}$], Tns, [NEG]]. There are no manifestations of an adult C. So the inventory of adult functional categories seems to be just {I}.

Child h, with MLU 3.39, produced an example with a phrase structure complexity of 7, shown in (6a) below, and child b produced the example in (6b), with a chain of length 6; the associated selectional chains are indicated. Both of these examples contain two functional categories, but only one functional category per clause.

(6)	a.	*He's trying to climb up the tree.*	(I-V-I-V-P-D-N)
	b.	*I want to leave the door open.*	(I-V-I-V-D-N)

Examples with one functional category produced by child h include15 examples of *BE* V-*ing*, 23 of infinitival *to*, and 1 modal Aux (*can*). Child b produced 39 instances of *BE* V-*ing*, 22 of infinitival *to*, 1 modal *can*, and 4 instances of *I'm*. These count as paradigms for one functional category, but, as with the other children considered to this point, they are curiously sparse paradigms, dominated to an extent not seen with ND children by instances of the progressive form *BE* V-*ing*, and infinitival *to*. The sparseness of the paradigms for exemplification of I(nfl) in child i through child b (as sequenced by MLU in Table 5) will be discussed in section 4 below. Turning to negation, children h and b produced multiple examples such as *That one's not eating*, and *It's not working*, which seem to exhibit clausal negation, but only with *BE* V-ing in third singular. The negation seems productive for these forms, but not the inflection; thus they are best classified as exhibiting Neg, but not I. Thus, the inventory of functional elements for children h and b is at least {I, Neg}. Some fledgling *wh*-questions in (9) below suggest that child h may have C as well.

Candidate examples with two functional categories per clause for children h and b included those in (7)–(9) below, cited to demonstrate their limited variability.

(7)	a.	*That one's not eating.*	(child h)
	b.	*It's not working.*	(child h)
	c.	*The person's not driving.*	(child h)
	d.	*The baby's not crawling.*	(child h)
	e.	*I not play army.*	(child b)

f. *I not know where the castle's at.* (child b)
g. *I not put it on her.* (child b)
h. *I not see something.* (child b)
i. *They not go here.* (child b)

(8) a. *Can't get it in.* (child h)
b. *Can't get it off.* (child h)
c. *I don't know that one.* (child b)
d. *I don't see him.* (child b)
e. *I don't know his name.* (child b)
f. *I don't know.* (multiple) (child b)

(9) a. *Why are you leaving this here?* (child h)
b. *I know how to fix it.* (child h)
c. *How many stickers do you have?* (child h)

The prospective [I+Neg] combinations are all of the form shown in (7)–(8). The lack of productivity suggests that (on a conservative count) I is not productive in (7), and that *can't* and *don't* are adjoined in (8). The questions in (9) uttered by child h seem more productive and could reasonably be considered incipient instances of two functional categories per clause.

On the feature-based account, if children h and b do not yet project I and Neg as separate functional categories which can occur together within a clause, the examples in (7a–d) and (8) can be regarded as the result of projecting ^[NEG], or possibly the non-adult category ^[Tns, NEG], and those in (7e–i) as the result of projecting ^[[NOM], [NEG]]. The need to resort to these is explicable if these children are still in the one functional category stage, as seems clearly to be the case for child b, and for child h in all but *wh*-question formation.

Child f (MLU 3.65) is the first (in order of increasing MLU) to show a full paradigm of two productive adult functional categories occurring together within a clause, as discussed below. Thus, the example in (10a) counts along with that in (10b) as evidence of a selectional chain of length 6.

(10) a. *He won't live in the jungle.* (I-Neg-V-P-D-N)
b. *I need to open the door garage.* (I-V-I-V-D-N)

The 69 examples of clauses with exactly one functional category produced by child f exhibited a greater variety of I-elements than any of the other children considered so far; these included auxiliaries *can*, *will*, *'ll*, *'m*, as well as infinitival *to*, and *BE* V-*ing*. But child f also presents good evidence for clauses with two functional categories, combining Neg with auxiliaries rather productively. In addition to (10a), other examples of two functional categories per clause include those in (11).

(11) a. *He doesn't stand very well.*
b. *It doesn't close.*
c. *I can't talk anymore.*
d. *He won't go to school.*
e. *What are we doing?*
f. *What do you get that for?*

Child f clearly displays the full {C, I, Neg} inventory of functional elements, as do all the remaining children in this study, with MLU's above those of child f.

The case for productive use of nominative case improves quickly with increasing MLU across the children with SLI: child k (MLU = 3.07), like child i, has a large number of examples with nominative subject, but all but 2 are first person singular; however, with child h (MLU = 3.39), a quarter of the 44 examples with nominative subject are person-number combinations other than first person singular, and this continues through the children with higher MLUs.

Child a (MLU = 4.00) has a good paradigm of clauses with two functional elements, including [C+I] as well as [I+Neg]. This remains the case for the children with larger MLUs (child e through child g). But child a also shows an interesting late avoidance of nominative case in examples which otherwise exhibit I and C elements, such as the following.

(12) a. *Them are all good.*
b. *Them are hanging.*

These appear to result from the projection of the non-adult category ^[Tns]. Likewise, child c (MLU 4.40) exhibits very late avoidance of nominative case in examples such as those in (13).

(13) a. *Them can't be upside down.*

b. *Me don't want it.*
c. *Them can't go in there.*
d. *Can them come in the ark?*

The examples in (13a–c) appear to result from the projection of the non-adult category ^[Tns, [NEG]], while (13d) results from projection of ^[Tns], followed by head movement of Aux, out of VP, to ^[Tns].

Finally, the counts of clauses with three functional categories turn up a striking fact: none of the children with SLI have any such clauses, except child g, with MLU = 4.78. The examples for child g consisted of the following.

(14) a. *I know because I don't want anymore.*
b. *Because I'm not driving it.*
c. *So it can't get in the pool.*
d. *I gotta put it right there because I don't have enough room.*
e. *So the baby won't fall off.*
f. *Because I didn't get the dinosaur, did I?*

Child j (MLU = 4.26) and child c (MLU = 4.40) do not exhibit such examples, despite the fact that they have ample phrase structure complexity and they exhibit paradigms of C-elements, I-elements, and negation, occurring singly or in combinations of two at a time. Child j demonstrates command of C-elements *because*, *if*, *till*, *so*, and I-elements *can('t)*, *don't*, *should*, *would*, *will*, *won't*, *must*, *might*, as well as clausal negation, and has phrase structure complexity of at least 6 (cf. *I can't wait till I'm done*). Child c demonstrates command of C-elements *if*, *so*, *for*, and I-elements *do(n't)*, *can('t)*, *will*, *won't*, and infinitival *to*, as well as negation, and exhibits selectional chains of length 6 and 7 with two or three functional categories straddling clausal boundaries, as in (15) below.

(15) a. *See if I get him to stand up.* (V-C-I-V-I-V-(Prt))
b. *I didn't know he wanted the house with the bell.*
(I-Neg-V-I-V-D-N)

But neither child j nor child c uses one functional element from each category together in a single clause, nor do any of the children with lower MLUs. As in Chapter 7, the transition from two to three functional categories per clause seems to be regulated by growth in the grammatical resources for representing functional categories, not by the acquisition of associated elements instantiating these categories.

The results in this section are summarized in Table 6 below. For each transcript, the number in the second column is the MLU computed across child utterances in the transcript; the number in the third column is the phrase structure complexity exhibited, measured as the length of the largest selectional chain observed in child utterances in the transcript; the number in the fifth column is the maximum number of functional categories which were represented within a clause within the transcript. The number in the last column, before the slash, is the frequency of occurrence of examples with the maximum number of functional categories per clause; the number after the slash is the number of child utterances in the file. The numbers in parentheses for children with only one functional category are modified frequencies of occurrence, in case nominative case is not taken to be productive for these children, and therefore should not be counted as evidence of the presence of Infl. The paradigms of functional elements instantiating the single functional category manifested by child i, child k, child h, and child b were rather partial; thus, the attribution of one functional category to these children was not as secure as with the files for larger MLUs. All of the children had phrase structure complexity sufficient to represent up to three functional categories per clause, indicating that phrase structure complexity is not an obstacle to the representation of functional elements within a clause for any of these children.

Table 6. Children with SLI studied

Child	MLU	PS compl.	Inventory of FC's	max #FC's	Freq. occurrence of max #FC's
i	3.06	4	I	1	70 (22) / 466
k	3.07	5	I	1	71 (41) / 500
h	3.39	7	(C), I, Neg	1 or 2	99 (50) / 924
b	3.51	6	I, Neg	1	98 (55) / 829
f	3.64	6	C, I, Neg	2	21 / 959
a	4.00	6	C, I, Neg	2	24 / 1233
e	4.135	6	C, I, Neg	2	68 / 1030
d	4.14	7	C, I, Neg	2	36 / 817
j	4.26	6	C, I, Neg	2	32 / 1087
c	4.40	7	C, I, Neg	2	56 / 1218
g	4.78	7	C, I, Neg	3	6 / 1035

3.2. Comparison with language-matched ND children

In Figure 1 below (p.302), the maximum number of functional categories per clause is plotted against MLU for all 11 of the children with SLI. For comparison, the MLU ranges for the ND children Peter, Nina, and Naomi given in Table 4 are also plotted, labelled ND1. The initial point of the *n* functional category stage (*n* = 1, 2, 3) from Table 4 is plotted on the line for *n* functional categories in Figure 1, while the final point of the *n* functional category stage (*n* = 1, 2) is plotted as the initial point of the *n*+1 functional category stage, on the line for *n*+1. In contrast, the figures for children with SLI given in Table 6 are from some unknown point of the *n* functional category plateau, not necessarily its initial point, since there are no longitudinal data regarding the number of functional categories per clause for these children. Thus, the comparison of SLI data in Table 6 with the ND data in Table 4 must really be a comparison of the SLI data for *n* functional categories (*n* = 1, 2) with ND data for the *n* functional category plateau, whose initial point is on the line numbered *n* in Figure 1, and whose final point is on the line numbered *n*+1. To provide more directly equivalent data points for ND children to be plotted in Figure 1, six additional points were randomly chosen among files for three additional ND children, Sarah and Eve (Brown 1973), and Shem (Clark 1978, 1979). Information for these additional data points is given in Table 7 below.[4]

Table 7. Additional ND data points

Child	Age	MLU	PS compl.	Inventory of FC's	Max #FC's	Freq. occurrence of max #FC's
Sarah	3;5-7	2.75	6	C, I, Neg	2	19 / 447
Sarah	4;3-13	3.18	7	C, I, Neg	3	4 / 258
Eve	1;10-0	2.71	5	I	1	28 (8) / 477
Eve	2;3-0	2.83	7	C, I, Neg	2	8 / 434
Shem	2;2-16	2.81	7	C, I, Neg	2	3 / 401
Shem	3;2-2	3.56	7	C, I, Neg	3	5 / 282

Figure 1 plots MLU on the horizontal axis, and the maximum number of functional categories per clause on the vertical axis. The points for the 11 children with SLI are plotted as circles; the beginnings of the functional category stages for Peter, Nina, and Naomi (ND1) are plotted as squares, and the randomly selected points for Sarah, Eve, and Shem (ND2) are plotted as triangles.[5]

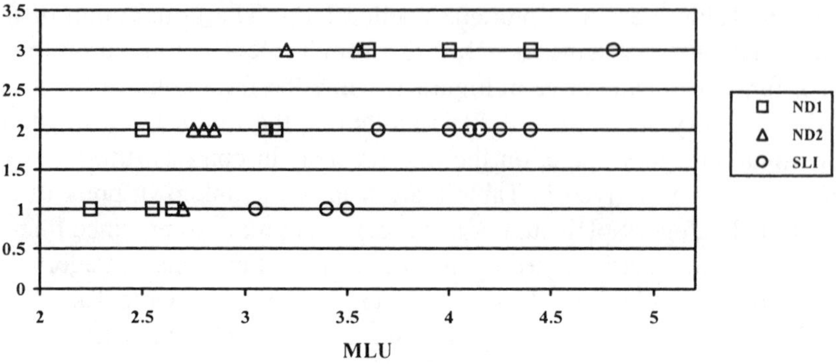

Figure 1. Maximum number of functional categories per clause, versus MLU

This graph reveals two major points. First, for any given MLU value at which a child with SLI exhibits *n* functional categories per clause (*n* = 1, 2, or 3), all of the ND children plotted exhibit use of *n* functional categories per clause at a lower MLU value. Specifically, all the ND children exhibit one functional category per clause at MLU values less than 3.06, which is the lowest value at which a child with SLI does; they all exhibit 2 functional categories at MLUs less than 3.64, the lowest value at which a child with SLI does; and they all exhibit 3 functional categories at MLUs less than 4.78, the only value at which a child with SLI does. This comparison is straightforward for the SLI points and the ND2 points, since both are randomly chosen points with respect to the onset of the *n* functional category plateaus. For comparison with Peter, Nina and Naomi, the SLI points should be compared to the initial and final points of the *n* functional category plateaus for Peter, Nina, and Naomi.

The second major point revealed by this graph is that, for any given MLU value, *m*, at which a child with SLI exhibits a maximum of *n* functional categories per clause (*n* = 1 or 2), most or all of the ND children attained *n*+1 functional categories per clause at some MLU ≤ *m*, and those who did not do so are on the verge of doing so, in that they attain *n*+1 functional categories at a MLU value *m′* just slightly higher than *m*. For example, at MLU = 3.06, the lowest MLU value at which children with

SLI exhibit 1 functional category, 4 of the ND children have attained 2 functional categories at lower MLU values than this, and the remaining 2 will do so at just slightly higher MLU values, at MLU = 3.14 and 3.15. Furthermore, at MLU = 3.64 (child f), the lowest MLU value at which the children with SLI attain 2 functional categories per clause, 3 of 5 ND children attain 3 categories at lower MLU values. But child f is early among children with SLI in attaining 2 categories. At more typical MLU values for the attainment of two functional categories by the children with SLI, around MLU = 4.14, all but one of the ND children has attained 3 functional categories per clause.

Thus, in a couple of different ways, this graph illustrates that the children with SLI attain the capacity to represent n functional categories per clause (for each $n = 1, 2, 3$) at distinctly higher MLU values than ND children.

4. Discussion

To begin with, referring to Table 6, we can observe that from child b though child c (in order of increasing MLU), the maximum number of functional categories per clause displayed, using conservative counts to count adult manifestations of the functional categories, lags behind what the child should be capable of producing given the phrase structure complexity attained and the inventory of functional elements which the child exhibits in adult form on an individual basis. As in the discussion of language acquisition by ND children in Chapter 7, phrase structure complexity can be regarded as a control on verbal working memory and processing capacity. If a child is capable of producing a sentence with a selectional chain of length of at least 4, and in fact produces chains of length 5, 6, or 7, and if the child has acquired an inventory of functional categories which includes adult manifestations of C, I, and Neg, used individually (or two at a time), then there is no evident reason why there should be limits of working memory and processing capacity which would prevent the projection of three functional categories together within a clause. A further structural constraint on the projection of functional categories seems to be implicated.

Furthermore, given such limitations on the projection of functional categories, the projection of non-adult combinations of features becomes explicable. In the one functional category stage, there is evidence that children i and k project ^[Tns, [NEG]]. Children h and b seem to project ^[[NOM], [NEG]] in the one functional category stage, even though child h seems to be on the verge of projecting two functional categories together. Even when children have the capacity to project enough functional categories to express adult combinations of features, they sometimes show non-adult combinations of those features. It was noted that children a and c show evidence of projecting [Tns] by itself as ^[Tns], even though they show ample evidence of being able to project an adult I category, and child c exhibits examples resulting from the projection of ^[Tns, [NEG]] even though child c has productive adult-like combinations of I+Neg.

So far, this just shows that children with SLI share in the aspects of functional category acquisition detailed for ND children in Chapter 7. This helps broaden the empirical base of phenomena in the acquisition of functional categories which (as argued in Chapter 7) are explained by the feature-based theory of functional categories, but which cannot be explained by theories of functional category acquisition based on a fixed stock of functional categories.

The main purpose of the present chapter is to compare the development of the functional category system in the grammar of children with SLI with its development in ND children, specifically, to determine how children with SLI compare to ND children in the number of functional categories which can be represented within a single clause at comparable points of development. The result obtained through the longitudinal study of ND children in Chapter 7 was that the capacity to represent functional categories within a clause increases incrementally, from 0, to 1, to 2, to 3, in a way indicative of the growth of basic representational resources of the grammar. This result is explicable on the theory of functional categories presented in Chapter 2. If functional categories are formed by combining functional features matching or instantiating those on lexical items in the numeration for a clause, then the capacity to represent functional elements depends on the acquisition of very particular resources, including the lexical items and their features, but it also depends on the development of a more general representational ability, the capacity to form feature matrices projected into the phrase structure as merged functional heads. This raises the possibility that SLI might be characterized (not exclusively, but in part) by an overall limitation in the number of feature matrices which can be projected into syntax, or by a developmental lag, relative to that displayed by ND children, in the capacity to form *n* feature matrices, for each successive value of *n* (1, 2, 3), and thus a developmental lag in the capacity to project *n* functional categories.

In Figure 1, it was found that the children with SLI studied here exhibited *n* functional categories, for each *n* = 1, 2, 3, at higher MLU values than any of the data points for ND children, including most of the MLU ranges for Peter, Nina and Naomi, but also the randomly chosen points for Sarah, Eve, and Shem. Furthermore, in Figure 1, if we project vertically upward from the SLI points at *n* functional categories (for *n* = 1 or 2) to a point on the line for *n*+1 categories, at the same MLU value, we see that the ND children at a given MLU typically have one more functional category than the children with SLI, or are on the verge of acquiring it.

These results indicate that children with SLI lag behind ND children in the development of the capacity to represent *n* functional categories within a single clause, for each *n* = 1, 2, 3. At sufficient MLU values, the children with SLI can generate quite long sentences with multiple clausal embeddings and with multiple functional elements appearing in different clauses. But at a given level of attainment in utterance length and phrase structure complexity, the children with SLI do not match their ND peers in the number of functional categories they can represent within a single clause. This is true even in files in which the children with SLI demonstrate command of negation and inventories of I-elements and C-elements which are comparable to those of their MLU-matched ND peers, and fully adequate for performance to match normal levels (as was the case with child a, child e, child d, child j and child c). Thus, the developmental lag manifested by the children with SLI is not attributable entirely to a lag in the acquisition of lexical items and their features. There is at least a component of developmental difference between the ND children and children with SLI which consists of a lag in the development of resources for the representation of functional structure on the part of the children with SLI relative to their ND counterparts. This is true even though the ND children themselves were shown to exhibit a lag in the number of functional categories which they could project together within a clause, given the phrase structure complexity they had attained and inventories of functional elements which they had acquired.

The more restricted inventories of I-elements exhibited by children with SLI with lower MLU values among those studied do not compromise this result. The preponderance of present tense progressive forms (*BE* V-*ing*) and infinitival *to* among these children suggests a lack of variety in their I-inventories, which might say something about their representation of finite tense of relevance to the Extended Optional Infinitives hypothesis (discussed further below). But it does not change the conclusions reached here regarding the capacity to represent functional categories per clause. If it has any impact on that issue, it would be to question the fullness of the paradigm of I-elements demonstrated by these children, so that we might withhold attribution of one functional category to children i and k. But this would mean that these children acquire functional categories at even higher MLU values than assumed here, which would merely strengthen the conclusion that children with SLI lag relative to MLU-matched ND counterparts in the development of the capacity to represent functional categories.

The results obtained here are consistent with observations of slow development of functional categories by Eyer and Leonard (1995) and the account proposed here provides a structural grounding for that developmental lag. However, the result obtained here regarding the development of the functional category systems is not predicted by, and cannot be subsumed under, existing accounts of the mechanics of the deficits of children with SLI, reviewed in section 1 above. Consider first the Extended Optional Infinitive (EOI) hypothesis of Rice and Wexler (1996) and Rice, Wexler and Cleave (1995). On this account, all children (learning non-null subject languages) optionally use root infinitives in an early developmental stage, but children with SLI use them beyond the point at which age-matched and MLU-matched ND peers have left this phase. On this hypothesis, we would expect children with SLI to instantiate Infl with fewer tense elements. Indeed, the results of the present study can be interpreted as supporting this prediction. If one effect of the EOI phase is to limit the productive expression of auxiliaries, then the results obtained here for children i, k, h, and b, might reflect this restriction, with root I largely confined to expressing present tense forms of *be* through over-use of the simple present progressive. But at comparable MLU values, when the children with SLI are exhibiting these effects on the instantiation of Infl, there is no reason according to this account why they should lag behind MLU-matched ND children in the representation of Neg. These children have subordinate clauses, and their phrase structure complexity is fully adequate to the expression of C-elements and Neg, and children h and b show adult use of Neg, in addition to I (though not in the same clause together). Furthermore, since the optional infinitive stage is characterized by the optionality of finite forms, not their complete absence, the child with SLI with one functional category should sometimes express Infl, as well as Neg (and

C, if C-elements have been acquired). Thus, even during the EOI phase, the child with SLI should not lag in the instantiation of one functional category by Neg, nonfinite I-elements, C-elements (if available) and the occasional (optional) expressions of tense. And at higher MLU values, where children with SLI do not exhibit such a difference in their inventories of I-elements relative to MLU-matched ND peers, the EOI hypothesis has no impact on the representation of functional categories. Therefore, the EOI hypothesis in itself provides no reason why the maximum number of functional categories per clause exhibited by children with SLI should lag behind that of ND children with comparable MLUs, as observed here.

This argument holds even for formulations of the EOI which appeal to structural impoverishment of the I-systems, which might seem, at first glance, to subsume the results obtained in the present study. Schütze and Wexler (1996) and Wexler (1999) propose that one of T and Agr_S will be missing in the OI and EOI phase. But this shouldn't produce the lag in the development of functional categories observed here. Even if the child with SLI is subject to the EOI phase, once the capacity to represent one functional category has developed, it should be manifested by Neg, C-elements (if available), and sometimes by I-elements (when T is present). Thus, while the paradigm of T-elements may be less frequently, or even less fully, instantiated under EOI, there should be no major impediment to the expression of one functional category.

On the account of Clahsen (1989), children with SLI have a deficit in the expression of structural agreement relations. This proposal has potential ramifications for the structural representation of functional categories, in particular, if a failure to fully express subject-verb agreement in the clausal system were due to the absence of Agr_S. However, such a condition, even if it were the case, would not be detected by the present study. The present study counted clauses with *n* functional categories (for each *n* = 1, 2, 3), and for this purpose did not distinguish Agr_S and T, instead counting I as manifested by any (sufficiently productive paradigm of) auxiliary verbs, as well as by infinitival *to*. This was due to the choice made in connection with the work of Chapter 7 to count only lexical manifestations of functional categories, not morphological manifestations.[6] A deficit in expressing structural agreement relations, even if realized by the absence of the category Agr_S in the clausal system, would not affect counts that were made in this study.

On the account proposed by Morehead and Ingram (1973), children with SLI have deficits in the consistency, productivity and creativity of the application of grammatical principles. As they put it (344), "once the linguistic systems are developed, deviant children [i.e., children with SLI – M.H.] do not use them as creatively as normal children for producing highly varied utterances." [quoted by Leonard (1998: 229)]

This certainly describes the manifestation of I-elements in the transcripts for children i, k, h, and b. Child k, for example, in clauses with exactly one functional category, exhibits 23 examples of infinitival *to*, 16 examples of present progressive *BE* V-*ing*, and 2 instances of modal auxiliary *can*, as the entire inventory of I-elements, and shows a lack of productivity in the manifestation of nominative case, which is almost entirely in the first person singular. The principal impression one gets in counting these elements, in contrast to performing the same task with transcripts of ND children, is exactly one of a lack of variety and a more limited productivity or creativity of the SLI productions of I-elements at this stage.

The possibility that children with SLI generally have limited inventories of functional elements poses an issue for the interpretation of the results of the present study. Children i, k, h, and b each exhibit a set of examples with I and Neg apparently co-present within a single clause, but these were dismissed as evidence of two functional categories per clause, in large part because the inventories of functional elements involved in these sets were very limited. But if we can assume that limited inventories are a general feature of SLI, as an instance of Morehead and Ingram's proposal, then we might be inclined to suppose that these sets of examples of clauses with two functional categories are really evidence of two functional categories in the transcripts of children i, k, h, and b, at MLU values 3.06, 3.07, 3.39, and 3.51, respectively. At two functional categories per clause, these would be respectable values relative to ND peers under MLU-matching, as revealed by Table 4 and Figure 1. If this were right, then the data for these four children with SLI would not exhibit a lag in the development of one functional category relative to MLU-matched peers. There would still be SLI effects, involving restricted inventories of functional elements and a lag in the growth of MLU relative to age for children with SLI in comparison to ND children, but there would be no particular lag in the development of the functional category systems such as that claimed here.

This proposal might have some force for children i and k since these two children exhibit adult use of only one functional category, I, and this only barely. So the lack of functional projections for these two children could follow from limitations in the inventory of functional elements. But children h and b exhibit adult use of I and Neg, even though the I-inventory is sparse. The failure to project two functional categories (at least for child b) must then follow from some further deficit, beyond the limited inventories of functional elements. Furthermore, the suggestion that the present study has failed to attribute higher counts of functional categories per clause to children with SLI due to limited inventories of functional elements has no force, even prima facie, with respect to the development of the three functional category stage from the two functional category stage, since the children with SLI in the two functional category stage have substantial inventories of I-elements and C-elements, and show robust use of Neg: they just never happen to combine all three types of element within a single clause. This fact would not follow from the supposition that children with SLI have limited inventories of functional elements, and is instead strongly indicative of a structural deficit in the representation of functional categories.

Finally, even to the extent that it is the case that initial inventories of classes of functional elements are weaker for children with SLI than for ND children, and that the inventories remain weak considerably longer for children with SLI, we still shouldn't allow that children with SLI might have the structural resources for representations for which they don't exhibit strong paradigms. We shouldn't embrace the supposition that they could have the functional phrase structure, but lack even partial paradigms of the associated functional elements with which to instantiate the functional structure, for this supposition undermines the rationale for positing functional structure. Structural representations of functional categories are posited in order to capture generalizations, namely, to account for the co-occurrence of productive inventories of functional elements in a given syntactic position within the clause. Absent at least a partial inventory of functional elements instantiating a functional category, there is no generalization to capture: the data, in that case, are consistent with ad hoc adjunction structures, or memorized collocations. The attribution of functional structure is not well motivated without at least partial paradigms of associated functional elements. Only in the context of the feature-based theory of functional elements is it reasonable to analyze early functional categories with non-adult combinations of features as products of the processes which compose functional categories, and not as ad hoc adjunction structures.

So we should reject an interpretation of the present results as not revealing a lag in the development of *n* functional categories per clause for children with SLI relative to MLU-matched ND counterparts, and as, instead, merely confirming that children with SLI have weak inventories of functional elements. Nevertheless, we can appeal to weak inventories of functional elements, on Morehead and Ingram's proposal, as an account of why the inventories of I-elements for children i, k, h, and b are so weak. This application of Morehead and Ingram's proposal seems to be real and to be especially active or in force for children with SLI with MLUs up to 3.5.

Finally, the proposal of Gopnik (1990a,b), Gopnik and Crago (1991), and Gopnik and Goad (1997) that children with SLI have deficits in implicit rule systems required to produce regular morphology does not have an impact on the present study, for the reasons given in section 1.3 above. The expression of C is not morphological, nor is the expression of I by auxiliaries, or Neg by *not*. Thus there are plenty of elements with which to instantiate the clausal functional categories quite apart from morphological competence.

5. Conclusion

The work reported in this chapter confirms the standard result that children with SLI lag behind age-matched ND children in their development of functional categories, and that they particularly lag in the acquisition of tense elements. Additionally, it shows that the syntactic systems of children with SLI have a developmental lag relative to MLU-matched ND peers in more general representational resources of the syntax, namely, in the capacity to represent a given number of functional categories per clause. In both ND children and children with SLI, this capacity develops in discrete stages, from 0, to 1, to 2, then to 3. But for children with SLI, each of these stages (especially the last two) is achieved later – at a higher MLU value – than for ND children. Children with SLI, like their normally developing counterparts, project non-adult combinations of features as functional categories when they don't have the capacity to project the full adult feature matrices, including the target features along with all the features which normally accompany them in the adult grammar, as adult functional categories.

Notes

1. Some have argued that the impairment is not entirely specific to language, and instead rooted in some more general cognitive deficit in the capacity for serial ordering, temporal sequencing, or sequential memory. See Gillam, Cowan and Day (1995), their summary of the literature, and the sources they cite.
2. The MLU of Naomi's utterances in the file in which she first exhibited two functional categories per clause (at age 2;1-17) was almost the same as in the file in which she first exhibited one functional category per clause (at age 1;11-6). That is, her MLU did not change significantly over the intervening two and a half months, while the complexity of her functional category system did change.
3. There are examples of nonclausal negation, as constituent negation of DP (*not that one*) or AP (*not hard*).
4. Frequencies of occurrence in Table 7 are considerably smaller than in Table 6, in large part because the files are much smaller. The frequencies in Table 7 are on a par with those for some of the small files for Naomi.
5. The data points for child i (MLU = 3.06) and child k (MLU = 3.07) are too close together to be resolved, and therefore appear as a single circle in this graph. Of course, the squares for the initial MLU values of the two and three functional category stages for Peter, Nina and Naomi are, ipso facto, squares for the final MLU values of the corresponding one and two functional category stages.
6. Nominative case was also counted as a possible manifestation of I, but this count was kept separate throughout in order that it could be subtracted out at will.

Chapter 9
Conclusion

The present work has pursued and developed a feature-based approach to the syntax of functional categories in natural language. The construction of functional categories proceeds from morpho-syntactic features matching those on lexical items in the numeration, together with features for mood, negation, and other semantic characteristics of the clause which are reflected in the grammar. A partial linear checking order is defined on these features. Following Giorgi and Pianesi (1996, 1997), the features are grouped into hierarchically structured matrices, on which a derivative linear order is defined, preserving the linear order defined on the component features. These matrices of features are merged into phrase structure as functional heads. As with Giorgi and Pianesi, different groupings of features into feature matrices derived from the same set of morpho-syntactic and semantic features can yield different constructions (in the traditional sense) from a given numeration.

Some basic constraints were then motivated to regulate the set of morpho-syntactic and semantic features out of which functional categories are defined, and to regulate the distribution of these features into matrices which are projected as functional categories. These constraints include the Economy of Feature Projection, which constrains the suite of matching features entered into a numeration for projection onto functional categories to be a minimal one, given the morpho-syntactic features present on lexical items in the numeration. This prevents the spurious generation of redundant functional structure. Another constraint, the Economy of Projection of Infl-Categories, requires that a functional category in the Infl-system of a clause have at least one clause-defining feature (V-feature or A-feature, or [EPP]) at its core. This distinguishes Infl-categories in the clausal system from functional categories which might be generated as projections of a nominal head. A third constraint, the Minimal Feature Ordering principle, restricts initial specification of the checking order on features to be defined only for features which occur together within a clause, and for features at the boundaries of clauses (and complex nominals), and it makes the ordering of N-features with respect to one another parasitic on the ordering of the associated V-features. This comes into play when N-features are present in a numeration without their associated V-features, and are therefore required by the Economy of Projection of Infl-Categories to project with other V-features in the numeration.

A major source of cross-linguistic syntactic variation is in feature co-occurrence restrictions on the features from which functional categories are constructed, whether these are morpho-syntactic features matching features on lexical items in the numeration, or features encoding basic semantic characteristics of the clause. In Chapter 3, it was shown that different sets of co-occurrence restrictions on mood, topic, and Infl-features across the Germanic languages result in the projection of different groups of features cross-linguistically, driving different combinations of movement of a verb and "topic" element, yielding different patterns of verb-second across these languages. Furthermore, the difference between the ordering $F < F'$ and $F \leq F'$, for feature bundles F and F′, were found to yield different syntactic constructions (such as subject-V2 versus non-subject-V2) within a language.

In the analysis of clitic placement given in Chapter 4, the absence of V-features, $F_{V\text{-}o}$, in infinitives resulted in different feature groupings than when these features are present, in finite clauses. Given the Economy of Projection of Infl-Categories, the associated N-features, $F_{N\text{-}o}$, had to be grouped and projected differently than in the case when $F_{V\text{-}o}$ are present, resulting in a different "construction" of the language – enclisis of an object pronoun, rather than proclisis. The status of $F_{N\text{-}o}$ when $F_{V\text{-}o}$ are absent, and the need to project into phrase structure with V-features, makes clitic climbing possible as a result of association of $F_{N\text{-}o}$ with a matrix of V-features associated with a higher verb.

The analysis of the tenseless clauses examined in Chapter 5 shows the paucity of features which can be projected under special circumstances. The possibility of clauses with such restricted functional structure is expected when functional categories are derived from matching features which are introduced, bundled, and projected as needed, as opposed to the projection of functional categories in an invariable suite such as {C, Neg, I}, or {C, Agr_S, T, Neg, Agr_O}. Before this chapter, the applications of the theory developed here had been confined to providing compact accounts of paradigms of data discussed extensively in the literature. In this chapter, it was used to elucidate new data concerning a little known construction.

The acquisition studies in Chapters 6 and 7 show that the acquisition of functional categories, beyond the acquisition of the lexical items involved, depends on the structure of the functional category system according to the feature-based derivation of functional categories. The results in these chapters were interpreted as showing that the development of the system of functional categories is a maturational process, but not the maturation of a fixed stock of functional categories, whether all at once, as proposed by Radford (1990), or in a fixed sequence, as proposed by Vainikka (1993/94) and Guilfoyle and Noonan (1992). Rather, they were interpreted as showing the development of early child language proto-functional-categories, obtained by projecting feature matrices composed of individual features or non-adult combinations of features, followed by the development of adult functional categories under a representational constraint according to which the number of functional categories which can be represented together within a single clause increases incrementally, from 0, to 1, to 2, to 3. It was argued that the best interpretation of this result is that functional categories do not consist of a fixed stock, {C, Neg, I}, or {C, Agr_S, T, Neg, Agr_O} but rather, that they are derived as feature matrices, with each feature matrix projected as a functional category. From this perspective, the results obtained here demonstrate that there is progressive development over time in the number of matrices of features which a child can construct and project as functional categories.

Finally, in Chapter 8, some standard data regarding Specific Language Impairment were examined and shown to exhibit a lag (with respect to language-matched peers) in the number of clausal functional categories which can be represented within a single clause. Using phrase structure complexity as a control for working memory limitations or processing limitations, it was argued that the observed lag reflects a deficit in representational resources for the projection of feature matrices as functional categories, which exists over and above any other deficits which these children might have relative to peers who are (otherwise) language-matched with them.

Appendix

At each age, the number of clauses with one functional category in the clausal system is indicated by a circle, the number of clauses with two clausal functional categories is indicated by a square, and the number of clauses with three clausal functional categories is indicated by a triangle. For each n = 1, 2, and 3, a count of zero clauses with n clausal functional categories is not indicated unless a nonzero number of such clauses has been obtained at an earlier age; that is, initial zeros are not depicted here.

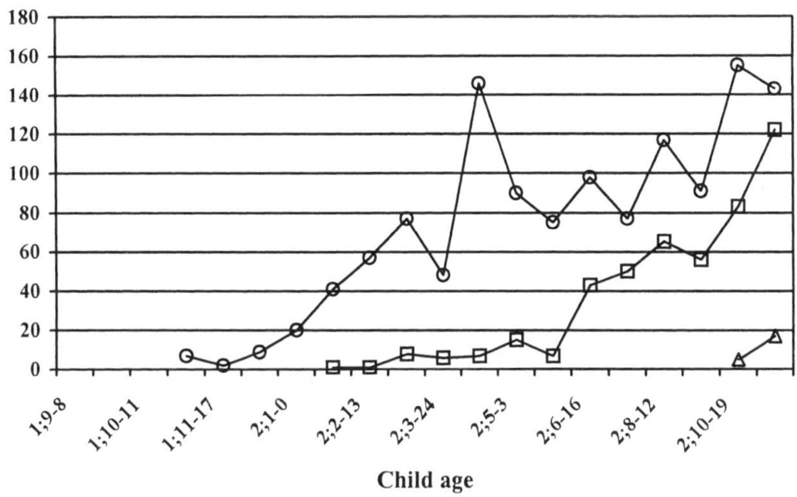

Figure 2. Peter's clauses with functional categories: first mention

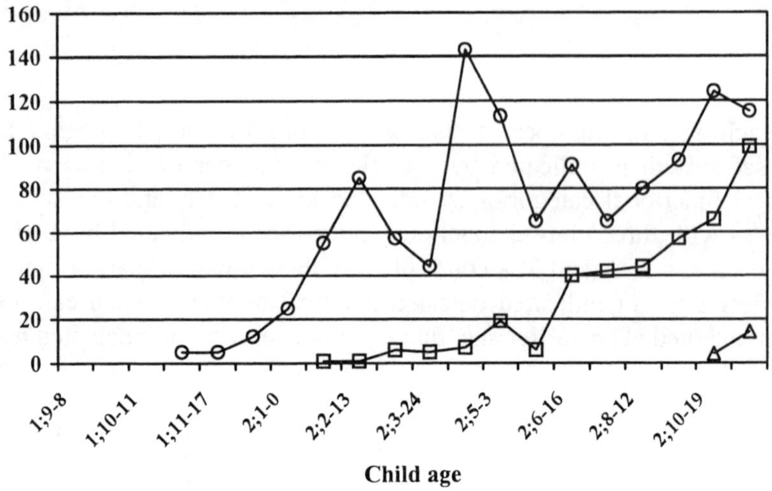

Figure 3. Peter's clauses with functional categories: normalized

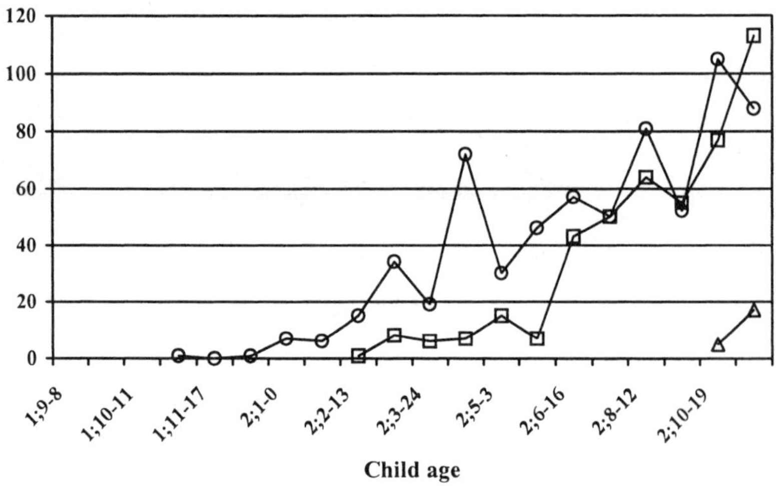

Figure 4. Peter's clauses with functional categories: first mention, without nominative case

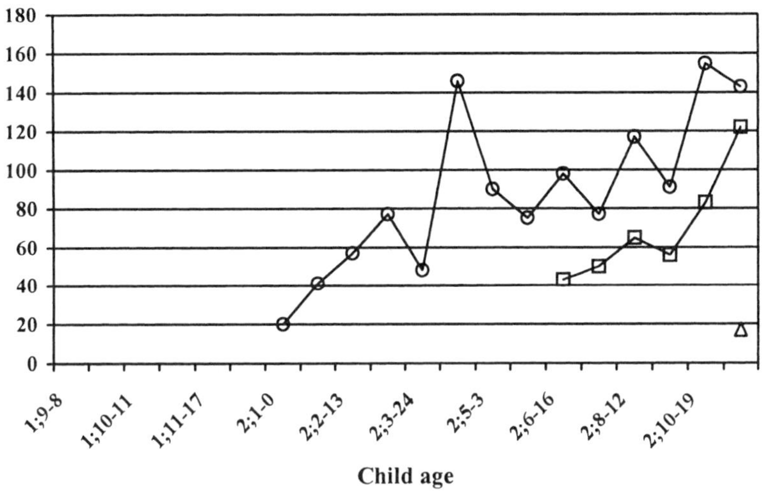

Figure 5. Peter's clauses with functional categories: paradigm

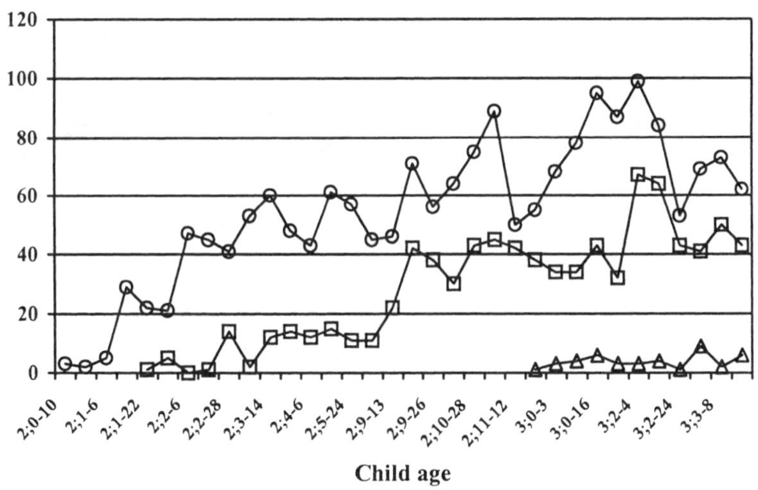

Figure 6. Nina's clauses with functional categories: first mention

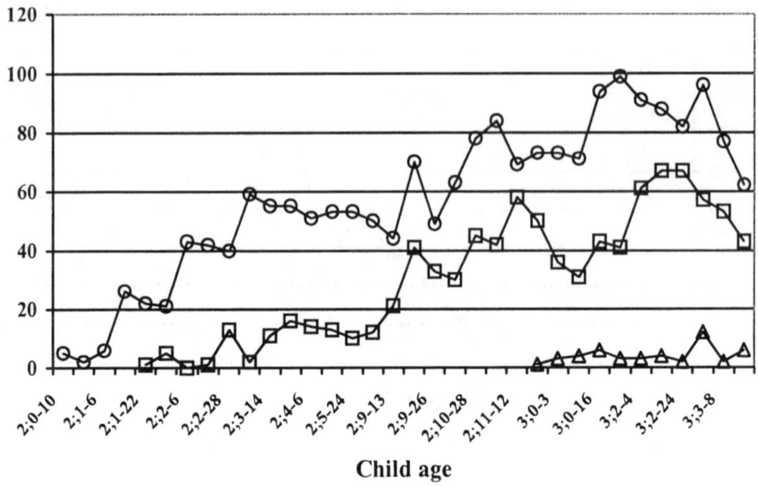

Figure 7. Nina's clauses with functional categories: normalized

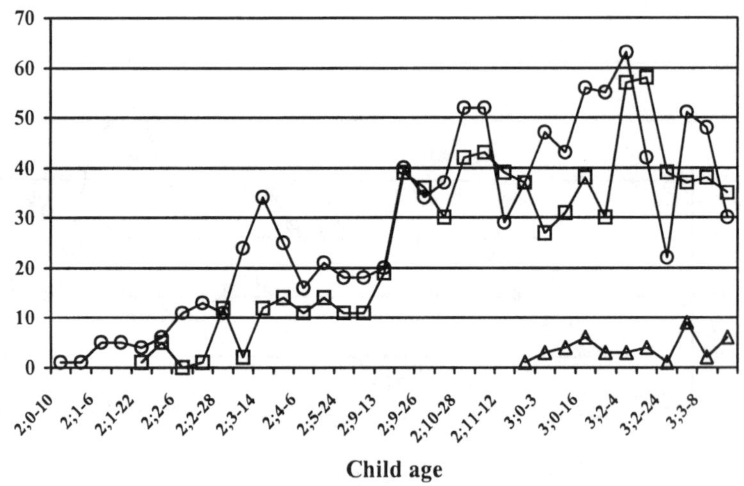

Figure 8. Nina's clauses with functional categories: first mention, without nominative case

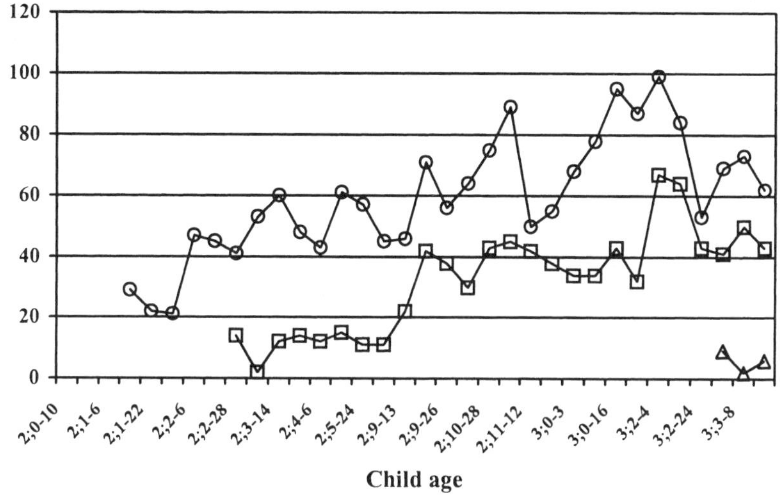

Figure 9. Nina's clauses with functional categories: paradigm

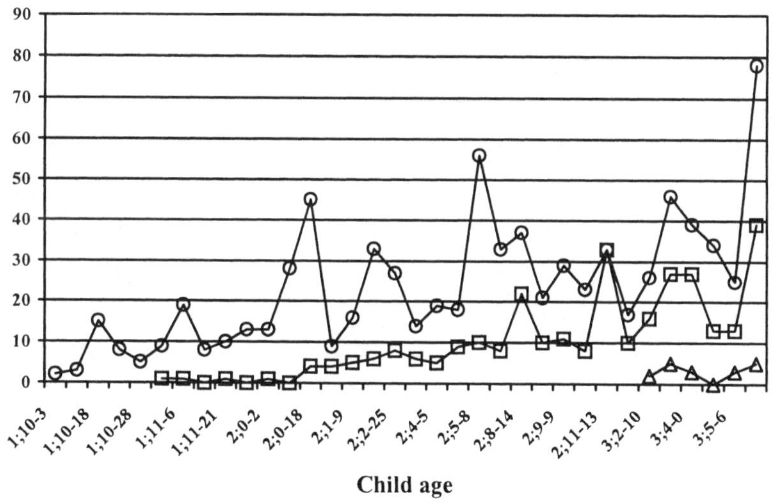

Figure 10. Naomi's clauses with functional categories: first mention

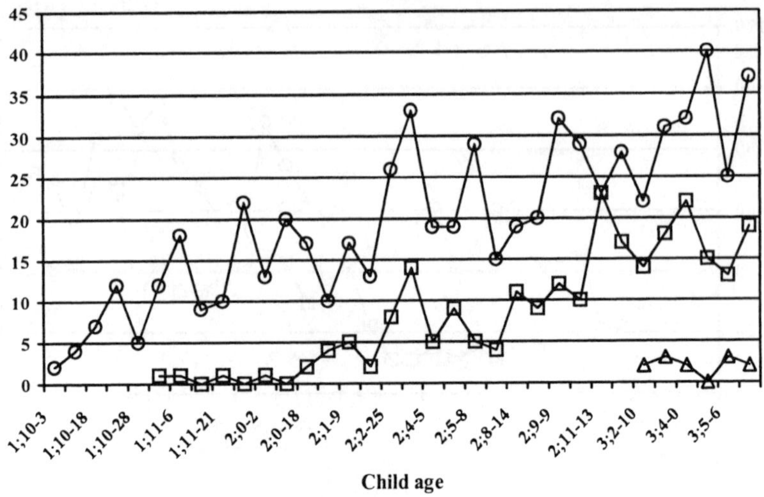

Figure 11. Naomi's clauses with functional categories: normalized

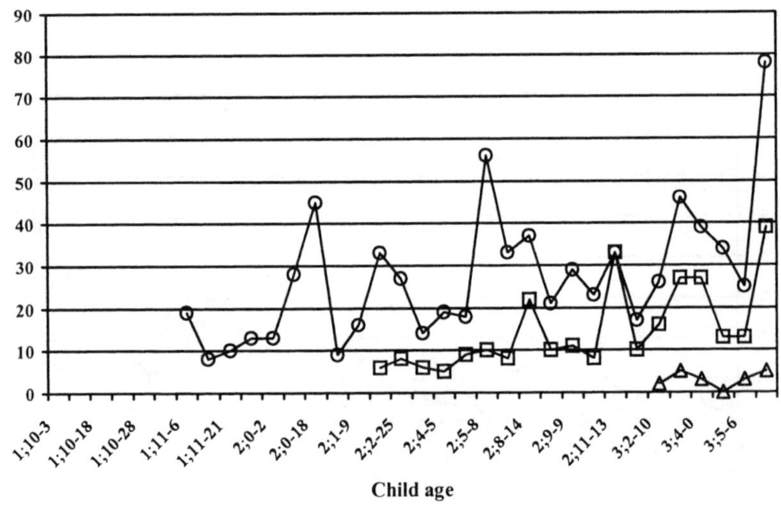

Figure 12. Naomi's clauses with functional categories: paradigm

References

Authier, J.-Marc
1992 Iterated CPs and embedded topicalization. *Linguistic Inquiry* 23: 329–336.

Baddeley, Alan
1986 Working memory and comprehension. In *Working Memory*, D. Broadbent, J. McGaugh, M. Kosslyn, N. Mackintosh, E. Tulving, and L. Weiskrantz (eds.), 75–107. Oxford: Oxford University Press.

Baddeley, Alan
2003 Working memory and language: an overview. *Journal of Communication Disorders* 36: 189–208.

Baker, C. L.
1991 The syntax of English *not*: The limits of core grammar. *Linguistic Inquiry* 22: 387–429.

Bean, Marian C.
1983 *The Development of Word Order Patterns in Old English*. London: Croom Helm.

Belletti, Adriana
1990 *Generalized Verb Movement*. Torino: Rosenberg and Sellier.

Belletti, Adriana
1999 Italian/Romance clitics: structure and derivation. In *Clitics in the Languages of Europe*, Henk van Riemsdijk (ed.), 543–579. Berlin: Mouton de Gruyter.

Benincá, Paola, and Cecilia Poletto
2004 Topic, focus, and V2: Defining the CP sublayers. In *The Structure of CP and IP: The Cartography of Syntactic Structures*, Vol.2, Luigi Rizzi (ed.), 52–75. Oxford: Oxford University Press.

den Besten, Hans
1983 On the interaction of root transformations and lexical deletive rules. In *On the Formal Syntax of the Westgermania*, Werner Abraham (ed.), 47–131. Amsterdam: John Benjamins. Originally distributed in 1977.

Bloom, Lois
1970 *Language Development: Form and Function in Emerging Grammars*. Cambridge, Mass.: MIT Press.

Bobaljik, Jonathan David, and Dianne Jonas
1996 Subject positions and the roles of TP. *Linguistic Inquiry* 27: 195–236.

Bonet, Eulalia
1991 Morphology after syntax: Pronominal clitics in Romance. Ph.D. diss., Department of Linguistics and Philosophy, Massachusetts Institute of Technology.

Borer, Hagit
1994 The projection of arguments. In *Functional Projections, University of Massachusetts Occasional Papers*, Vol. 17, Elena E. Benedicto and Jeffrey T. Runner (eds.), 19–47. Amherst, Mass.: GLSA.

Borer, Hagit, and Ken Wexler
1987 The maturation of syntax. In *Parameter Setting*, Thomas Roeper and Edwin Williams (eds.), 123-172. Dordrecht: D. Reidel Publishing Company.

Boser K., B. Lust, L. Santelmann, and J. Whitman
1992 The syntax of CP and V-2 in early child German (ECG): The strong continuity hypothesis. In *NELS 22: Proceedings of the Northeast Linguistic Society*, 51-65. Amherst, Mass.: GLSA.

Bošković, Željko
1995 Principles of economy in non-finite complementation. Ph.D. diss., Department of Linguistics, University of Connecticut.

Bošković, Željko
1996 Selection and the categorial status of infinitival complements. *Natural Language and Linguistic Theory* 14: 269–304.

Bošković, Željko
1997 *The Syntax of Non-finite Complementation: An Economy Account.* Cambridge, MA: MIT Press.

Bošković, Željko
2000 Sometimes in [Spec, CP], sometimes in situ. In *Step by Step: Essays on Minimalist Syntax in Honor of Howard Lasnik*, Roger Martin, David Michaels, and Juan Uriagereka (eds.), 53–87. Cambridge, Mass.: MIT Press.

Bouchard, Denis, and Paul Hirschbüler
1986 French *quoi* and its clitic allomorph *que*. In *Studies in Romance Languages*, Carol Neidle and Rafael Nuñez Cedeño (eds.), 39–60. Dordrecht: Foris Publications.

Brandi, Luciana, and Patrizia Cordin
1989 Two Italian dialects and the Null Subject Parameter. In *The Null Subject Parameter*, Osvaldo Jaeggli and Kenneth J. Safir (eds.), 111–142. Dordrecht: Kluwer Academic Publishers.

Brandner, Ellen
2004 Head-movement in minimalism, and V2 as FORCE-marking. In *The Syntax and Semantics of the Left Periphery*, Horst Lohnstein and Susanne Trissler (eds.), 97–138. Berlin: Mouton de Gruyter.

Brown, Roger
1973 *A First Language: The Early Stages*. Cambridge, Mass.: Harvard University Press.

Burzio, Luigi
1986 *Italian Syntax: A Government-Binding Approach*. Dordrecht: D. Reidel Publishing Company.

Chenal, A.
1986 *Le franco-provençal valdôtain*. Aoste: Musumeci.

Chomsky, Noam
1991 Some notes on economy of derivation and representation. In *Principles and Parameters in Comparative Grammar*, Robert Freidin (ed.), 417–454. Cambridge, Mass.: MIT Press. Reprinted in Chomsky (1995b: 129–166).

Chomsky, Noam
1993 A minimalist approach to linguistic theory. In *The View from Building 20*, Kenneth Hale and Samuel Jay Keyser (eds.), 1–52. Cambridge, Mass.: MIT Press. Reprinted in Chomsky (1995b: 167–217).

Chomsky, Noam
1995a Bare phrase structure. In *Government and Binding Theory and the Minimalist Program*, Gert Webelhuth (ed.), 383–439. Oxford: Blackwell Publishers.

Chomsky, Noam
1995b Categories and transformations. In *The Minimalist Program*, Noam Chomsky, 219–394. Cambridge, Mass.: MIT Press.

Chomsky, Noam
2000 Minimalist inquiries: The framework. In *Step by Step: Essays on Minimalist Syntax in Honor of Howard Lasnik*, Roger Martin, David Michaels, and Juan Uriagereka (eds), 89–155. Cambridge, Mass.: MIT Press.

Chomsky, Noam
2001 Derivation by phase. In *Ken Hale: A Life in Language*, Michael Kenstowicz (ed.), 1–52. Cambridge, Mass.: MIT Press.

Chomsky, Noam, and Howard Lasnik
1995 The theory of principles and parameters. In *The Minimalist Program*, Noam Chomsky, 13–127. Cambridge, Mass.: MIT Press.

Christensen, Kirsti Koch
1991 AGR, adjunction, and the structure of Scandinavian existential sentences. *Lingua* 84: 137–158.

Cinque, Guglielmo
1990 *Types of A'-Dependencies*. Cambridge, Mass.: MIT Press.

Cinque, Guglielmo
1999 *Adverbs and Functional Heads: A Cross-Linguistic Perspective.* Oxford: Oxford University Press.

Cinque, Guglielmo (ed.)
2002 *Functional Structure in DP and IP: The Cartography of Syntactic Structures*. Vol. 1. Oxford: Oxford University Press.

Clahsen, Harald
1989 The grammatical characterization of developmental dysphasia. *Linguistics* 27: 897–920.

Clahsen, Harald
1991 *Child Language and Developmental Dysphasia. Linguistic Studies in the Acquisition of German*. Amsterdam: John Benjamins.

Clahsen, H., S. Bartke, and S. Göllner
1997 Formal features in impaired grammars: A comparison of English and German SLI children. *Journal of Neurolinguistics* 10: 151–171.

Clahsen, Harald, Martina Penke, and Teresa Parodi
1993/94 Functional categories in early child German. *Language Acquisition* 3 (4): 395–429.

Clamons, Robbin, Ann E. Mulkern, Gerald Sanders, and Nancy Stenson
1999 The limits of formal analysis: Pragmatic motivation in Oromo grammar. In *Functionalism and Formalism in Linguistics. Vol. II: Case Studies*, Michael Darnell, Edith Moravcsik, Frederick Newmeyer, Michael Noonan, and Kathleen Wheatley (eds.), 59–76. Amsterdam: John Benjamins Publishing Company.

Clark, Eve V.
1978 Awareness of language: Some evidence from what children say and do. In *The Child's Conception of Language*, A. Sinclair, R. J. Jarvella, and W. J. M. Levelt (eds.), 17–43. Berlin: Springer Verlag.

Clark, Eve V.
1979 Building a vocabulary: Words for objects, actions and relations. In *Language Acquisition: Studies in First Language Development*, P. Fletcher and M. Garman (eds). Cambridge: Cambridge University Press.

Diesing, Molly
1990 Verb movement and the subject position in Yiddish. *Natural Language and Linguistic Theory* 8: 41–79.

Diesing, Molly
1991 *Indefinites*. Cambridge, Mass.: MIT Press.

Emonds, Joseph E.
1976 *A Transformational Approach to English Syntax*. New York: Academic Press.

Emonds, Joseph
1978 The verbal complex V′-V in French. *Linguistic Inquiry* 9: 151–175.

Eyer, Julia A., and Laurence B. Leonard
1995 Functional categories and specific language impairment: A case study. *Language Acquisition* 4 (3): 177–203.

Felix, Sascha W.
1992 Language acquisition as a maturational process. In *Theoretical Issues in Language Acquisition: Continuity and Change in Development*, Jürgen Weissenborn, Helen Goodluck, and Thomas Roeper (eds.), 25–51. Hillsdale, New Jersey: Lawrence Erlbaum.

Fischer, Olga, Ans van Kemenade, Willem Koopman, and Wim van der Wurff
2000 *The Syntax of Early English*. Cambridge: Cambridge University Press.

Frampton, John
1997 Expletive insertion. In *The Role of Economy Principles in Linguistic Theory*, Chris Wilder, Hans-Martin Gärtner, and Manfred Bierwisch (eds), 36–57. Berlin: Academie-Verlag.

Friedemann, Marc-Ariel, and Tali Siloni
1993 AgrO is not AgrP: A comparative study of complex tenses. *GenGenP* 1: 41–53.

Garrett, Merrill
1988 Processes in language production. In *Linguistics: The Cambridge Survey*, Vol. 3, Frederick J. Newmeyer (ed.), 69–96. Cambridge: Cambridge University Press.

van Gelderen, Elly
1993 *The Rise of Functional Categories*. Amsterdam: John Benjamins.

van Gelderen, Elly
1996 Restraining functional projections: Auxiliaries and participles. In *The Proceedings of the Fourteenth West Coast Conference on Formal Linguistics*, José Comacho, Lina Choueiri, and Maki Watanabe (eds.), 111–122. Stanford: CSLI

Gillam, Ronald B., Nelson Cowan, and Linda S. Day
1995 Sequential memory in children with and without language impairment. *Journal of Speech and Hearing Research* 38: 393–402.

Giorgi, Alessandra, and Fabio Pianesi
1996 Verb movement in Italian and syncretic categories. *Probus* 8: 137–160.

Giorgi, Alessandra, and Fabio Pianesi
1997 *Tense and Aspect: From Semantics to Morphosyntax*. Oxford: Oxford University Press.

Giorgi, Alessandra, and Fabio Pianesi
2004 Complementizer deletion in Italian. In *The Structure of CP and IP: The Cartography of Syntactic Structures*, Vol.2, Luigi Rizzi (ed.), 190–210. Oxford: Oxford University Press.

Gopnik, M.
1990a Feature-blind grammar and dysphasia. *Nature* 344: 715.

Gopnik, M.
1990b Feature-blindness: A case study. *Language Acquisition* 1: 139– 164.

Gopnik, M., and Martha B. Crago
1991 Familial aggregation of a developmental language disorder. *Cognition* 39: 1–50.

Gopnik, M., and H. Goad
1997 What underlies inflectional error patterns in genetic dysphasia? *Journal of Neurolinguistics* 10: 109–137.

Grimshaw, Jane
1991 Extended projection. Ms., Brandeis University.

Grimshaw, Jane
1997 Projection, heads, and optimality. *Linguistic Inquiry* 28: 373–422.

Grootveld, M.
1992 On the representation of coordination. In *Linguistics in the Netherlands 1992*, R. Bok-Bennema and R. van Hout (eds.), 61–73. Amsterdam: John Benjamins.

Grünberg, M.
1967 *The West Saxon Gospels: A Study of the Gospel of St. Matthew with Text of the Four Gospels*. Amsterdam: Scheltema & Holkema.

Guasti, Maria Teresa
2002 *Language Acquisition: The Growth of Grammar*. Cambridge, Mass.: MIT Press.

Guilfoyle, Eithne, and Máire Noonan
1992 Functional categories and language acquisition. *Canadian Journal of Linguistics* 37 (2): 241–272.

Haider, Hubert
1985 V-second in German. In *Verb Second Phenomena in Germanic Languages*, Hubert Haider and Martin Prinzhorn (eds.), 49–75. Dordrecht: Foris Publications.

Hegarty, Michael
1993 The derivational composition of phrase structure. Ms., University of Pennsylvania.

Heycock, Caroline, and Anthony Kroch
1993 Verb movement and coordination in a dynamic theory of licensing. *The Linguistic Review* 11: 257–283.

Heycock, Caroline, and Beatrice Santorini
1993 Head movement and the licensing of non-thematic relations. In *Proceedings of the Eleventh West Coast Conference on Formal Linguistics*, Jonathan Mead (ed.), 262–276. Stanford: CSLI.

Higginbotham, James
1983 The logic of perceptual reports: An extensional alternative to situation semantics. *The Journal of Philosophy* 80: 100–127.

Hoekstra, Teun, and Nina Hyams
1996 The syntax and interpretation of dropped categories in child language: A unified account. In *The Proceedings of the Fourteenth West Coast Conference on Formal Linguistics*, José Comacho, Lina Choueiri, and Maki Watanabe (eds.), 123–136. Stanford: CSLI.

Hoekstra, Teun, and Peter Jordens
1994 From adjunct to head. In *Language Acquisition and Studies in Generative Grammar*, Teun Hoekstra and Bonnie D. Schwartz (eds.), 119–149. Amsterdam: John Benjamins.

Höhle, Tilman
1983 Subjektlücken in Koordinationen. Ms., Cologne University.

Höhle, Tilman
1990 Assumptions about asymmetric coordination in German. In *Grammar in Progress: A Festschrift for Henk van Riemsdijk*, Joán Mascaro and Marina Nespor (eds.), 221–235. Dordrecht: Foris Publications.

Holmberg, Anders
1986 Word order and syntactic features in the Scandinavian languages and English. Ph.D. diss., University of Stockholm.

Holmberg, Anders, and Christer Platzack
1995 *The Role of Inflection in Scandinavian Syntax*. Oxford: Oxford University Press.

Hornstein, Norbert
1995 *Logical Form: From GB to Minimalism*. Oxford: Blackwell Publishers.

Hornstein, Norbert
1999 Minimalism and quantifier raising. In *Working Minimalism*, Samuel David Epstein and Norbert Hornstein (eds.), 45–75. Cambridge, MA: MIT Press.

Iatridou, Sabine
1990 About Agr(P). *Linguistic Inquiry* 21: 551–577.

Iatridou, Sabine
1993/94 On the contribution of conditional *then*. *Natural Language Semantics* 2: 171–199.

Iatridou, Sabine
1994 Comments on the Paper by Roberts. In *Verb Movement*, David Lightfoot and Norbert Hornstein (eds.), 243–260. Cambridge: Cambridge University Press.

Iatridou, Sabine, and Anthony Kroch
1992 The licensing of CP-recursion and its relevance to the Germanic verb-second phenomenon. In *Working Papers in Scandinavian Linguistics* 50: 1–25.

Johannessen, Janne Bondi
1998 *Coordination*. Oxford: Oxford University Press.

Johnson, Kyle
1991 Object positions. *Natural Language and Linguistic Theory* 9: 577–636.

Jonas, Dianne, and Jonathan David Bobaljik
1993 Specs for subjects: The role of TP in Icelandic. In *Papers on Case and Agreement 1: MIT Working Papers in Linguistics*, Vol. 18, Jonathan D. Bobaljik and Colin Phillips (eds.), 59–98. Cambridge, Mass.: Department of Linguistics and Philosophy, MIT.

Jones, Michael Allan
1996 *Foundations of French Syntax*. Cambridge: Cambridge University Press.

Kayne, Richard S.
1989a Null subjects and clitic climbing. In *The Null Subject Parameter*, Osvaldo Jaeggli and Kenneth J. Safir (eds.), 239–261. Dordrecht: Kluwer Academic Publishers.

Kayne, Richard S.
1989b Facets of Romance past participle agreement. In *Dialect Variation and the Theory of Grammar*, Paola Benincà (ed.), 85–103. Dordrecht: Foris Publications.

Kayne, Richard S.
1991a Romance clitics, verb movement, and PRO. *Linguistic Inquiry* 22: 647–686.

Kayne, Richard S.
1991b Italian negative infinitival imperatives and clitic climbing. Ms., City University of New York.

Kayne Richard S.
1994 *The Antisymmetry of Syntax*. Cambridge, Mass.: MIT Press.

Kehler, Andrew
2002 *Coherence, Reference, and the Theory of Grammar*. Stanford: CSLI.

Kemenade, Ans van
1997 V2 and embedded topicalization in Old and Middle English. In *Parameters of Morphosyntactic Change*, Ans van Kemenade and Nigel Vincent (eds.), 326–352. Cambridge: Cambridge University Press.

Kitahara, Hisatsugu
1996 Raising quantifiers without quantifier raising. In *Minimal Ideas: Syntactic Studies in the Minimalist Framework*, Werner Abraham, Samuel David Epstein, Höskuldur Thráinsson, and C. Jan-Wouter Zwart (eds.), 189–198. Amsterdam: John Benjamins Publishing Company.

Klima, Edward S.
1964 Negation in English. In *The Structure of Language*, Jerry Fodor and J. J. Katz (eds.), 246–323. Englewood Cliffs, New Jersey: Prentice Hall.

Koizumi, Masatoshi
1993 Object agreement phrases and the split VP hypothesis. In *Papers on Case and Agreement I: MIT Working Papers in Linguistics*, Vol. 18, Jonathan D. Bobaljik and Colin Phillips (eds.), 99–148. Cambridge, Mass.: Department of Linguistics and Philosophy, MIT.

Koizumi, Masatoshi
1994 Layered specifiers. In *NELS 24: Proceedings of the North East Linguistic Society*, Mercè Gonzàlez (ed.), 255–269. Amherst, Mass.: GLSA.

Koizumi, Masatoshi
1995 Bare phrase structure in minimalist syntax. Ph.D. diss., Department of Linguistics and Philosophy, Massachusetts Institute of Technology.

Kratzer, Angelika
1994 On External Arguments. In *Functional Projections, University of Massachusetts Occasional Papers*, Vol. 17, Elena E. Benedicto and Jeffrey T. Runner (eds.), 103–130. Amherst, Mass.: GLSA.

Krazter, Angelika
1995 Stage-level and individual-level predicates. In *The Generic Book*, Gregory Carlson and Francis Jeffry Pelletier (eds.), 125–175. Chicago: The University of Chicago Press. Originally distributed in 1989.

Kroch, Anthony
1989 Reflexes of grammar in patterns of language change. *Language Variation and Change* 1: 199–244.

Kroch, Anthony, and Ann Taylor
1997 Verb movement in Old and Middle English: Dialect variation and language contact. In *Parameters of Morphosyntactic Change*, Ans van Kemenade and Nigel Vincent (eds.), 297–325. Cambridge: Cambridge University Press. Originally published in *University of Pennsylvania Working Papers in Linguistics*, Vol. 1, Roumyana Izvorski, Miriam Meyerhoff, Bill Reynold, and Victoria Tredinnick (eds.), 45–68. University of Pennsylvania, 1994.

Laenzlinger, Christopher
1993 A syntactic view of Romance pronominal sequences. *Probus* 5: 241–270.

Laka, Itziar
1990 Negation in syntax: On the nature of functional categories and projections. Ph.D. diss., Department of Linguistics and Philosophy, Massachusetts Institute of Technology.

Lakoff, George
1986 Frame semantic control of the coordinated structure constraint. In *CLS 22, Part 2: Papers from the Parasession on Pragmatics and Grammatical Theory*, A. M. Farley et al. (eds.), 152–167. Chicago: Chicago Linguistic Society.

Langacker, Ronald W.
1972 *Fundamentals of Linguistic Analysis*. New York: Harcourt Brace Jovanovich, Inc.

LaPolla, Mark Vincent
1988 Clitic movement in Spanish and the Projection Principle. In *Advances in Romance Linguistics*, David Birdsong and Jean-Pierre Montreuil (eds.), 217–231. Dordrecht: Foris Publications.

Lasnik, Howard
1999 *Minimalist Analysis*. Oxford: Blackwell Publishers.

Law, Paul
1991 Effects of head movement on theories of subjacency and proper government. Ph.D. diss., Department of Linguistics and Philosophy, Massachusetts Institute of Technology.

Leonard, Laurence B.
1995 Functional categories in the grammars of children with specific language impairment. *Journal of Speech and Hearing Research* 38: 1270–1283.

Leonard, Laurence B.
1998 *Children with Specific Language Impairment*. Cambridge, Mass.: MIT Press.

Leonard, L., U. Bortolini, M. C. Caselli, K. McGregor, and L. Sabbadini
1992. Morphological deficits in children with specific language impairment: The status of features in the underlying grammar. *Language Acquisition* 2: 151–179.

Lepschy, Anne Laura, and Giulio Lepschy
1988 *The Italian Language Today*. New York: New Amsterdam Books.

Levelt, William
1989 *From Intention to Articulation*. Cambridge, Mass.: MIT Press.

Li, Charles N., and Sandra A. Thompson
1976 Subject and topic: A new typology of language. In *Subject and Topic*, Charles N. Li (ed.), 457–489. New York: Academic Press.

Loeb, Diane Frome, and Laurence B. Leonard
1991 Subject case marking and verb morphology in normally developing and specifically language-impaired children. *Journal of Speech and Hearing Research* 34: 340–346.

Luján, Marta
1980 Clitic Promotion and Mood in Spanish Verbal Complements. *Linguistics* 18: 381–484.

Lust, Barbara
1994 Functional projection of CP and phrase structure parameterization: An argument for the strong continuity hypothesis. In *Syntactic Theory and First Language Acquisition: Cross-Linguistic Perspectives*, Vol. 1, *Heads, Projections, and Learnability*, Barbara Lust, Margarita Suñer, and John Whitman (eds.), 85–118. Hillsdale, New Jersey: Lawrence Erlbaum.

MacWhinney, Brian
1995 *The CHILDES Project: Tools for Analyzing Talk*. Second Edition. Hillsdale, New Jersey: Lawrence Erlbaum.

Madeira, Ana Maria
1993 Clitic second in European Portuguese. *Probus* 5: 155–174.

Maling, Joan
1987 Existential sentences in Swedish and Icelandic: Reference to thematic roles. *Working Papers in Scandinavian Syntax* 28: 1–21.

Maling, Joan
1988 Variations on a theme: Existential sentences in Swedish and Icelandic. In *McGill Working Papers in Linguistics: Special Issue on Comparative Germanic Syntax*, Denise Fekete and Zofia Laubitz (eds.), 168–191. Montréal: Department of Linguistics, McGill University.

Manzini, Maria Rita
1994 Triggers for verb-second: Germanic and Romance. *The Linguistic Review* 11: 299–314.

Manzini, M. Rita, and Leonardo M. Savoia
2004 Clitics: Cooccurrence and mutual exclusion patterns. In *The Structure of CP and IP: The Cartography of Syntactic Structures*, Vol.2, Luigi Rizzi (ed.), 211–250. Oxford: Oxford University Press.

Martin, Roger
1996 A minimalist theory of PRO and control. Ph.D. diss., Department of Linguistics, University of Connecticut.

Martin, Roger
2001 Null case and the distribution of PRO. *Linguistic Inquiry* 32: 141–166.

Martins, Ana-Maria
1994 Enclisis, VP-deletion and the Nature of Sigma. *Probus* 6: 173–205.

May, Robert
1985 *Logical Form: Its Structure and Derivation*. Cambridge, Mass.: MIT Press.

McKee, Cecile, and Noriko Iwasaki
2001 Lemma structure in language learning: Comments on representation and realization. In *Approaches to Bootstrapping: Phonological, Lexical, Syntactic and Neurophysiological Aspects of Early Language Acquisition*, Vol. 1, Jürgen Weissenborn and Barbara Höhle (eds.), 125–144. Amsterdam: John Benjamins.

Meisel, Jürgen M.
1994 Getting FAT: Finiteness, agreement and tense in early grammars. In *Bilingual First Language Acquisition: French and German Grammatical Development*, Jürgen M. Meisel (ed.), 89-129. Amsterdam: John Benjamins.

Montgomery, James W.
2003 Working memory and comprehension in children with specific language impairment: What we know so far. *Journal of Communication Disorders* 36: 221–231.

Morehead, Donald M., and David Ingram
1973 The development of base syntax in normal and linguistically deviant children. *Journal of Speech and Hearing Research* 16: 330–352.

Mulkern, Ann Elizabeth
2003 Cognitive status, discourse salience, and information structure: Evidence from Irish and Oromo. Ph.D. diss., Program in Linguistics, University of Minnesota.

Müller, Gereon, and Wolfgang Sternefeld
1993 Improper movement and unambiguous binding. *Linguistic Inquiry* 24: 461–507.

Munn, Alan
1987 Coordinate structure and X-bar theory. *McGill Working Papers in Linguistics* 4. Montreal: McGill University.

Munn, Alan
1993 Topics in the syntax and semantics of coordinate structures. Ph.D. diss., Department of Linguistics, University of Maryland.

Napoli, Donna Jo
1981 Semantic interpretation vs. lexical governance: Clitic climbing in Italian. *Language* 57: 841–887.

Oetting, Janna B., and Janice E. Horohov
1997 Past-tense marking by children with and without specific language impairment. *Journal of Speech, Language, and Hearing Research* 40: 62–74.

Oetting, Janna B., and Mabel L. Rice
1993 Plural acquisition in children with specific language impairment. *Journal of Speech and Hearing Research* 36: 1236–1248.

Pintzuk, Susan
1991 Phrase structures in competition: Variation and change in Old English word order. Ph.D. diss., Department of Linguistics, University of Pennsylvania.

Pintzuk, Susan
1993 Verb seconding in Old English: Verb movement to Infl. *The Linguistic Review* 10: 5–35.

Platzack, Christer
1983 Existential sentences in English, German, Icelandic and Swedish. In *Papers from the Seventh Scandinavian Conference of Linguistics*, Fred Karlsson (ed.), 80–100. Helsinki: Department of General Linguistics, University of Helsinki.

Platzack, Christer
1986 The position of the finite verb in Swedish. In *Verb Second Phenomena in Germanic Languages*, Hubert Haider and Martin Prinzhorn (eds.), 27–47. Dordrecht: Foris Publications.

Platzack, Christer, and Anders Holmberg
1989 The role of AGR and finiteness in Germanic VO languages. *Working Papers in Scandinavian Syntax* 43: 51–76.

Poeppel, David, and Kenneth Wexler
1993 The Full Competence Hypothesis of clause structure in early German. *Language* 69: 1–33.

Poletto, Cecilia
1993 Subject clitic/verb inversion in North Eastern Italian Dialects. In *Syntactic Theory and the Dialects of Italy*, Adriana Belletti (ed.), 204–251. Torino: Rosenberg and Sellier.

Poletto, Cecilia
1996 Three kinds of subject clitics in Basso Polesano and the theory of pro. In *Parameters and Functional Heads*, Adriana Belletti and Luigi Rizzi (eds.), 269–300. Oxford: Oxford University Press.

Poletto, Cecilia
1999 The internal structure of AgrS: Subject clitics in Northern Italian. In *Clitics in the Languages of Europe*, Henk van Riemsdijk (ed.), 581–620. Berlin: Mouton de Gruyter.

Poletto, Cecilia, and Jean-Yves Pollock
2004 On the left periphery of some Romance wh-questions. In *The Structure of CP and IP: The Cartography of Syntactic Structures*, Vol.2, Luigi Rizzi (ed.), 251–296. Oxford: Oxford University Press.

Pollock, Jean-Yves
1989 Verb movement, universal grammar, and the structure of IP. *Linguistic Inquiry* 20: 365–424.

Pollock, Jean-Yves
1997 Notes on clause structure. In *Elements of Grammar: Handbook of Generative Syntax*, Liliane Haegeman (ed.), 237–279. Dordrecht: Kluwer Academic Publishers.

Pope, John C.
1968 *Homilies of Ælfric: A Supplementary Collection*. Vols. I, II. Oxford: Oxford University Press.

Postal, Paul M.
1974 *On Raising: One Rule of English Grammar and its Theoretical Implications*. Cambridge, Mass.: MIT Press.

Prince, Ellen
1992 The ZPG letter: Subjects, definiteness, and information status. In *Discourse Description: Diverse Analyses of a Fundraising Text*, William C. Mann and Sandra A. Thompson (eds.), 295–325. Amsterdam: John Benjamins.

Radford, Andrew
1990 *Syntactic Theory and the Acquisition of English Syntax: The Nature of Early Child Grammar of English*. Oxford: Basil Blackwell.

Radford, Andrew
1996 Towards a structure-building model of acquisition. In *Generative Perspectives on Language Acquisition*, Harald Clahsen (ed.), 43-89. Amsterdam: John Benjamins.

Rambow, Owen
1994 Mobile heads and strict lexicalization. M.A. Thesis, University of Pennsylvania.

Rambow, Owen, and Beatrice Santorini
1995 Incremental phrase structure generation and a universal theory of V2. In *NELS 25: Proceedings of the North East Linguistic Society*, Jill N. Beckman (ed.), 373-387. Amherst, Mass.: GLSA.

Rice, Mabel L., and Janna B. Oetting
1993 Morphological deficits in children with SLI: Evaluation of number marking and agreement. *Journal of Speech and Hearing Research* 36: 1249–1257.

Rice, Mabel L., and Kenneth Wexler
1995 Extended optional infinitive (EOI) account of specific language impairment. In *Proceedings of the 19th Annual Boston University Conference on Language Development*, Vol. 2, Dawn MacLaughlin and Susan McEwen (eds.), 451-462. Somerville, Mass.: Cascadilla Press.

Rice, Mabel L., and Kenneth Wexler
1996 Toward tense as a clinical marker of specific language impairment in English-speaking children. *Journal of Speech and Hearing Research* 39: 1239–1257.

Rice, Mabel L., Kenneth Wexler, and Patricia L. Cleave
1995 Specific language impairment as a period of extended optional infinitive. *Journal of Speech and Hearing Research* 38: 850–863.

Rivero, Maria-Luisa
1994 Clause structure and V-movement in the languages of the Balkans. *Natural Language and Linguistic Theory* 12: 63–120.

Rivero, Maria-Luisa, and Arhonto Terzi
1995 Imperatives, V-movement and logical mood. *Journal of Linguistics* 31: 301–332.

Rizzi, Luigi
1982 *Issues in Italian Syntax*. Dordrecht: Foris Publications.

Rizzi, Luigi
1986 On the status of subject clitics in Romance. In *Studies in Romance Syntax*, Osvaldo Jaeggli and C. Silva-Corvalàn (eds.), 391–419. Dordrecht: Foris Publications.

Rizzi, Luigi
1994 Early null subjects and root null subjects. In *Language Acquisition and Studies in Generative Grammar*, Teun Hoekstra and Bonnie D. Schwartz (eds.), 151–176. Amsterdam: John Benjamins.

Rizzi, Luigi
1996 Residual verb second and the wh-criterion. In *Parameters and Functional Heads*, Adriana Belletti and Luigi Rizzi (eds.), 63–90. Oxford: Oxford University Press. Distributed in 1990.

Rizzi, Luigi
1997 The fine structure of the left periphery. In *Elements of Grammar: Handbook of Generative Syntax*, Liliane Haegeman (ed.), 281–337. Dordrecht: Kluwer Academic Publishers.

Rizzi, Luigi (ed.)
2004 *The Structure of CP and IP: The Cartography of Syntactic Structures*, Vol.2. Oxford: Oxford University Press.

Rizzi, Luigi, and Ian Roberts
1996 Complex inversion in French. In *Parameters and Functional Heads*, Adriana Belletti and Luigi Rizzi (eds.), 91–116. Oxford: Oxford University Press. Originally published in *Probus* 1, 1989.

Roberts, Ian
1994a Two types of head movement in Romance. In *Verb Movement*, David Lightfoot and Norbert Hornstein (eds.), 207–242. Cambridge: Cambridge University Press.

Roberts, Ian
1994b Past-participle agreement and object clitics in Franco-Provençal Valdôtain. In *Paths Towards Universal Grammar: Studies in Honor of Richard S. Kayne*, Guglielmo Cinque, Jan Koster, Jean-Yves Pollock, Luigi Rizzi, and Raffaella Zanuttini (eds.), 377–394. Washington, D.C.: Georgetown University Press.

Roberts, Ian
1997 Restructuring, head movement, and locality. *Linguistic Inquiry* 28: 423–460.

Roberts, Ian
2004 The C-system in Brythonic Celtic languages, V2, and the EPP. In *The Structure of CP and IP: The Cartography of Syntactic Structures*, Vol.2, Luigi Rizzi (ed.), 297–328. Oxford: Oxford University Press.

Roeper, Thomas, and Bernhardt Rohrbacher
1995 Null subjects in early child English and the theory of economy of projection. In *University of Pennsylvania Working Papers in Linguistics*, Vol.2, Roumyana Izvorski and Victoria Tredinnick (eds.), 83–119. University of Pennsylvania.

Roeper, Thomas, and Bernhardt Rohrbacher
2000 True pro-drop in child English and the principle of economy of projection. In *The Acquisition of Scrambling and Cliticization*, C. Hamann and S. Powers (eds.). Dordrecht: Kluwer Academic Publishers.

Rögnvaldsson, Eiríkur, and Höskuldur Thráinsson
1990 On Icelandic word order once more. In *Modern Icelandic Syntax, Syntax and Semantics*, Vol. 24, Joan Maling and Annie Zaenen, (eds.), 3–40. San Diego: Academic Press.

Rohrbacher, Bernhardt
1993 The Germanic VO languages and the full paradigm: A theory of V to I raising. Ph.D. diss., Department of Linguistics, University of Massachusetts, Amherst.

Rooryck, Johan
1992 Romance enclitic ordering and universal grammar. *The Linguistic Review* 9: 219–250.

Rooryck, Johan
1994 Against optional movement for clitic climbing. In *Issues and Theory in Romance Linguistics: Selected Papers from the Linguistic Symposium on Romance Languages XXIII*, Mike L. Mazzola (ed.), 415–441. Washington, D.C.: Georgetown University Press.

Ross, John Robert
1967 Constraints on variables in syntax. Ph.D. diss., Department of Linguistics and Philosophy, Massachusetts Institute of Technology.

Sabel, Joachim
2002 A minimalist analysis of syntactic islands. *The Linguistic Review* 19: 271–315.

Sachs, Jacqueline
1983 Talking about the there and then: The emergence of displaced reference in parent-child discourse. In *Children's Language*, Vol. 4. , K. E. Nelson (ed.). Hillsdale, N.J.: Lawrence Erlbaum.

Safir, Ken
1993 Perception, selection, and structural economy. *Natural Language Semantics* 2: 47–70.

Santorini, Beatrice
1992 Variation and change in Yiddish subordinate clause word order. *Natural Language and Linguistic Theory* 10: 595–640.

Schönenberger, Manuela
2001 *Embedded V-to-C in Child Grammar: The Acquisition of Verb Placement in Swiss German*. Dordrecht: Kluwer Academic Publishers.

Schütze, Carson T., and Kenneth Wexler
1996 Subject case licensing and English root infinitives. In *Proceedings of the 20th Annual Boston University Conference on Language Development*, Vol. 2, Andy Stringfellow, Dalia Cahana-Amitay, Elizabeth Hughes, and Andrea Zukowski (eds.), 670–681. Somerville, Mass.: Cascadilla Press.

Selkirk, Elisabeth O.
1984 *Phonology and Syntax: The Relation between Sound and Structure*. Cambridge, Mass.: MIT Press.

Sportiche, Dominique
1990 Movement, agreement and case. Ms., University of California, Los Angeles.

Sportiche, Dominique
1996 Clitic constructions. In *Phrase Structure and the Lexicon*, Johan Rooryck and Laurie Zaring (eds.), 213–276. Dordrecht: Kluwer Academic Publishers.

Suppes, Patrick
1973 The semantics of children's language. *American Psychologist* 88: 103–114.

Terzi, Arhonto
1993 Clitic climbing from finite clauses. Ms., University of Ottawa.

Terzi, Arhonto
1994 Clitic climbing from finite clauses and long head movement. *Catalan Working Papers in Linguistics* 3: 97–122.

Thráinsson, Höskuldur
1985 V1, V2, and V3 in Icelandic. In *Verb Second Phenomena in Germanic La*nguages, Hubert Haider and Martin Prinzhorn (eds.), 169–194. Dordrecht: Foris Publications.

Travis, Lisa de Mena
1984 Parameters and effects of word order variation. Ph.D. diss., Department of Linguistics and Philosophy, Massachusetts Institute of Technology.

Travis, Lisa
1988 The syntax of adverbs. In *McGill Working Papers in Linguistics, Special Issue on Comparative Germanic Syntax*, 280–310. Department of Linguistics, McGill University.

Tsimpli, Ianthi
1990 The clause structure and word order of Modern Greek. In *University College London Working Papers in Linguistics*, Vol. 2, John Harris (ed.), 228–255, University College London.

Tunstall, Susannne
1994 Case in aspectual perception complements. In *Functional Projections, University of Massachusetts Occasional Papers*, Vol. 17, Elena E. Benedicto and Jeffrey T. Runner (eds.), 227–251. Amherst, Mass.: GLSA.

Ura, Hiroyuki
1996 Multiple feature checking: A theory of grammatical function splitting. Ph.D. diss., Department of Linguistics and Philosophy, Massachusetts Institute of Technology.

Uriagereka, Juan
1995a An F position in Western Romance. In *Discourse Configurational Languages*, Katalin É. Kiss (ed.), 153–175. Oxford: Oxford University Press.

Uriagereka, Juan
1995b Aspects of the syntax of clitic placement in Western Romance, *Linguistic Inquiry* 26: 79–123.

Vainikka, Anne
1993/94 Case in the development of English syntax. *Language Acquisition* 3 (3): 257–325.

Vikner, Sten
1995 *Verb Movement and Expletive Subjects in the Germanic Languages*. Oxford: Oxford University Press.

Ward, Gregory, and Betty Birner
1995 Definiteness and the English existential. *Language* 71: 722–742.

Watanabe, Akira
1992 Subjacency and S-structure movement of *wh*-in-situ. *Journal of East Asian Linguistics* 1: 255–291.

Watanabe, Akira
1993a AGR-based case theory and its interaction with the A′-system. Ph.D. diss., Department of Linguistics and Philosophy, Massachusetts Institute of Technology.

Watanabe, Akira
1993b Larsonian CP recursion, factive complements and selection. In *NELS 23: Proceedings of the North East Linguistics Society*, Amy J. Schafer (ed.), 523–537. Amherst, Mass.: GLSA.

Webelhuth, Gert
1992 *Principles and Parameters of Syntactic Saturation*. Oxford: Oxford University Press.

Wexler, Ken
1994 Optional infinitives, head movement and the economy of derivations. In *Verb Movement*, David Lightfoot and Norbert Hornstein (eds.), 305–350. Cambridge: Cambridge University Press.

Wexler, Ken
1999 Very early parameter setting and the unique checking constraint: A new explanation of the optional infinitive stage. In *Language Acquisition: Knowledge, Representation and Processing*, Antonella Sorace, Caroline Heycock, and Richard Shillcock (eds.), 23–79. Amsterdam: North Holland. Originally published in *Lingua* 106, 1998.

Williams, Edwin
1994 A reinterpretation of evidence for verb movement in French. In *Verb Movement*, David Lightfoot and Norbert Hornstein (eds), 189–205. Cambridge: Cambridge University Press.

Wurmbrand, Susanne
2001 *Infinitives: Restructuring and Clause Structure*. Berlin: Mouton de Gruyter.

Zanuttini, Raffaella
1991 Syntactic properties of sentential negation: A comparative study of Romance Languages. Ph.D. diss., Department of Linguistics, University of Pennsylvania.

Zanuttini, Raffaella
1997 *Negation and Clausal Structure: A Comparative Study of Romance Languages*. Oxford: Oxford University Press.

Zepeda, Ofelia
1983 *A Tohono O'odham Grammar*. Tucson: The University of Arizona Press.

Zwart, Jan-Wouter
1993 Dutch syntax: A minimalist approach. Ph.D. diss., Rijksuniversiteit Groningen.

Index of names

Index of subjects